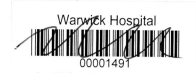
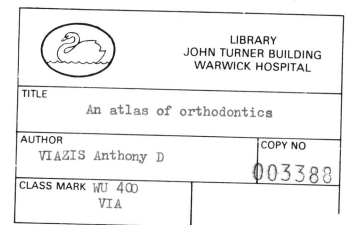

Atlas of
Orthodontics

Principles and
Clinical Applications

003388

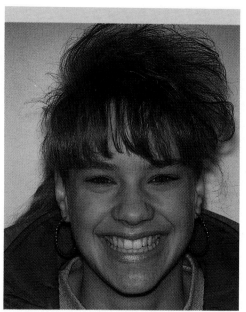

The smile that makes it all worthwhile.

Atlas of
Orthodontics

Principles and
Clinical Applications

Anthony D. Viazis, DDS, MS
Assistant Professor
Department of Orthodontics
Baylor College of Dentistry
Dallas, Texas

W.B. Saunders Company
A Division of
Harcourt Brace & Company
Philadelphia London Toronto
Montreal Sydney Tokyo

W.B. SAUNDERS COMPANY
A Division of
Harcourt Brace & Company
The Curtis Center
Independence Square West
Philadelphia, Pennsylvania 19106

Library of Congress Cataloging-in-Publication Data

Viazis, Anthony D.
    Atlas of orthodontics: principles and clinical applications /
Anthony D. Viazis.
       p.   cm.
    Includes index.
    ISBN 0-7216-6643-4
    1. Orthodontics — Atlases.   I. Title.
    [DNLM: 1. Orthodontics — atlases.   WU 17 V623a]
RK521.V5   1993
617.6'43'00222 — dc20
DNLM/DLC   92-48199

Atlas of Orthodontics: Principles and Clinical Applications   ISBN 0-7216-6643-4

Printed in the United States of America.

Last digit is the print number: 9   8   7   6   5   4   3   2   1

To my family, Damianos, Georgia, Angelo, and the memory of Panos.

Preface

Atlas of Orthodontics: Principles and Clinical Applications was written with the intention to introduce to the world of clinical orthodontics its first illustrated text. This colorful, methodological presentation of the most up-to-date information and direct clinical application aims to aid the students of orthodontics in understanding the logical sequence from diagnosis to a successful treatment. In addition, as the innovations and revolutionary improvements in clinical orthodontics over recent years have widened the scope of diagnosis and broadened the horizons of treatment, this work aims to serve as the most updated illustrated reference of all these new advances. Thus, the atlas can very easily serve as a guide to students, dentists, and orthodontists alike.

Atlas of Orthodontics is an array of original photographs and drawings that highlight the state-of-the-art modern practice of orthodontics with fresh, new ideas on diagnosis, treatment planning, and, above all, therapy and its clinical application. It provides the reader with a step-by-step decision-making approach to the practice of orthodontics. The comprehensive yet easily readable text and the legends that accompany the illustrations span the breadth of the references. The clinician learns various techniques from photographic material (in color) directly from the patient's mouth. This atlas offers a system that gives the best results while disclosing invaluable tips on preventing clinical blunders that would lead to complications. It methodically explains the reasons for all the clinical techniques used based on fundamental biological and biomechanical principles, so that the reader will easily understand the orthodontic thinking process. Furthermore, it will give the practitioner the satisfaction of being able to apply clinically all that he reads. While reflecting the most current accepted treatment methods, its structured outline and continuity provide all the information in an easy, commonsense format. No other book in the field of orthodontics focuses on the clinical side of day-to-day practice with such an abundance of illustrations that educate the reader on critical judgment and clinical modalities that give the best treatment results. It is an invaluable educational source of the art and science of clinical orthodontics for the graduate and undergraduate student, for the general dentist, and even for the most experienced orthodontist.

My sincere appreciation is addressed to the following individuals for their significant contributions to my education and academic endeavors in orthodontics: from Baylor College of Dentistry, Drs. Richard Ceen, Robert Gaylord, Tom Matthews, and Peter Buschang, Rohit Sachdeva, Doug Crosby, Monte Collins, Joe Jacobs, Richard Aubrey, Moody Alexander, Wick Alexander, Ed Genecov, Larry Wolford, Mr. Stan Richardson, and Mr. Chris Semos; from the University of Minnesota, Drs. William Liljemark, Richard Bevis, Gerald Cavanaugh, T. Michael Speidel, Kevin Denis, Mark Holmberg, James Swift, Robert Feigal, Robert Gorlin, William Douglas, and the former President of the American Board of Orthodontics, Lloyd Pearson; from the University of Maryland, Dr. Dianne Rekow; from Tufts University, Drs. Nicholas Darzenta and Anthi Tsamtsouris; from the University of North Carolina, Dr. William

Proffit; from the University of Southern California, Dr. Peter Sinclair; from the University of Iowa, Drs. John Casko and Samir Bishara; from the University of Athens, Drs. Meropi Spyropoulos, Paul Apostolopoulos, and George Vouyouklakis; from the Medical College of Virginia, Dr. Robert Isaacson; and from Louisiana State University, Dr. Jack Sheridan; and from the University of Toronto, Dr. Angelo Metaxas.

A special acknowledgment is addressed to one man who is an inspiration to many in the field of orthodontics: Dr. T.M. Graber, Editor-in-Chief of the *American Journal of Orthodontics and Dentofacial Orthopedics.* I am deeply grateful to him for his advice, recommendations, endless energy and enthusiasm, and the wonderful support that all my academic endeavors have enjoyed from him.

I am also grateful to all the students with whom I have had the distinct pleasure of working, from the undergraduate junior dental class at the University of Minnesota that presented me with the greatest honor of my academic life, the "Teacher of the Year Award" after my very first year in teaching, to the graduate students at the same school and at Baylor College of Dentistry for their excellent work on all the cases that we treated together. Their critical thinking and quest for knowledge have certainly influenced me and the way I teach.

ANTHONY D. VIAZIS, DDS, MS

Contents

Preliminary Examination of the Patient

Chief Complaint

The examination of the patient in the office should always start with the medical history, as is done in any dental office.[1-3] The dental clinical evaluation should follow, where general notes, as well as an evaluation of the intraoral soft tissue, teeth, and oral function, and panoramic radiograph are made.[2,3] Any operative, periodontal, and endodontic work (if needed) should be completed before initiation of orthodontic treatment, whereas any temporomandibular joint (TMJ) pain or dysfunction should be addressed before the onset of orthodontic treatment (Table A1.1). Permanent prosthetic work should be done afterward.

Inquiring about the patient's chief complaint, *i.e.,* the reason he or she seeks orthodontic treatment, is of utmost importance. The chief complaint must have been met by the end of treatment, otherwise the patient will not be happy, even if the orthodontic therapy is of the highest standards. If the patient or guardian has unrealistic expectations that may not be met with treatment, the clinician ought to educate him or her so that he or she understands the limitations of the various therapeutic modalities in modern orthodontics. A good example is the change of the soft tissue (lips) as a result of extraction therapy. A patient will not be satisfied if, after 2 years of orthodontics, he or she has a beautiful occlusion accompanied by late nasal growth that makes the lips appear more retrusive.[4] In addition, the low degree of predictability associated with the upper lip in response to orthodontic tooth movement, possibly caused by the complex anatomy or dynamics of the upper lip,[1] might cause undesirable changes in the soft-tissue profile in crowded cases that involve extractions of permanent teeth. Nonorthodontic measures (*i.e.,* rhinoplasty or genioplasty) should be discussed with the patient before the start of the orthodontic treatment.[1]

Table 1.1 Clinical Information Form (Dental)

General Information

Parent name	Guardian name		Date
Address			Telephone
Patient name	Grade	Hobbies	Chief complaint
Patient height	Father's height	Mother's height	Patient motivation
Prepubertal	Circumpubertal	Postpubertal	Habits
Family history of malocclusion			

Intraoral Soft-Tissue Evaluation

Pathology	Oral hygiene	Attached gingiva	Gingival recession
Attachment	Pocket depth > 3mm		Frenum

Intraoral Dental Evaluation and Panoramic Radiograph

Decay	Extracted	Root length
Hypocalcification	Fractured crown	Crown/bridge
Missing	Fractured root	Supernumerary
Impacted	Stained	Wisdom teeth
Ankylosed	Endodontically treated	Bone pathology
Unerupted	Condylar outline	Alveolar bone

Functional Evaluation

Speech pathology	Muscle tenderness	Internal derangement
Breathing	Clenching	Stage I (early or late clicking)
Swallowing	Bruxism	Stage II (morning lock)
Tongue size	Deviation upon opening	Stage III (acute lock)
Lip tonicity	Deviation upon closing	Stage IV (function off disk)
Tonsil size	Range of motion (ROM)	Stage V (pain, grating sound)
CO/CR discrepancy	TMJ pain	TMJ dysfunction

References

1. Talass MF, Tallas L, and Baker RC: Soft tissue profile changes resulting from retraction of maxillary incisors. Am J Orthod Dentofacial Orthop 91:385–394, 1987.
2. Proffit WR, and White RP, Jr.: *Surgical-Orthodontic Treatment.* St. Louis, MO: Mosby Year Book, 1991.
3. Proffit WR: *Contemporary Orthodontics.* St. Louis, MO: C.V. Mosby Co., 1986.
4. Buschang PH, Viazis AD, DelaCruz R, and Oakes C: Horizontal growth of the soft-tissue nose relative to maxillary growth. J Clin Orthod 26:111–118, 1992.

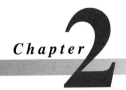

Dental Development

The development of teeth begins *in utero,* but it is not until 2 to 3 years of age that all deciduous teeth appear in the toddler's mouth.[1,2] The most common sequence of eruption starts with the lower central incisors, followed by the upper centrals in the first 6 months of life; the upper lateral and lower incisors erupt by the end of the first year of age; the upper and lower first deciduous molars, followed by the cuspids, appear by 18 months, and the lower and upper second deciduous molars erupt by the end of the second year or as late as the third year of life[1,2] (see Fig. F1.15). Past this point, very little increase in dental arch width occurs. Spacing is desirable in the primary dentition; lack of spacing means large teeth or small arches and is strongly suggestive of crowding in the permanent dentition.

The eruption of the permanent dentition starts around the age of 5 or 6 years with the first permanent molars distal to the second deciduous molar teeth.[1,2] The periods 5 to 8 years of age and 9 to 12 years of age are called early and late mixed dentition stages, respectively. Around 6.5 years of age, the lower central incisors erupt, followed by the upper centrals by 7 years of age.[1,2] The lower laterals erupt by age 7.5 years, followed by their maxillary counterparts at age 8 years or as late as 9 years of age[1,2] (see Fig. F1.16). At approximately 10 years of age, the lower permanent cuspids make their appearance in the child's mouth, followed by the upper first bicuspids at age 10.5 years and the lower first bicuspids at age 11 years.[1,2] The upper and lower second bicuspids erupt very close to each other at age 11.5 years, followed by maxillary cuspids and the second permanent molars by the age of 12 years or as late as age 13 years.[1,2] One must keep in mind that there is one significant variation of tooth eruption in the population: teeth may erupt as early or as late as 2 years in relation to the average ages mentioned above and still be considered normal.

Teeth usually erupt when the roots are one half to three quarters formed.[2] After the end of the early mixed dentition stage, the upper incisors may have substantial spacing as their crowns are inclined toward the distal. This is called the "ugly ducking stage" and is considered a normal condition that will self-correct later on; it happens due to the eruption path of the permanent cuspids as they come into position for eruption along the roots of the lateral incisors (Fig. A2.1).

The sum of the mesiodistal width of the deciduous cuspid and molar teeth is 1.3 and 3.1 mm greater than the permanent cuspid and bicuspid teeth in the maxilla and the mandible, respectively (leeway space).[2] This space is generally used in the permanent dentition to permit improvement of possible crowding of anterior teeth and also to allow a slight mesial migration of the first permanent mandibular molar into a solid class I occlusion.[2,3] The leeway space may be quickly lost from premature exfoliation of teeth and quick mesial movement of the permanent molar to an extent that the lower second bicuspid may be blocked out toward the lingual[2] (see Fig. D6.7). It should be noted that the last increase in dental arch width occurs as the permanent cuspid teeth erupt into their position in the arch. Expansion of the arches in this area is questionable past this stage.

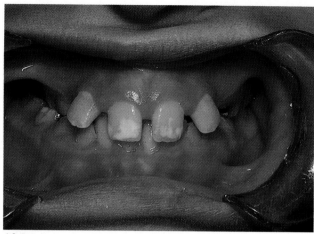

A2.1

Figure A2.1 The "ugly duckling" stage of tooth development.

In a study on the changes in the molar relation between the deciduous and permanent dentitions, it was concluded that 61.6%, 34.3%, and 4.1% of patients end up with a class I, class II, and class III permanent molar relationship, respectively.[3] Patients who start with a full distal step in the deciduous dentition develop into a class II molar relationship; thus, treatment should be initiated in these cases as early as possible. Conversely, almost half (50%) of patients who have a 50% class II primary molar relation (end-to-end flush plane) develop a class I permanent molar occlusion.[3] Close observation of these patients is needed until a class I relation occurs.

References

1. Mohl ND, Zarb GA, Carlsson GE, and Rugh JD: *A Textbook of Occlusion.* Chicago: Quintessence Publishing, 1988.
2. Undergraduate syllabus. University of Minnesota, Department of Orthodontics, Minneapolis, MN, 1989.
3. Bishara SE, Hoppens BJ, Jacobsen JR, and Kohout FJ. Changes in the molar relationship between the deciduous and permanent dentition: A longitudinal study. Am J Orthod Dentofacial Orthop 93:19–28, 1988.

Chapter 3

Articulated Casts

The most supero-anterior position of the condyle is musculoskeletally the most stable position of the joint (centric relation).[1-3] In this position, the condyles are resting against the posterior slopes of the articular eminences with the articular disks properly interposed and all of the muscles that coordinate joint movement at rest.[1-3] During rest and function, this position is both anatomically and physiologically sound. A posterior force to the mandible can displace the condyle to an unstable posterior (or retruded) position. Because the retrodiscal tissues are highly vascularized, well supplied with sensory nerve fibers, and not structured to accept forces, there is great potential for eliciting pain or causing breakdown.[1,3]

The position of the mandible where the relation of opposing teeth provides for maximum occlusal intercuspation is called centric occlusion.[1-4] This, ideally, should coincide with centric relation[4]; this is what the clinician should strive for during orthodontic treatment. In most cases, a slight discrepancy of about 1 mm also can be acceptable, where the position of the mandible in centric relation is slightly behind its position in centric occlusion.

In contrast to craniometric variables, which have high heritabilities, almost all of the occlusal variability is acquired rather than inherited.[5] Thus, a careful examination of the patient's malocclusion is essential. This is best done from a set of articulated casts in centric relation (CR) (Fig. A3.1).

The following wax bite registration technique is suggested for proper recording of the patient's bite[6]: the right thumb is placed on top of the patient's chin with the right index finger under the patient's left gonial angle and the right second finger under the patient's right gonial angle (Fig. A3.2). The mandible is allowed to close (Fig. A3.3) in such a manner that the lower incisors contact the anterior wax, until a 2-mm posterior opening in the molar area is obtained (Fig. A3.4). When the patient squeezes, the muscle contractions seat the condyles in a superior and slightly anterior position against the eminence.[6] The objective is to gain an index of both maxillary and mandibular incisal edges without making any tooth contacts. The anterior wax is cooled down and removed while a soft posterior wax is placed against the maxillary posterior teeth (first molar and second premolar area) (Fig. A3.5). The hard anterior wax is secured in the anterior region (Fig. A3.6) and the mandible is gently manipulated into centric relation as described above (Fig. A3.7). After the mandibular closure has been stopped by the limit of the indexes in the anterior section (Fig. A3.8), both pieces of wax are removed after they are cooled down with air-spray (Fig. A3.9). A centric occlusion wax bite is also taken as the patient opens widely and bites all the way through the wax until the teeth touch fully.

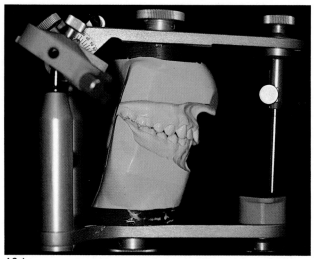

A3.1

Figure A3.1 Articulated casts on SAM 2 (Great Lakes, NY) articulator. Only by mounting the casts are we able to notice any prematurities, functional shifts, and the exact relationship of teeth in centric relation. Hand-articulating polished casts cannot capture initial tooth contacts.

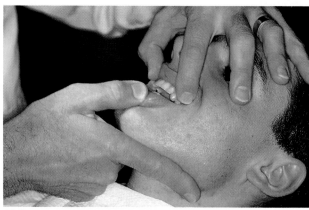

A3.2

Figure A3.2 Hand manipulation for recording centric relation (CR) position: the clinician's right thumb is placed on top of the patient's chin, the right index finger under the patient's left gonial angle, and the right second finger under the patient's right gonial angle.

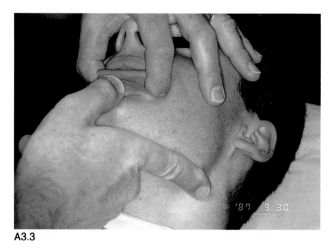

A3.3

Figure A3.3 The patient's mandible is allowed to close gently.

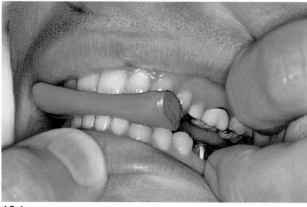

A3.4

Figure A3.4 The closing motion is stopped when the lower incisors come in contact with the anterior wax. Note the bite opening in the bicuspid/molar area. No posterior teeth are allowed to contact.

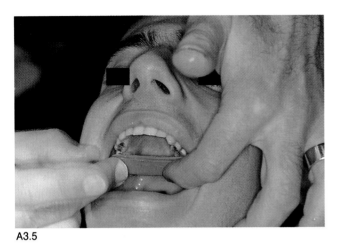

A3.5

Figure A3.5 A soft posterior piece of wax is pressed lightly against the posterior teeth.

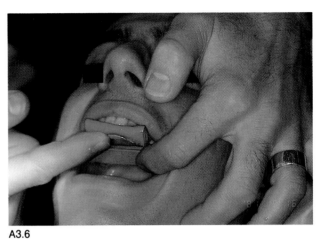

A3.6

Figure A3.6 While gently holding the posterior wax in place, the hard anterior wax is secured in its position. Note the indentations of the lower incisors recorded previously.

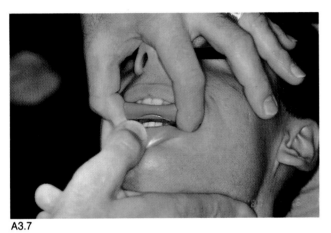

A3.7

Figure A3.7 The mandible is again very gently manipulated into CR. Note that the anterior wax is held against the upper anterior teeth during the closing motion of the mandible.

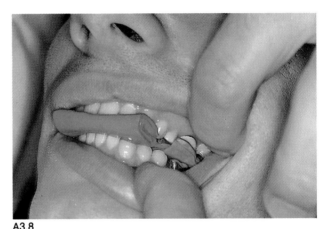

A3.8

Figure A3.8 The mandibular closing motion is stopped as soon as the lower anterior teeth come in contact with the hard anterior wax. The posterior teeth made their cusp indentations in the posterior wax, without even coming in contact with their counterparts. This way, the muscles have guided and seated the condyles in the most supero-anterior position against the eminence.

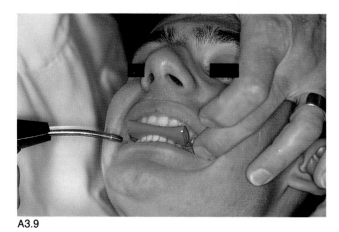

A3.9

Figure A3.9 The wax pieces are cooled down with air-spray before they are removed from the mouth.

Once mounted on the articulator, the dental casts are used to evaluate the following[7]:

Angle Classification

A class I molar relation exists when the mesiobuccal cusp tip of the upper first molar occludes in the buccal groove of the lower first molar (see Fig. E3.7). Similarly, a class I cuspid relation exists when the upper cuspid occludes in the embrasure between the lower first bicuspid and the lower cuspid (see Fig. F4.72). A full cusp width ahead of the class I position is defined as a full-step class II (see Figs. F4.84, F4.92, F4.96). A full cusp width back of the class I position is a full class III (see Fig. C1.15). An end-to-end relation is termed as a 50% class II (see Fig. D11.1) or 50% class III (see Fig. D9.33), depending on the direction of discrepancy.

Overbite

The vertical overlap of teeth is the overbite (OB). The OB in the incisor area should be approximately 2 mm (see Fig. C1.18).

Overjet

The horizontal overlap of teeth is the overjet (OJ). The OJ in the incisor area should be 1 to 2 mm (see Fig. C1.18).

Crowding

The best and most accurate way to evaluate the existing arch length discrepancy is by measuring the width of all the teeth in the arch with a campus, as well as measuring the actual arch length.[7] A clinical way to assess crowding is by "eyeballing" it, taking into consideration the average width of various major teeth (bicuspids—7 mm; cuspids—8 mm; lower incisors—6 mm; upper centrals—10 mm). By subtracting how much tooth material is blocked out of the arch or is in a crowded position, one may very quickly evaluate the space that is needed to obtain good tooth alignment. This is undoubtedly a very crude method, but one that clinical experience has shown to approximate (±1 mm) to the exact discrepancy (see Figs. D6.6, D6.7, D9.18, D9.19, F4.62, F4.63, F5.3, F5.4, F5.11, F5.12, F5.24, F5.25). The cause of crowding may differ from one subject to another, or there may be more than one factor contributing to the development of crowding in any one individual.[8]

Crossbite

Crossbite occurs when one or more teeth are in an abnormal buccolingual relationship.[7] Single-tooth crossbites are usually dental in nature (see Figs. E4.1, E4.2). Multiple-tooth crossbites are anterior (see Fig. C1.13) or posterior (see Figs. C1.13, C1.26, C1.30) and usually skeletal in nature.[7] Anterior tooth crossbites may be "pseudo class III" (due to a shift) (see Figs. F1.16, F1.17) or "true class III" (true skeletal) (see Fig. C1.13).[7] Posterior crossbites are unilateral or bilateral. Unilateral, multiple-tooth crossbites are usually the result of a side shift to one side from a bilateral skeletal crossbite. The vast majority of multiple-tooth crossbites are bilateral and are due to a constricted maxilla (see Fig. F4.105). Multiple-tooth crossbites should be corrected as soon as possible (the youngest known patient is 3 years old) to avoid the possible development of a skeletal malocclusion or abnormal eruption of teeth, as well as to improve the patient's esthetics[9] (see Figs. F1.12 through F1.15).

Dental Midlines

The facial midline (see Fig. B1.1) (middle of eyebrows, tip of the nose, cupid's bow) should coincide with the upper dental midline (between the upper centrals) and the lower dental midline (between the lower centrals) (see Fig. D9.27). If a compromise must be made due to the patient's malocclusion, it may be best to leave the lower midline off by 1 to 2 mm (a lot of patients do not show their lower teeth upon smiling). The upper dental midline should coincide with the facial midline for an esthetically pleasing smile (see Fig. A8.3).

Tooth-Size Discrepancy

A tooth-size discrepancy (TSD) exists when the size of the lower or the upper teeth is not in proportion with that of their counterparts.[10-12] An anomaly in the size of the upper lateral incisors is the most common cause, but variations in bicuspids or other teeth may be present[7] (see Figs. A3.10, F3.7, F5.22). In such a case, it would be impossible to obtain an ideal OB/OJ relation of 2 mm when the cuspids are in a class

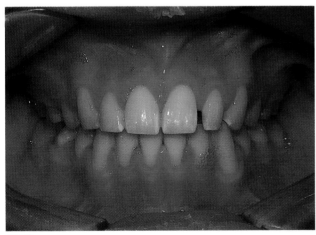

A3.10

Figure A3.10 Small upper left lateral. Spaces were left next to it for prosthetic work.

I occlusion. If there is excess maxillary tooth material, we will end up with an excessive OJ (see Fig. F5.8); if the excess is in the mandibular arch, then minimal OB/OJ will exist and the cuspids will occlude in a slight class III relation.

A large percentage of patients have mesial–distal tooth-size discrepancies, approximately 13.8% and 9.2% for the mandibular and maxillary dentitions, respectively.[11] Such discrepancies, if left untreated, could lead to future posttreatment relapse, especially in the mandibular incisor area. Interproximal reduction will, in most cases, alleviate such discrepancies.

A method used to assess TSD is Bolton's analysis.[7,12] If alterations of tooth size are to be done in the upper arch, the sum of the width of the lower anterior teeth is multiplied by 1.3 to give the dimensions of the ideal upper arch for these particular lower anteriors.[10] If alterations of tooth size are to be done in the lower arch, then the width of the upper anterior teeth is multiplied by .775 to give the ideal lower arch.[10] If the TSD is in the posterior teeth, then they may be selectively reduced in width, enough to obtain a class I cuspid relation (see Figs. F3.7, F3.8). Interproximal reduction should be done in the upper or lower arch in order to make these teeth fit in relation to their counterparts.

References

1. Okeson JP: *Management of Temporomandibular Disorders and Occlusion,* 2nd ed. St. Louis, MO: C.V. Mosby Co., 1989.
2. Mohl ND, Zarb GA, Carlsson GE, and Rugh JD: *A Textbook of Occlusion.* Chicago: Quintessence Publishing, 1988.
3. American Academy of Craniomandibular Disorders: *Craniomandibular Disorders: Guidelines for Evaluation, Diagnosis and Management.* McNeill C, ed. Chicago: Quintessence Publishing, 1990.
4. Parker WS: Centric relation and centric occlusion—An orthodontic responsibility. Am J Orthod Dentofacial Orthop 74:481–500, 1978.
5. Harris EF, and Johnson MG: Heritability of craniometric and occlusal variables: A longitudinal sib analysis. Am J Orthod Dentofacial Orthop 99:258–268, 1991.
6. Carlson G: Advances in Orthodontics: Seminar Series (Course Syllabus). Minneapolis, MN, 1988.
7. Proffit WR: *Contemporary Orthodontics.* St. Louis, MO: C.V. Mosby Co., 1986.
8. Richardson ME: The role of the third molar in the cause of late lower arch crowding: A review. Am J Orthod Dentofacial Orthop 95:79–83, 1989.
9. Vadiakas G, and Viazis AD: Anterior crossbite connection in the primary dentition. Am J Orthod Dentofacial Orthop 102:160–162, 1992.
10. Wolford LM: Surgical–orthodontic correction of dentofacial and craniofacial deformities—Syllabus. Baylor College of Dentistry, Dallas, TX, 1990.
11. Crosby DR, and Alexander RG: The occurrence of tooth size discrepancies among different malocclusion groups. Am J Orthod Dentofacial Orthop 95:457–461, 1989.
12. Bolton WA: The clinical application of tooth size analysis. Am J Orthod Dentofacial Orthop 48:504–529, 1962.

Chapter 4

Radiographic Evaluation

A careful dental and radiographic (panoramic or periapical) evaluation may reveal a number of situations that need to be addressed before the initiation of orthodontic mechanotherapy.

Ankylosis

Ankylosis,[1] a localized fusion of alveolar bone and cementum, is the result of a defective or discontinuous periodontal membrane and is apparently caused by mechanical, thermal, or metabolic trauma to the periodontal membrane during or after tooth eruption. It occurs most often in the primary dentition (see Fig. D10.8) in the mandibular teeth, and in molars. It can sometimes be detected from radiographic evidence of periodontal membrane obliteration or by a sharp or ringing sound upon percussion and by lack of tooth mobility or soreness, even with heavy, continuous orthodontic forces.[1]

In the primary dentition, ankylosis is usually treated by simple neglect, restoration, or extraction.[1] Ankylosis of a permanent tooth, however, is more complicated if orthodontic treatment is planned. Intervention can include luxation, corticotomy, or ostectomy.[1]

Most infra-occluded and ankylosed primary molars with a permanent successor exfoliate normally.[2] The decreased height of the alveolar bone level at the site of the infra-occluded primary molar has been reported to normalize after the eruption of the permanent successor. Infra-occlusion and ankylosis of primary molars does not constitute a general risk of future alveolar bone loss mesial to the first permanent molars.

Primary Failure of Eruption

Primary failure of eruption describes a condition in which nonankylosed, usually posterior teeth fail to erupt, either fully or partially, because of failure of the eruption mechanism.[3-5] The teeth most commonly involved are the deciduous and permanent molars, although premolars and cuspids may also be affected.[5] There appears to be no mechanical impediment to eruption in these cases.[5] Unilateral situations occur more frequently than bilateral ones. A posterior open bite, caused by a primary failure of eruption, will not respond to orthodontic treatment; a segmental alveolar osteotomy offers the only possible treatment modality.

Diastemas

Midline diastemas are quite common among individuals (see Fig. F4.11). Closing them poses no problem orthodontically, but in many patients they tend to re-open, especially if caused by an abnormal labial frenum.[6]

It is important to close the space orthodontically as soon as possible and then perform the surgical procedure of abnormal labial frenum, thus allowing healing of the tissues to occur with the teeth in their newly established positions.[6] It is suggested that when the frenum is wide and attached below the mucogingival junction in keratinized tissue, it often will regenerate after frenectomy.[7] To prevent this from occurring, epithelial graft from the palate is placed over the area on removal of the frenum, preventing its ingrowth.[7]

Root Resorption

Root resorption occurs in every patient who undergoes orthodontic treatment. In the majority of cases, it is a mere blunting of the root apices. In some patients, it is more severe for reasons that seem to be idiopathic, with the exception of previously traumatized teeth, which are more susceptible to resorption and loss of vitality (Fig. A4.1).[8] Around 16.5% of patients have approximately 1 mm of resorption of the maxillary incisor teeth.[8] Maxillary incisors have been reported to be the most susceptible to this severe resorption, with other teeth less affected. A recent study showed that 3% of patients have severe resorption (greater than one quarter of the root length) of both maxillary central incisors (Fig. A4.2).

Less resorption is observed in patients treated before age 11 years, perhaps due to a preventive effect of the thick layer of predentin on young, undeveloped roots.[9] Contact of maxillary incisors with the lingual cortical plate may predispose to resorption.[9] Class III patients are overrepresented in the group with severe resorption.[9]

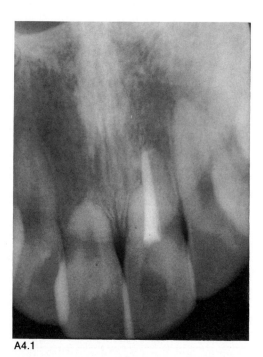

A4.1

Figure A4.1 Trauma to these central incisors from a bicycle accident led to their severe root resorption and loss of vitality.

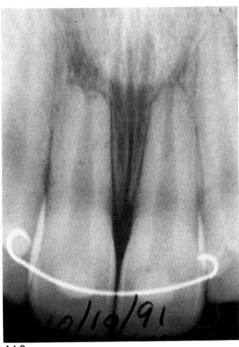

A4.2

Figure A4.2 Resorption of central incisor teeth after 2 years of orthodontic treatment. One quarter to one third of these roots have been lost.

The longer the active treatment time, the greater the chance of severe resorption. Obviously, a patient with small, rounded roots is not a good candidate for excessive tooth movement. Iatrogenic root resorption is caused by jiggling teeth over long periods of time, indecisive treatment that causes changes in the direction of tooth movement, and proximating of the cortical plate.[10] No relation has been found between the amount of root shortening and degree of intrusion achieved.[11] In general, treatment time is the most significant factor for occurrence of root shortening. In a recent long-term evaluation of root resorption occurring during orthodontic treatment, it was shown that there are no apparent changes after appliance removal except remodeling of rough and sharp edges.[12]

Impacted Cuspids

Impaction of the cuspid teeth[13-20] is caused primarily by the rate of root resorption of the deciduous teeth, disturbances in tooth eruption, tooth size/arch length discrepancies, rotation or trauma of tooth buds, premature root closure, ankylosis, cystic or neoplastic formation, clefts, and idiopathic causes. Most of the impactions are unilateral and on the palatal side.[16] The evidence of maxillary impaction ranges from 0.92% to 2.2%; maxillary impaction is twice as common in females than in males.[16] The incidence of mandibular impaction is much less, 0.35%.[16] Impacted cuspids may cause resorption of the adjacent incisor teeth; thus, their extraction or uncovering and movement into the dental arch is necessary (Fig. A4.3). Potential incisor resorption cases from impacted cuspids are those in which the cuspid cusp in periapical and panoramic films is positioned medially to the midline of the lateral incisor (0.71%).[16] The risk of resorption also increases with a more mesial horizontal path of eruption.[21]

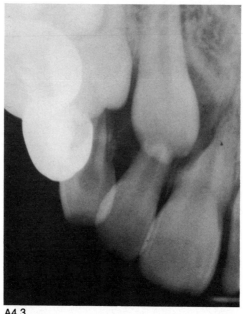

A4.3

Figure A4.3 An impacted cuspid has caused almost complete resorption of the lateral incisor tooth and significant destruction of the central incisor tooth.

Surgical uncovering of these teeth is the standard treatment procedure, followed by direct bonding of an orthodontic bracket onto the tooth and mechanical traction with elastics or springs to bring the teeth into the arch (see Fig. F4.58). An apically repositioned flap for labially situated cuspids is recommended.[14] Adequate attached gingiva need be present (or surgically placed) to avoid mucogingival problems. Wire ligation ("lasso" type) instead of direct bracket placement onto the uncovered tooth is prohibited because it leads to loss of attachment and to external root resorption and ankylosis.[15] In addition, any surgical exposure beyond the cement–enamel junction leads to bone loss.

Treatment of cases with impacted cuspids is quite lengthy, depending on the position and orientation of the impacted tooth in the bone.[16,17] It may take between 12 and 30 months. Also, at the end of treatment, these teeth will show the presence of a 5- to 7-mm pocket, usually on the distal side. They display significantly more loss of periodontal support on the buccal and palatal surfaces than do normal teeth.[17] Excellent oral hygiene will preserve these teeth throughout life without further sequelae.

An alternative to surgical uncovering and lengthy orthodontic treatment of impacted teeth is the autotransplantation of these teeth. Autotransplantation should be performed at a stage when optimal root development of the transplant may be expected; namely, one half to three quarters of the full root length.[18] When transplantation is performed at an earlier stage of root development, the final root length may be shorter than desirable. If autotransplantation is performed at a later stage of root development, the risk of root resorption increases. The surgical procedure should be as atraumatic as possible and requires a surgeon well acquainted with the method.

Teeth transplanted with incomplete and complete root formation show 96% and 15% pulp healing, respectively.[19] The size of the apical foramen and possibly the avoidance of bacterial contamination during the surgical procedure are explanatory factors for pulpal healing. Trauma to the periodontal ligament (PDL) of the transplant is the explanatory factor for the development of root resorption.[19]

A fairly new technique, transalveolar transplantation, is used to remove large amounts of bone with a bur except for a thin layer close to the root surface.[20] This bone is then very gently removed with an elevator to avoid damage to the cementum. The tooth is stored in the socket throughout the operative procedure. Finally, the cuspid is moved through the alveolar process into its determined position. A sectional arch wire is used to stabilize but not immobilize the transplanted cuspid. Sometimes, grinding of the antagonist tooth is required to avoid traumatic occlusion. A postoperative orthodontic appliance check is performed 1 week later, when the sutures are removed. Further orthodontic controls are performed every 2 weeks for 6 to 8 weeks.

Tooth Transpositions

Transposition has been described as an interchange in the position of two permanent teeth within the same quadrant of the dental arch.[22-25] The maxillary permanent cuspid is the tooth most frequently involved in transposition with the first bicuspid,[22,25] less often with the lateral incisor (Fig. A4.4).[22,24] The retained deciduous cuspid may be the primary cause for deviation of the permanent cuspid from its normal path of eruption.

If the mandibular cuspid and lateral incisor have already erupted in their transposed position, correction to their normal position should usually not be attempted.[22] Alignment in their transposed position with reshaping of their incisal surfaces will not damage the teeth or supporting structures and will present an acceptable esthetic result. If one of the transposed or adjacent teeth is severely affected by caries or trauma or if there is a severe lack of space, extraction of that tooth should be considered.[22,23] If tooth movement is undertaken to correct the transposition, in order to avoid root interference or resorption during treatment and to prevent bony loss at the cortical plate of the labially positioned cuspid, the transposed tooth (premolar or lateral incisor) should first be moved palatally, enough to allow for a free movement of the cuspid to its normal place.[22,23] This last method is the least desirable treatment of choice.

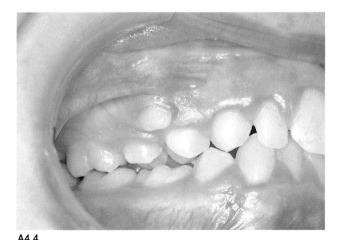

A4.4

Figure A4.4 Transposed maxillary right cuspid, as it is erupting distal to the first bicuspid. Note the retained primary cuspid.

Supernumerary Teeth

Supernumerary (extra teeth) or congenitally missing teeth occur quite frequently among patients.[26] The most common situation of a supernumerary tooth is a mesodens between the central incisors, which may prevent their normal eruption. The most frequent missing teeth are the upper laterals (see Fig. F5.30), followed by the lower second bicuspids, the upper second bicuspids, and lower incisors. Of course, the third molars (wisdom teeth) are missing in a large percentage of the population.

Third Molars

The role of mandibular third molars in the relapse of lower anterior crowding after the cessation of retention in orthodontically treated cases has provoked much speculation in the dental literature over many years.[27] Most practitioners are of the opinion that third molars sometimes produce crowding of the mandibular anterior teeth.[28] A number of studies over recent years have substantiated very clearly that the presence of third molars does not appear to produce a greater degree of lower anterior crowding than that which occurs in patients with no third molars.[27-29] Therefore, the recommendation for mandibular third molar removal with the objective of relieving interdental pressure and thus alleviating or preventing mandibular incisor crowding is not justified.[28,29]

References

1. Phelan MK, Moss RB Jr., Powell RS, and Womble BA: Orthodontic management of ankylosed teeth. J Clin Orthod 24:375–378, 1990.
2. Kurol J, and Olson L: Ankylosis of primary molars—A future periodontal threat to the first permanent molars? Eur J Orthod 13:404–409, 1991.
3. Proffit WR, and Vig KWI: Primary failure of eruption: A possible cause of posterior open bite. Am J Orthod 80:173–190, 1981.
4. Ireland AJ: Familial posterior open bite: A primary failure of eruption. Br J Orthod 18:233–237, 1991.
5. Nashed RR, and Holmes A: Case report—A posterior open bite. Br J Orthod 17:47–53, 1990.
6. Bishara SE: Management of diastemas in orthodontics. Am J Orthod 61:55–63, 1972.
7. Takei H: Periodontal problem-solving for orthodontics. Summarized by Turley PK. Pacific Coast Society of Orthodontists Bulletin, Spring, 34–36, 1991.
8. Linge L, and Linge BO: Patient characteristics and treatment variables associated with apical root resorption during orthodontic treatment. Am J Orthod Dentofacial Orthop 99:35–43, 1991.
9. Kaley J, and Phillips C: Factors related to root resorption in edgewise practice. Angle Orthod 61:125–131, 1991.
10. Hickham JH: Directional forces revisited. J Clin Orthod 20:626–637, 1986.
11. McFadden WM, Engstrom C, Engstrom H, and Anholm JM: A study of the relationship between incision intrusion and root shortening. Am J Orthod Dentofacial Orthop 96:390–396, 1989.
12. Remington DN, Joondeph DR, Artun J, Riedel RA, and Chapko MK: Long-term evaluation of root resorption occurring during orthodontic treatment. Am J Orthod Dentofacial Orthop 96:43–46, 1989.
13. Bishara SE, Kommer DD, McNeil MH, Mantagana LN, Oestler LJ, and Youngquist HW: Management of impacted cuspids. Am J Orthod 69:371–387, 1976.
14. Vanarsdall RL, and Corn H: Soft-tissue management of labially positioned unerupted teeth. Am J Orthod 72:53–64, 1977.
15. Boyd RL: Clinical assessment of injuries in orthodontic movement of impacted teeth. Am J Orthod 82:478–486, 1982.
16. Bishara SE: Impacted maxillary canines: A review. Am J Orthod Dentofacial Orthop 101:159–171, 1992.
17. Wisth PJ, Norderal K, and Boe OE: Periodontal status of orthodontically treated impacted maxillary cuspids. Angle Orthod 46:69–76, 1976.
18. Lagerstom L, and Kristerson L: Influence of orthodontic treatment on root development of autotransplanted premolars. Am J Orthod 89:146–150, 1986.
19. Andreasen JO, Paulsen HV, Yu Z, Ahlquist R, Bayer T, and Schwartz O: A long-term study of 370 autotransplanted premolars. Eur J Orthod 12:3–50, 1990.
20. Sagne S, and Thilander B: Transalveolar transplantation of maxillary cuspids. A follow-up study. Br J Orthod 12:140–147, 1990.
21. Ericson S, and Kurol J: Resorption of maxillary lateral incisors caused by ectopic eruption of the cuspids. Am J Orthod Dentofacial Orthop 94:503–513, 1988.
22. Shapira Y, and Kuftinek MM: Tooth transpositions—A review of the literature and treatment considerations. Angle Orthod 59:271–276, 1989.

23. Laptook T, and Silling G: Cuspid transposition—Approaches to treatment. J Am Dent Assoc 107:746–748, 1983.
24. Gholston LR, and Williams PR: Bilateral transposition of maxillary cuspids and lateral incisors: A rare condition. Journal of Dentistry for Children 51:58–63, 1984.
25. Joshi MR, and Bhatt NA: Cuspid transposition. Oral Surg Oral Med Oral Pathol 31:49–54, 1971.
26. Undergraduate Syllabus. University of Minnesota, Orthodontic Department, Minneapolis, MN, 1989.
27. Kaplan RG: Mandibular third molars and postretention crowding. Am J Orthod 66:411–430, 1974.
28. Ades AG, Joondeph DR, Little RM, and Chapko MK: A long-term study of the relationship of third molars to changes in the mandibular dental arch. Am J Orthod Dentofacial Orthop 97:323–335, 1990.
29. Southard TE, Southard KA, and Weeda LW: Mesial force from unerupted third molars. Am J Orthod Dentofacial Orthop 99:220–225, 1991.

Chapter 5

The Temporomandibular Joint

The key to understanding temporomandibular disorders (TMDs) is in the differential diagnosis of joint (internal derangement) versus muscle pathology (myofacial pain) or a combination of the two.[1-6] Internal derangement of the temporomandibular joint (TMJ) refers to any abnormal anatomic relation between the three parts of the TMJ, namely, the condyle, the disk, and the articular fossa.[1,4,6] The most common internal derangement is that of anterior disk displacement, which results in the clinical sign of "clicking" or "popping" as the condyle snaps over the posterior band of the disk and on to it during mandibular movements[1] (stage I). The click may again be audible in a closing movement as the condyle slips off the back of the disk, and this is termed a reciprocal click.[1,4,6] This clicking on and off the disk is called anterior disk displacement with reduction.[1]

Anterior disk displacement also may occur without reduction (the condyle functions off the disk—stage II). Extracapsular muscle pain (myofacial pain) with no internal derangement usually presents with bilateral or unilateral soreness in the muscles of mastication and restricted mandibular motion due to muscle spasm[1,6] (but not due to internal derangement—no joint sounds should be present and radiographs should reveal normal osseous contours).

One should keep in mind that as much as 50%, if not more, of the population has one sign of joint dysfunction (noise, tenderness, etc.); the female to male ratio ranges from 3:1 to 9:1, and only 5% of the patients with signs and symptoms are in need of TMJ therapy.[6] During the TMJ examination of the patient, the clinician should look for possible sore muscles (in the neck and mouth area) and any "clicking" noises (with the use of a stethoscope or digital palpation), as well as any deviation on opening and closing[7-9] (the mandible will deviate toward the side of an anteriorly dislocated disk), any signs of bruxism and clenching (it is nighttime clenching that in many cases results in morning headaches), and the overall strain-level status of the patient.

The mouth should be able to open anywhere between 35 to 45 mm. Often, the patient may have a "closed lock" where he or she cannot open the mouth because the displaced disk is hindering mouth opening (stage III). At other times, the patient cannot close the mouth, "open lock," because a posteriorly displaced disk may not allow the condyle to return to its position in the fossa.[7-9] This may occur in the orthodontic office during bracket placement, where the patient's mouth remains open for a long period of time. If the joints demonstrate a high level of mobility ("loose joint"), it should be noted in order to avoid overstretching the already compromised ligaments.[4] Any crepitus joint sound (a cracking sound indicating a rough condyle, disk, or eminence surface) may be the result of direct, long-term bone contacts between the fossa and the condyle[1,4] (stage IV). Unless the condition stabilizes at this point, pain and degeneration of tissues may develop, resulting in severe dysfunction[4] (stage V).

The management of TMJ disorders ranges from behavior modification, pharmacotherapy, and palliative home care to physical therapy, orthopedic appliance therapy, and surgical treatment.[4,6] The description of these is beyond the scope of this text.

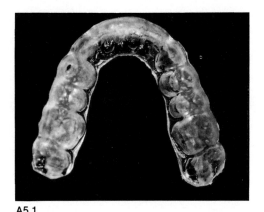

A5.1

Figure A5.1 An interocclusal appliance (splint).

Excellent sources are available in the literature on such treatment modalities.[4-6,10] Self-care, including a soft diet (no gum or caffeine), limited function, heat, and self-massage, should be instituted.[2] Disk displacement may be an adaptation to stability and should not necessarily be viewed as pathologic.[2] It is most probably due to a slow alteration and not to trauma.[2]

No orthodontic treatment should be initiated before possible TMJ pain or dysfunction is under control. Sometimes this can be addressed with simultaneous orthodontic therapy, but in no case should it be postponed until after orthodontic tooth movement. In most cases, an interocclusal appliance (splint) generally improves the TMJ status of the patient.[11] An interocclusal appliance is generally considered to be a removable device made of hard acrylic resin that fits between the maxillary and mandibular teeth (Fig. A5.1). It stabilizes and improves the function of the TMJ and the masticatory system and protects the teeth from attrition and the TMJ from traumatic loading. In some instances, however, TMJ surgery is the treatment modality of choice, which is sometimes combined with orthognathic surgery.[12]

The clinician must make every possible attempt to ensure that orthodontic mechanotherapy does not aggravate a patient's compromised TMJ status.[13-15] In the treatment of class II patients with deep bites and high cusps, a flat plate of acrylic that is placed over the occlusal surfaces of the lower posterior teeth in conjunction with fixed appliance therapy may prevent any unnecessary distal pressures on the condyles.[7] One must be careful, however, not to create posterior open bites. In the treatment of class III patients, chin-cap and class III elastics that exert distal pressure should not be used during sleeping hours, when the muscles are relaxed and therefore when there is more distal pressure on the condyles.[7] In the retention phase of a deep bite, one may consider the use of a Hawley bite plate to prevent the bite from getting deeper and thus exerting distal pressure on the condyle.[7]

TMJ dysfunction symptoms after orthodontic therapy may occur in an individual case, but in general there seems to be no connection between functional disturbances and well-planned orthodontic therapy.[16] Several good, scientific, controlled, long-term studies indicate that orthodontics is not a cause of TMJ dysfunction.[17-19] No data exist to support the notion that orthodontic treatment of children or adults prevents or lowers the risk of subsequently developing TMD.[20] Postorthodontic patients who were treated in various traditional ways of orthodontic treatment have no more TMD symptoms than do people with untreated malocclusion or people with normal occlusions.[20] If TMD symptoms arise during orthodontic treatment, observation and common sense are the best approaches.[20] If the symptoms are painful, it may be necessary

21. Sadowsky C, Theisen TA, and Sakols EI: Orthodontic treatment and TMJ sounds—A longitudinal study. Am J Orthod Dentofacial Orthop 99:441–447, 1991.
22. Dibbets JMH, and van der Weele LT: Extraction, orthodontic treatment, and craniomandibular dysfunction. Am J Orthod Dentofacial Orthop 99:210–219, 1991.
23. Kundinger KK, Austin BP, Christensen LV, Donegan SJ, and Ferguson DJ: An evaluation of TMJ and jaw muscles after orthodontic treatment involving premolar extractions. Am J Orthod Dentofacial Orthop 100:110–115, 1991.
24. Gianelly AA, Hughes HM, Wohlgemuth P, and Gildea G: Condylar position and extraction treatment. Am J Orthod Dentofacial Orthop 93:210–205, 1988.
25. Luecke PE III, and Johnston LE, Jr.: The effect of maxillary first premolar extraction and incisor retraction on mandibular position: Testing the central dogma of "functional orthodontics." Am J Orthod Dentofacial Orthop 101:4–12, 1992.
26. Egermark I, and Thilander B: Craniomandibular disorders with special reference to orthodontic treatment: An evaluation from childhood to adulthood. Am J Orthod Dentofacial Orthop 101:28–34, 1992.
27. Hirata RH, Heft NW, Hernandez B, and King GJ: Longitudinal study of signs of temporomandibular disorders (TMD) in orthodontically treated and nontreated groups. Am J Orthod Dentofacial Orthop 101:35–40, 1992.
28. Rendell JK, Norton LA, and Gay T: Orthodontic treatment and temporomandibular joint disorders. Am J Orthod Dentofacial Orthop 101:84–87, 1992.
29. Parker WS: Centric relation and centric occlusion—An orthodontic responsibility. Am J Orthod 74:481–500, 1978.
30. Andrews LF: The six keys to normal occlusion. Am J Orthod 62:296–309, 1972.

Chapter 6

Nasorespiratory Function

A thorough functional evaluation is an essential part of the development of the patient's stomatognathic problem list. Habits should be evaluated carefully, keeping in mind that approximately 50% of children without malocclusions have what is considered to be bad habits.[1] The duration and intensity may be more important than the actual presence of an abnormal condition.[1]

Nasal obstruction, causing mouth-breathing and a lowering of the mandible and tongue, may produce remarkable changes in the dental and facial relationships[2] (Figs. A6.1 and A6.2). If, after the age of 5 years, especially in the early mixed dentition stage of 6 to 8 years of age, the child has difficulty breathing through the nose, a referral to the otolaryngologist would be most appropriate. Although the literature is replete with statements that airway impairment alters facial and dental growth, there is substantial evidence to the contrary.[3]

In a recent study of mandibular and maxillary growth in boys after a changed breathing mode 5 years after adenoidectomy, it was found that there was almost a 4 mm greater mandibular growth (statistically significant) but no change in maxillary growth direction.[4] Conversely, there was also no change in the breathing mode in 20% of the sample. A concurrent study[5] on the relation between vertical dentofacial morphology and respiration in adolescents concluded that different breathing modes may be behaviorally based, rather than airway dependent, and that intervention to alter the nasal airway and thus to influence dentofacial growth is unjustified. What may be an excellent therapeutic modality for one patient does not indicate that it will have the same effect in the majority of patients. Although there seems to be a weak tendency among mouth breathers toward a class II skeletal pattern, increased anterior facial height, high mandibular plane angles, and retroclined incisors—all characteristics of a long face—a more thorough analysis of respiratory pattern is required to support the decision for clinical intervention.[6]

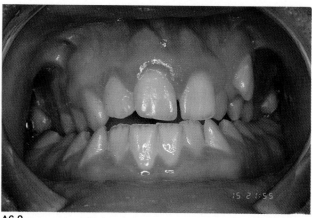

A6.2

Figure A6.2 Anterior view of the occlusion of the same patient as in Figure A6.1. Note the open bite, gingival inflammation, and constricted upper arch, all associated with a chronic mouth-breather.

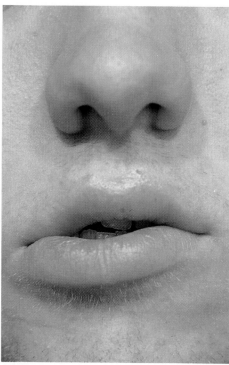

A6.1

Figure A6.1 Severe nasal obstruction has led to mouth-breathing and significant changes in this patient's facial characteristics, such as hypotonic rest position and lip incompetency.

References

1. Graber TM, Rakosi T, and Petrovic AG: *Dentofacial Orthopedics with Functional Appliances.* St. Louis: C.V. Mosby Co., 1985.
2. Linder-Aronson S: Nasorespiratory considerations in orthodontics. In: *Orthodontics—State of the Art.* Graber LW, ed. St. Louis: C.V. Mosby Co., 1986, 116–121.
3. Melsen B: *Current Controversies in Orthodontics.* Chicago: Quintessence Publishing, 1991.
4. Woodside DG, Linder-Aronson S, Lundstrom A, and McWilliams J: Mandibular and maxillary growth after changed mode of breathing. Am J Orthod Dentofacial Orthop 100:1–18, 1991.
5. Fields HW, Warren DW, Black K, and Phillips CL: Relationship between vertical dentofacial morphology and respiration in adolescents. Am J Orthod Dentofacial Orthop 99:147–154, 1991.
6. Ung N, Koenig T, Shapiro PA, Shapiro G, and Trask G: A quantitative assessment of respiratory patterns and their effects on dentofacial development. Am J Orthod Dentofacial Orthop 98:523–532, 1990.

Chapter 7

Oral Hygiene Considerations

Enamel demineralization (Fig. A7.1) is associated with fixed orthodontic therapy in an extremely rapid process that is caused by a high and continuous cariogenic challenge in the plaque developed around brackets and underneath ill-fitting bands[1] (Fig. A7.2). Because orthodontic appliances tend to increase the accumulation of plaque on the teeth, it is not surprising that gingival inflammation tends to increase in orthodontic patients as well.[2-6]

Careful inspection at every visit, preventive fluoride programs, and oral hygiene are very important throughout the duration of orthodontic treatment.[1-4] Proper brushing and flossing three times daily is recommended, followed by fluoride mouth rinses once a day.[5] The combination of daily brushing with a fluoridated dentifrice, coupled with daily rinsing with a fluoride wash provides complete protection for the orthodontic patient by inhibiting demineralization or by promoting remineralization of the surfaces at risk.[7] Toothbrushing with a relatively new electric, counterrotational power toothbrush is highly advisable. A rotary electric toothbrush is more effective than conventional toothbrushes for removing plaque and controlling gingivitis in adolescents during orthodontic treatment with fixed appliances.[8] A recent study that compared electric and manual toothbrushing found that the use of the electric system resulted in overall lower plaque scores.[2] Another study of the effectiveness of the new appliance concluded that plaque and gingival scores were significantly lower after brushing for 2 months with the electric counterrotational toothbrush than following brushing with the manual one.[3] The orthodontic treatment itself has an impact on oral hygiene in the long term as well; a study showed that children who received orthodontic treatment had a greater reduction of plaque and gingivitis than children who did not.[4] This was related more to behavior factors than to improved tooth alignment.[4]

Orthodontic treatment during adolescence has no discernible effect on late periodontal health.[9] In the absence of compromising conditions (*e.g.,* high decayed–missing–filled (teeth) [DMF] scores, periodontitis), adult patients are not inherently more likely than adolescents to lose dental support (*e.g.,* crestal bone height) during treatment.[10] In patients with passive-controlled periodontal disease, no increased progression of marginal periodontitis will occur due to orthodontic tooth movement provided that excellent oral hygiene is maintained throughout the orthodontic therapy and that the patient visits the periodontist every 3 to 4 months for check-ups.[11-13] Oral irrigators generally enjoy a high rate of compliance with adults.[11] Oral rinses, such as Listerine, can be effective adjuncts if compliance is good.[11] Cases with unmanageable gingival inflammation can be put on a 6-week regimen of rinsing with Peridex (Proctor & Gamble) twice daily[11] (Figs. A7.3 and A7.4). Dental cleaning will be needed at the end of the 6 weeks to remove stain.[11] Surgical treatment is generally employed for definitive pocket reduction postorthodontically. In addition, although grafting before orthodontics to prevent recession of prominent lower anteriors is highly recommended, there may be no need for grafting to prevent further recession in the post-treatment patient because most recession occurs quickly and then stabilizes.[6] Bony

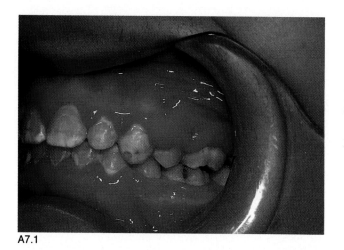

A7.1

Figure A7.1 Severe enamel demineralization and white spot formation due to lack of proper oral hygiene after 2 years of orthodontic therapy.

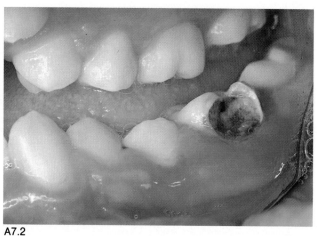

A7.2

Figure A7.2 Severe tooth decay underneath an ill-fitting band that was placed for space maintenance until the eruption of the bicuspid teeth.

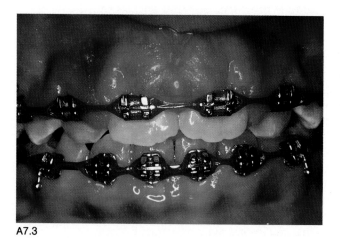

A7.3

Figure A7.3 Severe gingival inflammation, despite thorough brushing. This patient was placed on Peridex (Proctor and Gamble, Cincinnati, OH).

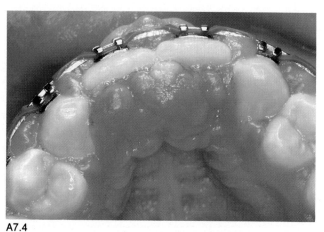

A7.4

Figure A7.4 Occlusal view of the same patient as in Figure A7.3. Note that the central incisors are almost buried underneath the soft-tissue overgrowth.

dehiscences can be created during the treatment phase, especially with a thin alveolar process, by inflammation or overzealous brushing[6] (Figs. A7.5 and A7.6).

During orthodontic treatment, forces should always be kept within physiological limits,[12] with the appliances and the mechanics used as simple as possible.[6] In general, the forces used in adults should be kept at a lower level than those used in children. Light, continuous, intrusive forces should be maintained during tooth displacement.[14,15] When dealing with teeth with bony defects, especially in the anterior regions (*i.e.,* flared upper incisors with palatal bony defects), it is advisable to consider mechanics that will intrude those teeth.[14,15] Even if no intrusion takes place, this intrusive force may negate the effects of the extrusive component.[14] If the orthodontist is contemplating bodily movement of teeth into areas of intrabony pockets, it is often prudent for the periodontist to do an open debridement procedure to prepare the root surface adjacent to the pocket.[16] Bodily movement of teeth can enhance bone growth and reattachment if the periodontium is properly prepared.[16]

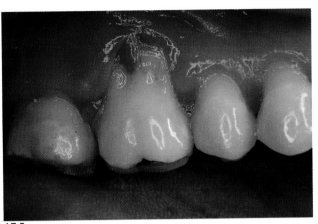

A7.5

Figure A7.5 This patient, who has extensive periodontal disease, would not be a good candidate for orthodontic treatment.

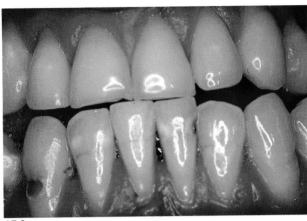

A7.6

Figure A7.6 Overzealous brushing in combination with a prominent occlusion and thin tissues has led to gingival recession, gingival clefts, and tooth abrasions.

Edentulous areas of the mouth need special attention during the treatment-planning phase, especially if attempting to move teeth through these spaces.[17,18] When attempting to close the edentulous space of a lost first molar by mesial and distal movements of the second molar and premolar, respectively, one should expect a definite loss of bone averaging more than 1 mm around the second molar and 0.5 mm around the premolar tooth.[17] As much as 4 to 5 mm of reduction in vertical bone height can occur.[17] Closed spaces are difficult to maintain in these patients as well.[18] In addition, the longer the treatment tenure, the greater the amount of root resorption of the second molar.[17,18] Although younger patients respond more favorably, older patients seem to resist the opposition of new alveolar bone.[17]

In cases of overerupted maxillary molars, where the use of conventional fixed appliances would lead to undesired extrusion of the adjacent teeth (extrusion happens much faster than intrusion), a single-stage osteotomy is used to reposition the involved tooth with its surrounding bone at the proper level.[19] Orthodontic tooth movement with sectional archwires will stabilize the result before the bone heals completely.[19] In cases where teeth need to be extruded, ample time needs to be given for "bone fill-in" around the new position of these teeth (1 mm/month).[20]

In patients with mild incisor irregularity or anterior tooth size discrepancies, interproximal enamel is removed during orthodontic treatment, and the roots are brought into closer proximity. In other patients with unusual crown/root morphology, root proximity is inevitable in order to produce alignment of the crown. The clinician need not be overly concerned, because these situations do not seem to result in a higher predilection for periodontal breakdown.[21]

Finally, one should be very careful in cases with a prominent dentition relative to the alveolar cortical plate with thin, overlying soft tissue and inadequate oral hygiene. Recession can occur quite rapidly. The donor site should be carefully evaluated for the existence of fenestration or dehiscence[22] (Figs. A7.7 and A7.8).

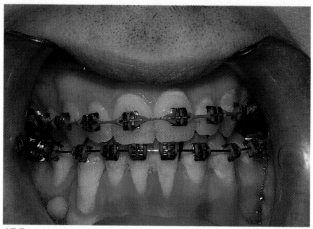

A7.7

Figure A7.7 Severe gingival recession of all the lower anterior teeth that was created within a few months of orthodontic treatment. This was a result of tooth movement in an environment with poor oral hygiene, prominent roots, and parafunctional habits.

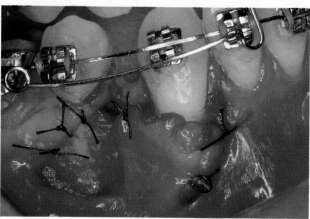

A7.8

Figure A7.8 A fenestration in the lower bicuspid area that was revealed.

References

1. Ogaard B, Rolla G, and Arends J: Orthodontic appliances and enamel demineralization. Am J Orthod Dentofacial Orthop 94:68–73, 1988.
2. Jackson CL: Comparison between electric toothbrushing and manual toothbrushing with and without oral irrigation, for oral hygiene of orthodontic patients. Am J Orthod Dentofacial Orthop 99:15–20, 1991.
3. Wilcoxon DB, Ackerman RJ, Killoy WJ, Love JW, Sakamura J, and Tira DE: The effectiveness of a counterrotational-action power toothbrush on plaque control in orthodontic patients. Am J Orthod Dentofacial Orthop 99:7–14, 1991.
4. Davies TM, Shaw WC, Worthington HV, Addy M, Dummer P, and Kingdon A: The effect of orthodontic treatment on plaque and gingivitis. Am J Orthod Dentofacial Orthop 99:155–162, 1991.
5. Shannon IL: Prevention of decalcification in orthodontic patients. J Clin Orthod 15:695–705, 1981.
6. Artun J: Long-term periodontal response to orthodontic treatment—Summary by Hawley B. Pacific Coast Society of Orthodontists Bulletin, Spring, 42–43, 1991.
7. O'Reilly MM, and Featherstone JDB: Demineralization and remineralization around orthodontic appliances: An in vitro study. Am J Orthod Dentofacial Orthop 92:33–40, 1987.
8. Boyd RL, Murray P, and Robertson PB: Effect of rotary electric toothbrush versus manual toothbrush on periodontal status during orthodontic treatment. Am J Orthod Dentofacial Orthop 96:342–347, 1989.
9. Polson AM, Subtenly JD, Heitner SW, Polson AP, Sommers EW, Iker HP, and Reed BE: Long-term periodontal status after orthodontic treatment. Am J Orthod Dentofacial Orthop 93:51–58, 1988.
10. Harris EF, and Baker WC: Loss of root length and crestal bone height before and during treatment in adolescent and adult orthodontic patients. Am J Orthod Dentofacial Orthop 98:463–469, 1990.
11. Boyd RL: Can adults with periodontitis be treated orthodontically? Summary by Quinn RS. Pacific Coast Society of Orthodontists Bulletin, Spring, 48–49, 1991.
12. Eliasson LA, Hugoson A, Kurol J, and Siwe H: The effects of orthodontic treatment on periodontal tissues in patients with reduced periodontal support. Eur J Orthod 4:1–9 1982.
13. Page R: Frontiers in periodontics. Summary by Nichols O. Pacific Coast Society of Orthodontists Bulletin, Spring, 39–41, 1991.
14. Kessler M: Interrelationships between orthodontics and periodontics. Am J Orthod 70:154–172, 1976.
15. Melsen B: Adult orthodontics. J Clin Orthod 22:630–641, 1988.
16. Hösl E, Zachrisson BV, and Baldauf A: *Orthodontics and Periodontics.* Chicago: Quintessence Publishing, 1985.

17. Goldberg D, and Turley PK: Orthodontic space closure of the edentulous maxillary first molar area in adults. International Journal of Adult Orthodontic and Orthognathic Surgery 4:255–266, 1989.
18. Stepovich ML: A clinical study on closing edentulous spaces in the mandible. Angle Orthod 49:227–233, 1979.
19. Mostafa YA, Tawfik KM, and El-Mangoury NH: Surgical orthodontic treatment for overerupted maxillary molars. J Clin Orthod 19:350–351, 1985.
20. Sperry TP: The role of tooth extrusion in treatment planning for orthognathic surgery. International Journal of Adult Orthodontic and Orthognathic Surgery 4:197–211, 1988.
21. Artun J, Kokich VG, and Osterberg SK: Long-term effect of root proximity on periodontal health after orthodontic treatment. Am J Orthod Dentofacial Orthop 91:125–130, 1987.
22. Viazis AD, Corinaldesi G, and Abramson MM: Gingival recession and fenestration in orthodontic treatment. J Clin Orthod 25:633–636, 1990.

Chapter 8

Periodontal Plastic Surgery

For years, covering exposed roots with soft-tissue grafting has been the ultimate goal in periodontal mucogingival surgery. Today that goal has been largely met with the use of various techniques.[1-4] The larger arena of esthetic enhancement now dominates our thought processes in dentistry. Periodontal plastic surgery is the term used to describe surgical procedures performed to correct or eliminate anatomic, developmental, or traumatic deformities of the gingiva and alveolar mucosa.[1] These procedures would also include treatment of marginal tissue recession, excessive gingival margins, and localized alveolar ridge deficiency, and exposure of unerupted teeth for orthodontic treatment.[3]

Excessive gingival display is a condition resulting from excessive exposure of maxillary gingiva during smiling, commonly called gummy smile or high lip line.[3] This condition may be caused by a skeletal deformity, a soft-tissue deformity, or a combination of the two. Another cause is short clinical crowns due to incomplete exposure of the anatomic crowns. If short clinical crowns result in a gummy smile, gingival contouring may be accomplished to achieve the desired esthetic result.

Periodontal plastic surgery may be used not only to enhance esthetics but also to aid in orthodontic treatment by a variety of means. The gummy smile can be managed to create proper clinical crown length and achieve pleasing gingival contours. Diagnosis of this problem can be made by the orthodontist early in treatment. Evaluation of the smile line, lip line, and tooth length can help differentiate between excessive gingival display due to vertical maxillary excess (Fig. A8.1) or insufficient crown length (Figs. A8.2 through A8.5). Furthermore, the establishment of the marginal tissue at the level of the cemento-enamel junction (CEJ) enhances esthetics and creates a situation in which the orthodontist can have a larger comfort zone when treating periodontally involved cases.

In addition, successful root coverage techniques can aid in the treatment of inadequate attached gingiva as well as root sensitivity and unesthetic appearance. Root coverage techniques for treatment of cuspid marginal tissue recession in the past have been relatively unpredictable procedures. Soft-tissue grafting was done primarily to increase the band on attached gingiva. In 1982, a predictable technique was described for covering roots using the free gingival graft following citric acid root conditioning.[1] In 1985, the subepithelial connective tissue graft for improved esthetics in root coverage grafting was introduced. Since then, it has proved especially useful in the treatment of gingival recession (Figs. A8.6 through A8.9).

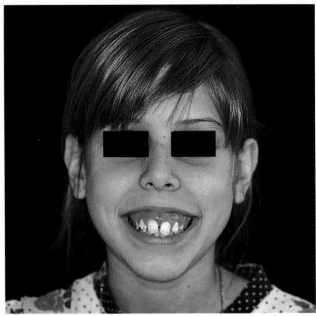

A8.1

Figure A8.1 Excessive gingival display due to vertical maxillary excess.

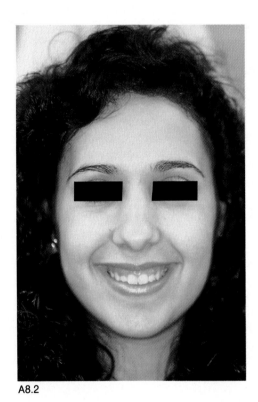

A8.2

Figure A8.2 Excessive gingival display due to insufficient crown length.

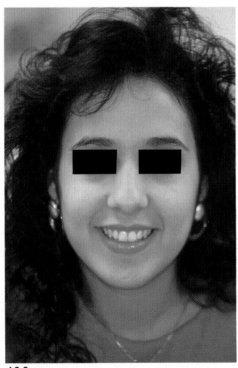

A8.3

Figure A8.3 The same patient as in Figure A8.2 after periodontal plastic surgery.

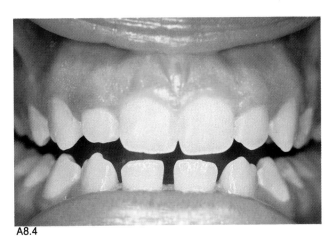

A8.4

Figure A8.4 Anterior view: lower incisor spacing and inadequate clinical crown length of the upper anterior teeth.

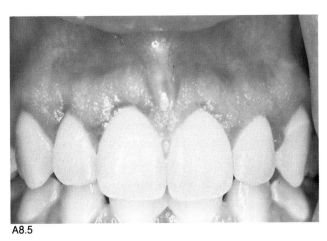

A8.5

Figure A8.5 The same patient as in Figure A8.4 after periodontal plastic surgery.

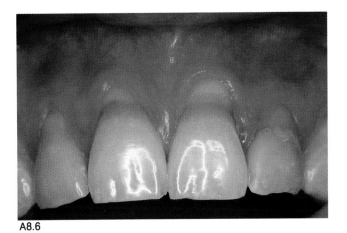

A8.6

Figure A8.6 Soft-tissue recession in the maxillary central incisor area that resulted in root exposure.

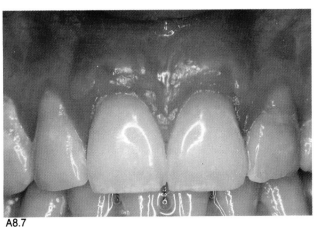

A8.7

Figure A8.7 The same patient as in Figure A8.6 1 month after a CT graft was placed over the exposed root surfaces in the CEJ area of the central incisors.

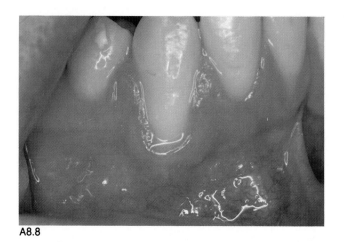

A8.8

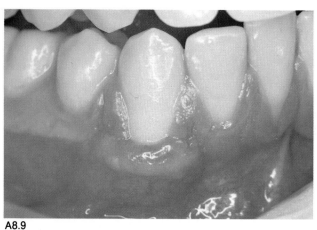

A8.9

Figure A8.8 Gingival recession of the mandibular right cuspid. Periodontal grafting is highly recommended to prevent further recession during tooth movement.

Figure A8.9 The same patient as in Figure A8.8 3 months after a CT graft covered the exposed root. Orthodontic treatment can now be attempted.

References

1. Miller PD, Jr.: Root coverage using a free soft tissue autograft following citric acid application: I. Technique. International Journal of Periodontics and Restorative Dentistry 2:65, 1982.
2. Langer B, and Langer L: Subepithelial connective tissue graft technique for root coverage. J Periodontol 56:715, 1985.
3. Allen EP: Use of mucogingival surgical procedures to enhance esthetics. Dent Clin North Am 32:307–330, 1988.
4. Jacoby B, Viazis AD, Abelson M, and Allen EP: Periodontal plastic surgery in orthodontics. J Clin Orthod (in press)

Facial and Cephalometric Evaluation

Natural Head Position

Facial examination is the key to diagnosis.[1] Orthodontic complications nearly always stem from errors in diagnosis, not from failures in execution of treatment. After the preliminary dental clinical information is obtained, the evaluation continues with the examination of the face from the frontal and profile views. The patient is instructed to sit upright and look straight ahead into the horizon or directly into a mirror on the wall. This position, called the *natural head position* (NHP), is the position in which the patient carries himself or herself in everyday life[2-8] (Figs. B1.1 and B1.2). Therefore, this is the reference position we should use in our examination. In this position the pupils of the eyes are centered in the middle of the eyes, defining the line of vision or *true horizontal* (TH).[6-8] The TH line should be parallel to the floor.[6]

Natural head position has been established over the past 30 years as the most appropriate reference position for cephalometric radiography.[2-8] It has been shown that it is related to the correct natural body posture and alignment with the cervical column, is based on the line of vision, and is determined by the overall head and body balance when the individual looks straight ahead.[3,4,9-15] The reproducibility of NHP has been shown to be within the clinically acceptable spectrum of variance of 4 degrees, which is certainly much better than the 26-degree variability of the Frankfurt horizontal and SN plane among different individuals.[4-6]

An NHP radiograph is taken with the patient in the cephalometer looking straight ahead into a mirror. The patient is observed from the side to ensure that the pupil is in the middle of the eye. In the event that the patient states that he or she is in NHP but the pupils are not centered in the middle of the eyes, the clinician should correct the head position.[6-8] Any habitual tendency for an individual to keep the head in an "unnatural" flexed or extended position must be observed, and it may be necessary to "correct" the registered head position.[16] Recently, using tracings of facial profiles, observers made independent, subjective estimations of NHP in 28 adults.[17] The results of these estimations were compared with recordings of NHP obtained through photographic registration of the same subjects. Only minor average differences (between 0 and 1.4 degrees) were found between the two methods. Estimation of NHP may, therefore, be performed with acceptable accuracy in most cases. Thus, it is the clinician, and not the patient, who determines the final position.[6-8]

The ear rods should be placed directly in front of the tragus so that they lightly contact the skin, establishing bilateral head support in the transverse plane. Lateral cephalostats with ear rods alter the position of the head and neck during postural recordings.[18] Subjects extend their heads and necks higher with ear rods in place than they do without ear rods.[18] The patient should be comfortable and relaxed, and the head should not be tilted or tipped. The correct position is confirmed by checking the patient from the front. The nose piece is then placed so that it lightly contacts the skin, to establish support in the vertical plane. The three light contact points secure the patient in NHP. After a final check, the x-ray is taken. The entire procedure should take only 1 to 3 minutes. The determination of an aesthetic true horizontal by visual inspection of the patient's face has been shown to be highly reproducible and to have more relevance to the soft tissue than does the Frankfort horizontal.[19-23]

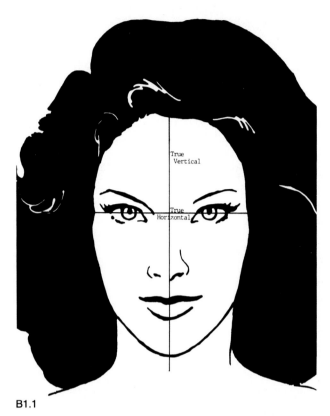

B1.1

Figure B1.1 Natural head position. The patient is looking straight ahead. The *true vertical* is perpendicular to the floor. The *true horizontal* is parallel to the floor and is defined from the pupil of the eyes.

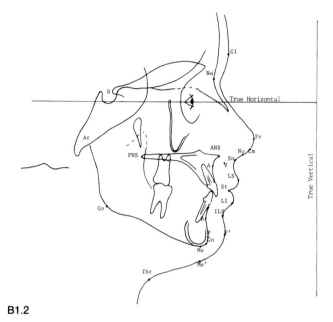

B1.2

Figure B1.2 The *true horizontal* coincides with the line of vision. The pupils of the eyes are centered in the middle of the eyes. The major cephalometric landmarks are also indicated.

References

1. Arnett GW: Excellent treatment results using ideal orthodontic/orthognathic treatment planning. Summarized by Nichols LO. PCSO Bulletin, 37–39, 1991.
2. Moorrees CFA, and Kean MR: Natural head position, a basic consideration in the interpretation of cephalometric radiographs. Am J Phys Anthropol 16:213–234, 1956.
3. Solow B, and Tallgren A: Head posture and craniofacial morphology. Am J Phys Anthropol 44:417–436, 1976.
4. Solow B, Siersbaek-Nielsen S, and Greeve E: Airway adequacy, head posture, and craniofacial morphology. Am J Orthod 86:495–500, 1983.
5. Cooke MS, and Wei SHY: A summary five-factor cephalometric analysis based on natural head posture and the true horizontal. Am J Orthod 93:213–223, 1988.
6. Viazis AD: A cephalometric analysis based on natural head position. J Clin Orthod 25:172–182, 1991.
7. Viazis AD: A new measurement of profile esthetics. J Clin Orthod 25:15–20, 1991.
8. Viazis AD: The cranial base triangle. J Clin Orthod 25:565–570, 1991.
9. Luyk NP, Whitfield PH, Ward-Booth RP, and Williams ED: The reproducibility of the natural head position in lateral cephalometric radiographs. Br J Oral Maxillofacial Surg 24:357–366, 1986.
10. Cannon J: Head posture—An historical review of the literature. Aust Orthod 9:234–237, 1985.
11. Solow B, Siersbaek-Nielsen S, and Greeve E: Airway adequacy, head posture, and craniofacial morphology. Am J Orthod 86:214–223, 1984.
12. Vig PS, Showfety KJ, and Phillips CP: Experimental manipulation of head posture. Am J Orthod 77:258–268, 1980.

13. Luyk NP, Whitfield PH, Ward-Booth RP, and Williams ED: The reproducibility of the natural head position in lateral cephalometric radiographs. Br J Oral Maxillofacial Surg 24:357–366, 1986.
14. Cole SC: Natural head position, posture, prognathism. Br J Orthod 15:227–239, 1988.
15. Michiels LYF, and Tourne LPM: Nasion true vertical: A proposed method for testing the clinical validity of cephalometric measurements applied to a new cephalometric reference line. Int J Adult Orthod Orthog Surg 5:43–52, 1990.
16. Lundstrom A: Guest editorial: Intercranial reference lines versus the true horizontal as a basis for cephalometric analysis. Eur J Orthod 13:167–168, 1991.
17. Lundstrom A, Fosberg CM, Westergren H, and Lundstrom F: A comparison between estimated and registered NHP. Eur J Orthod 13:59–64, 1991.
18. Greenfield B, Kraus S, Lawrence E, and Wolf SL: The influence of cephalostatic ear rods on the positions of the head and neck during postural recordings. Am J Orthod Dentofacial Orthop 95:312–318, 1989.
19. Bass NM: The aesthetic analysis of the face. Eur J Orthod 13:343–350, 1991.
20. Siersbaek-Nielsen S, and Solow B: Intra- and interexaminer variability in head posture recorded by dental auxiliaries. Am J Orthod 82:50–57, 1982.
21. Chang HP: Assessment of anteroposterior jaw relationship. Am J Orthod 92:117–122, 1987.
22. Showfety KJ, Vig PS, and Matteson SA: A simple method for taking natural-head-position cephalograms. Am J Orthod 83:495–500, 1983.
23. Lundstrom F, and Lundstrom A: Clinical evaluation of maxillary and mandibular prognathism. Eur J Orthod 11:408–413, 1989.

Bolton and Michigan Standards

A major disadvantage of most existing cephalometric analyses is that their differences in normative sample selection make direct comparisons among them scientifically unreliable, even though, in practice, many clinicians use measurements from various analyses to support their diagnoses.

In addition, most analyses offer only one mean for adolescents, regardless of the age or gender of the growing patient. Although patients should not be treated "by the numbers," a clinician using measurements from a particular analysis should be referred to a table appropriate to the patient's age. Such tables are available in the Bolton and Michigan standards.[1,2]

Many of the Bolton and Michigan standards are based on the Frankfort horizontal. Downs[3] has said that this plane could be considered level (that is, the same as the true horizontal) when the subject is standing and looking straight ahead. In the cases where he found a discrepancy between cephalometric measurements and his clinical impression, he noticed that the Frankfort horizontal deviated from the true horizontal plane (Fig. B2.1). When he included the degrees of deviation in his calculations (in other words, when he leveled the Frankfort horizontal), he found that his measurements agreed with his clinical findings.

In essence, Downs used a true horizontal plane in conjunction with the norms based on the Frankfort horizontal. We can follow this concept by taking radiographs in natural head position (NHP), basing the measurements on the true horizontal, and comparing them to the means and standard deviations of the Bolton and Michigan standards.

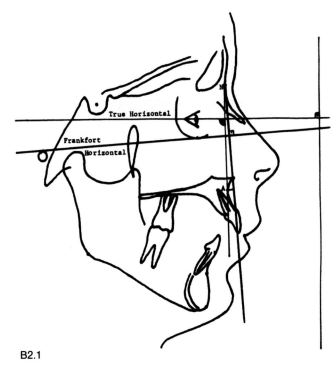

B2.1

Figure B2.1 Note the marked inclination of Frankfort horizontal (FH) relative to the true horizontal (TH). Although the maxilla is prognathic relative to the TH, it appears retrognathic relative to the FH. (See *Anteroposterior Skeletal Assessment.*)

References

1. Broadbent BH Sr, Broadbent BH Jr, and Golden WH: *Bolton Standards of Dentofacial Development Growth.* St. Louis: C.V. Mosby Co., 1975.
2. Riolo ML, Moyers RE, McNamara JA, and Hunter WS: *An Atlas of Craniofacial Growth: Cephalometric Standards.* Ann Arbor, MI: University School Growth Study, the University of Michigan. Monograph Number 2, Craniofacial Growth Series, Center for Human Growth and Development, 1972.
3. Downs WF: Analysis of the dento-facial profile. Angle Orthod 26:191–212, 1956.

Chapter 3

Cephalometric Landmarks

The following are some cephalometric landmarks most commonly used in cephalometric analyses[1-3] (Fig. B1.2):

A-point (A): An arbitrary point at the innermost curvature from the anterior nasal spine at the crest of the maxillary alveolar process.

Anterior nasal spine (ANS): The process of the maxilla that forms the most anterior projection of the floor of the nasal cavity.

Articulare: A constructed point at the intersection of the posterior cranial base and the ramus of the mandible.

B-point (B): An arbitrary point on the anterior profile curvature from the mandibular landmark, pogonion, to the crest of the alveolar process.

Columella (Cm): The most anterior and inferior point of the nose.

Glabella (Gl): The most anterior soft-tissue point of the frontal bone.

Gnathion (Gn): The most downward and forward point on the profile curvature of the symphysis of the mandible.

Gonion (Go): The most posterior and inferior point on the angle of the mandible that is formed by the junction of the ramus and the body of the mandible.

Hairline (Hr): The midpoint of the forehead where the hairline begins.

Inferior labial sulcus (ILS): A point at the innermost curvature of the lower lip.

Labialis inferioris (LI): An arbitrary point at the vermillion of the lower lip.

Labialis superioris (LS): An arbitrary point at the vermillion of the upper lip.

Menton (Me): The most inferior point on the symphysis of the mandible.

Middle of the nose (No): The midpoint between Sn and Pr on the true horizontal, projected on the inferior outline of the nose.

Nasion (N or Na): The most anterior point of the frontal suture.

Pogonion (P or Pg): The most anterior point on the symphysis of the mandible.

Posterior nasal spine (PNS): The process formed by the most posterior projection of the juncture of the palatine bones in the midline.

Pronasale (Pr): The tip of the nose.

Sella (S): A constructed point in the middle of the sella turcica.

Soft-tissue menton (Me′): The point on the lower contour of the chin opposite to the hard-tissue menton.

Soft-tissue pogonion (P′): The most anterior soft-tissue point of the chin.

Stomion (St′): A point at the interlabial junction of the mouth where the upper and lower lips connect.

Subnasale (Sn): The point at which the base of the nose meets the upper lip.

Th-point: The point at the junction of the neck and the submandibular soft tissue.

V-point: The midpoint of the distance between A-point and Sn.

Zygoma (Zy): The outermost point of the zygomatic processes on the soft tissue.

References

1. Proffit WR: *Contemporary Orthodontics.* St. Louis, MO: C.V. Mosby Co., 1986.
2. Viazis AD: Cephalometric analysis based on natural head position. J Clin Orthod 25:172–182, 1981.
3. Bass NM: The esthetic analysis of the face. Eur J Orthod 13:343–350, 1991.

Chapter 4

Soft-Tissue Evaluation

The significance of soft-tissue evaluation lies in the importance of the role that dentofacial attractiveness plays in our society.[1-4] As clinicians, we need to make sure that we do not compromise the soft tissue for a good occlusion and vice versa. A soft-tissue evaluation from the facial and profile view is essential in order to have a comprehensive understanding of the patient's esthetic characteristics.[5] See the previous chapter for a glossary of cephalometric landmarks used in abbreviations here.

Rules of Thirds[6,7]

The midline *true vertical,* as it passes through the middle of the forehead (Gl), tip of the nose (Pr), and the lips, divides the face into two halves and crosses perpendicular to the line of vision (true horizontal; TH) (see Fig. B1.1). A very slight asymmetry is normal and should be present in all individuals[6] (Fig. B4.1).

Along the true vertical, one may define the three equal vertical facial thirds[7] (Fig. B4.2) as the *upper facial third, middle facial third,* and *lower facial third.* The *main face* (eye to eye) may be divided into three equal thirds along the true horizontal (Fig. B4.3): *right eye width, nasal width,* and *left eye width.* According to this dimension, the eyes, intercanthal distance, and alar base should all be of approximately equal width. The whole face (ear to ear) may also be divided into equal thirds along the true horizontal (Fig. B4.3): *right facial width, mouth width,* and *left facial width.* The aforementioned thirds provide the clinician with a fairly good idea of the overall facial appearance and proportionality of the patient.

Facial Ratios[3,5,6]

We can define *facial height* as the distance between the glabella (Gl) and the soft-tissue menton (Me′) and *facial width* as the distance between the two most outer points of the malar prominences. Their ratio should be about 90%. The *pupil width* and *gonial width* should be around 50% and 75% of the facial width, respectively. The nasal width should be about 70% of nasal height (GlPr). Again, these ratios give a good impression of the patient's specific facial characteristics and proportions (Fig. B4.4).

Facial Taper

The facial taper may easily be determined from the *facial taper angle* that is formed by extending the right and left lines connecting the most lateral points of the orbits and the junction of the upper and lower lips at the corners of the mouth (Fig. B4.5). Their intersection forms an angle that, with a mean plus or minus one standard deviation (±SD), is 45 degrees ± 5 degrees. Larger values of this angle would indicate a wider, more square face, whereas lower ones indicate a longer, narrower face.

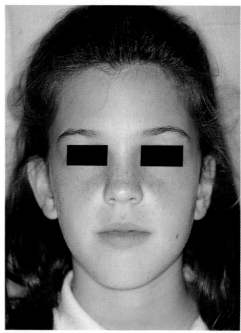

B4.1

Figure B4.1 A very slight asymmetry is normal in every individual.

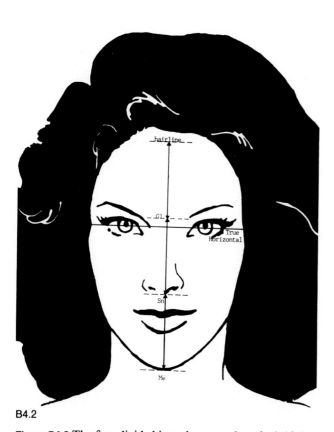

B4.2

Figure B4.2 The face divided into three equal vertical thirds.

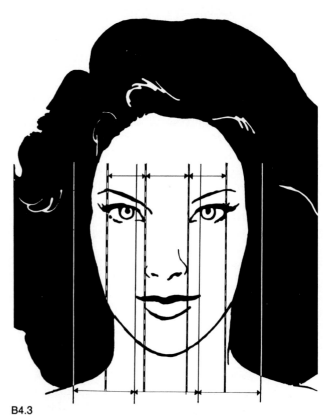

B4.3

Figure B4.3 The face divided into equal thirds along the true horizontal; the eye width should equal the nasal width; the mouth width should equal the distance from the ears to the corners of the eyes on each side.

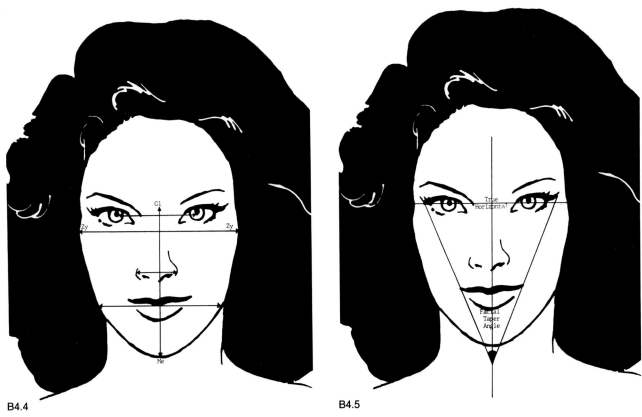

B4.4

B4.5

Figure B4.4 The facial ratios. Facial height:facial width = 9:10; pupil width:facial width = 1:2; nasal width:nasal height = 7:10; gonial width:facial width = 7.5:10.

Figure B4.5 The facial taper angle indicates a square, normal, or narrow face.

Evaluation of the Nose

The ratio of the *nasal width* to the *nasal height (Gl–Sn)* should be 70%. It gives us an overall estimate of nasal proportion.[3] A wider alar base appears to flatten the midface, and a narrow one lengthens the upper lip.

Two perpendicular lines to the TH from Sn and Pr define the *nasal length* as the distance of these two points on TH (Fig. B4.6). The mean ± SD is 18 ± 2 mm. If we locate the midpoint of Sn–Pr on TH and draw a vertical line to the lower contour of the nose, we may define the middle of the nose (No). Female profiles with smaller noses are considered more esthetically pleasing.[5] It is considered ideal for females to have less prominent noses and for males to have more prominent ones in relation to their chins.[5]

Convexity of the Profile

A parallel to the true vertical from No and the line NoPg′ define the *V-angle*[8] (Fig. B4.6). This angle denotes the convexity of the face.[8] The mean ± SD is −13 degrees ± 4 degrees. The NoPg′ line (Steiner's S-line)[9]—the line connecting the middle of the nose (No) and the chin (Pg)—should barely touch the upper and lower lips. Steiner's S-line[9] has been used for more than 25 years as a quick reference of the anteroposterior position of the lips relative to the nose and chin.

The V-angle is similar to the facial contour angle (FCA) (GlSn-SnPg′)[10,11] but provides a better indication of profile convexity because it concentrates on the lower half of the face and takes into account the size of the nose. It does not allow the size of the nose to affect the evaluation of lip position as much as the E-line (the line connecting the tip of the nose to the chin, PrPg′) does,[12-14] because it uses only half of the nose length.

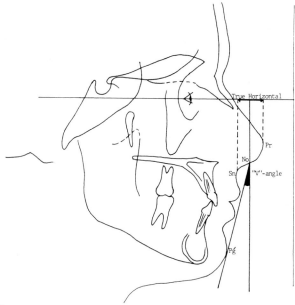

B4.6

Figure B4.6 The V-angle reveals the convexity of the profile. The nasal length is the distance of Sn to Pr on the true horizontal.

Evaluation of the Lips (Figs. B4.7 through B4.18)

The conventional *nasolabial angle* (LS–Sn–Cm) has a mean ± SD of 100 degrees ± 10 degrees.[5,10,11,15] It varies greatly among the different ethnic groups. More importantly, the *nasolabial angle ratio* defined by a line from Sn parallel to the TH, creating the upper and lower nasolabial angles, should be approximately 25% (upper to lower).[3] Ratios greater than 25% indicate either a protrusive upper lip or an upturned nose.[3] The opposite may denote a retrusive upper lip or a decreased nasal tip projection.

The *mentolabial angle* is similar to the nasolabial angle for the lower lip. It is defined by LI–ILS and a tangent from ILS to the soft-tissue chin. The mean ± SD is 130 degrees ± 10 degrees. A deeper mentolabial groove is preferred in men than in women.[5]

The *lip prominence angle* denotes the amount of lip protrusion. It is defined by the intersection of the lines Sn–LS and LI–ILS. The mean ± SD is 125 degrees ± 10 degrees. This angle is similar to the Sn–LS/IL–Pg′ angle,[5] but it takes into account the sulcus instead of the chin. The preference for a more acute lip prominence angle in women is statistically significant.[5] In other words, women with fuller dental areas and fuller lips look better and more esthetically pleasing to an independent panel of judges as compared to men. This may play a very important role in treatment planning and decision making of extraction versus nonextraction in females versus males, because lip protrusion is somewhat dependent on the amount of dentoalveolar protrusion.

Apart from the NoPg′ line mentioned above, the anteroposterior position of the lips may also be evaluated from their distance from a line parallel to the true vertical through Sn *(Sn perpendicular)*. The distance of the upper and lower lips, as well as of the chin, from this line should be 2 mm ± 2 mm, 0 mm ± 2 mm, −3.5 mm ± 2 mm, respectively. These numbers are similar to the ones suggested previously.[16–18] A perpendicular to the TH through *V*-point *(V perpendicular)* should pass through the soft-tissue pogonion.[19] The distances between the two perpendiculars to the TH from

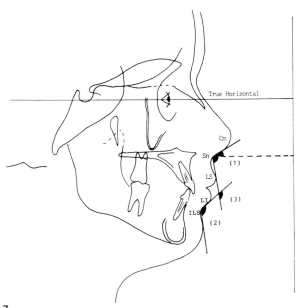

B4.7

Figure B4.7 **(1)** The nasolabial angle. Its ratio should be upper to lower = 1:4. **(2)** The mentolabial angle. **(3)** The lip prominence angle.

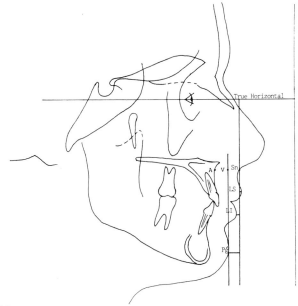

B4.8

Figure B4.8 The Sn and V perpendiculars.

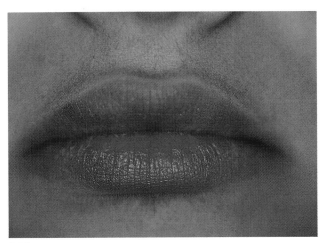

B4.9

Figure B4.9 Normal lip thickness (anterior view).

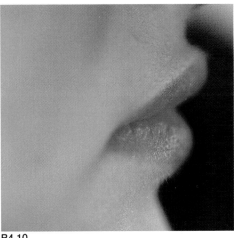

B4.10

Figure B4.10 Normal lip thickness (side view). Extraction of teeth should be avoided in order to preserve the lip contour.

V- and Sn-points provide the posterior and anterior limits of the harmonious soft-tissue chin position range.[19]

Patients with thin lips tend to have the greatest facial change relative to tooth movement, whereas those with thick lips have the least. The soft-tissue thickness of the upper lip, lower lip, and chin should be a 1:1:1 ratio.[16] The upper lip to the lower lip ratio (SnSt:StMe′) should be 50% or 1:1 if instead of stomion (St) we use LI. The lower anterior dental height (lower incisor tip to Me) should be approximately twice the upper lip length (Sn–St), *i.e.*, a 2:1 ratio.[16]

On smiling, the lips should reveal 0 to 2 mm of gingiva above the upper incisor teeth.[16-18] In repose, the amount of exposure of the maxillary incisors should be 2 to

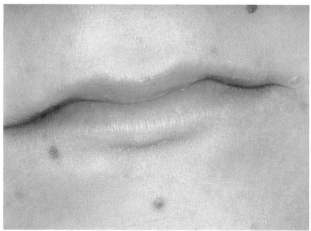

B4.11

Figure B4.11 Thin lips (anterior view).

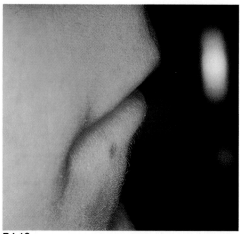

B4.12

Figure B4.12 Thin lips (side view). Extraction of teeth should be avoided in such patients.

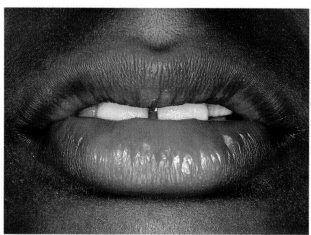

B4.13

Figure B4.13 Thick lips (anterior view).

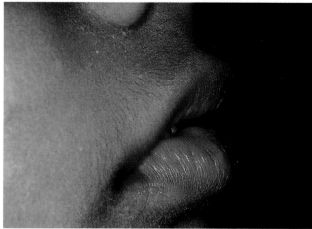

B4.14

Figure B4.14 Thick lips (side view). Extractions may not induce any significant lip changes.

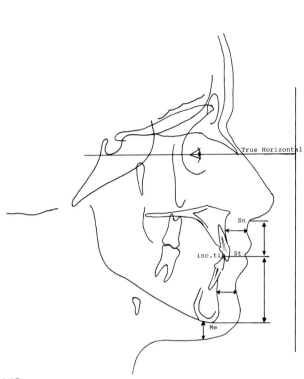

B4.15

Figure B4.15 A 1:1:1 ratio of upper lip:lower lip:chin thickness. A 2:1 ratio exists between lower anterior dental height and upper lip length.

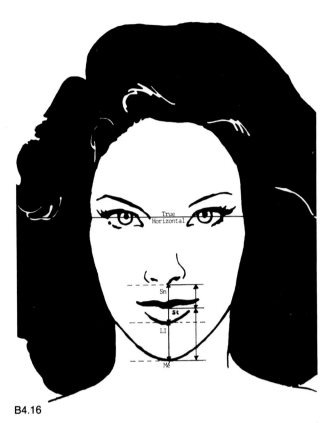

B4.16

Figure B4.16 The lip ratios (SnLi:LIMe' = 1:1 and SnSt:StMe' = 1:2).

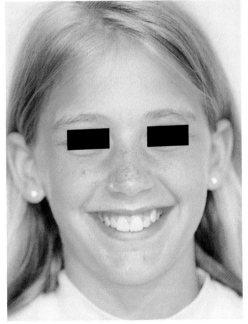

B4.17

Figure B4.17 Upon smiling, the lips should reveal 0 to 2 mm of gingiva above the incisors.

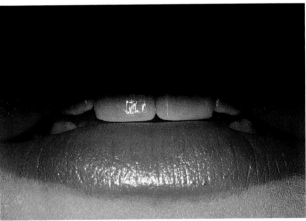

B4.18

Figure B4.18 Tooth exposure at rest should be in the range of 2 to 3 mm.

3 mm.[16-18] These are the most important observations from the facial view. The desire to have a beautiful smile is the primary reason patients seek orthodontic treatment, and we must ensure that we set our esthetic goals from the onset of therapy.

Evaluation of the Throat

We can define the throat line by Th and Me′ (see Fig. B4.15). As this line intersects the V-line (No perp), the *throat angle* is formed. The mean ± SD should be 105 degrees ± 5 degrees. The *throat length* (Th-Me′) should be approximately 40 mm ± 5 mm (Fig. B4.19). These measurements are important in planning mandibular orthognathic procedures; *i.e.,* a mandibular setback may not be possible when there is a short throat length.

A thorough evaluation of the soft tissue enables the clinician to develop a better understanding of the skeletal and dental problems of the individual patient (Figs. B4.20 and B4.21).

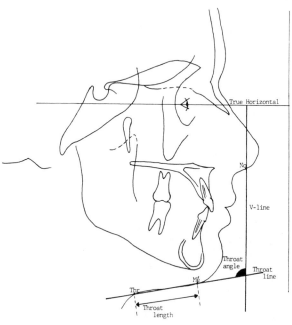

B4.19

Figure B4.19 The throat length and angle. These are very important measurements in cases of orthognathic surgery of the mandible.

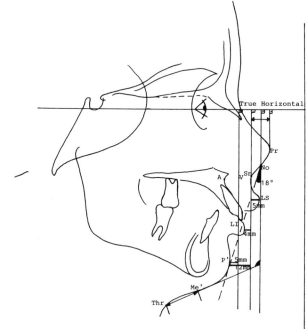

B4.20

Figure B4.20 This 10-year-old boy presents with a severe class II, division 1 malocclusion. It is obvious from the soft-tissue evaluation that this individual has significant discrepancies in the anteroposterior dimension. The increased convexity (V angle = 18°), the significant tooth exposure at rest (6 mm), the distances of the soft-tissue points LS, LI, and P from the Sn perpendicular, as well as the 5-mm posterior relationship of the chin in relation to the V perpendicular (normal = 0 mm) and the short throat length, are in accordance with the overall assessment of this patient as dentoalveolar maxillary protrusive and mandibular retrognathic.

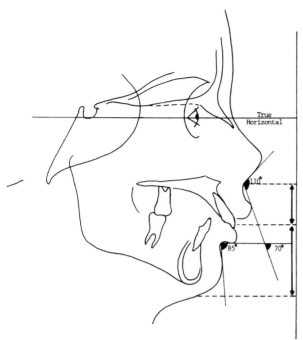

B4.21

Figure B4.21 The projection of the maxillary incisors results in a strong alteration of the soft tissue.

References

1. Tedesco LA, *et al.*: A dental-facial attractiveness scale. Am J Orthod 83:38–43, 1983.
2. Guyuron B: Precision rhinoplasty I: The role of life-size photographs and soft-tissue cephalometric analysis. Plast Reconstr Surg 81:489, 1988.
3. Stella JP, and Epker BN: Systematic aesthetic evaluation of the nose for cosmetic surgery. Oral Maxillofacial Surg Clin North Am 2:273, 1990.
4. Kerr WJS, and O'Donnell JM: Panel perception of facial attractiveness. Br J Orthod 17:299–304, 1990.
5. Lines PA, Lines RR, and Lines C: Profile metrics and facial esthetics. Am J Orthod 73:648, 1978.
6. Proffit WR: *Contemporary Orthodontics.* St. Louis, MO: C.V. Mosby Co., 1986.
7. Proffit WR, and White RP, Jr: *Surgical-Orthodontic Treatment.* St. Louis, MO: Mosby Year Book, 1991.
8. Viazis AD: A new measurement of profile esthetics. J Clin Orthod 25:15–20, 1991.
9. Steiner CC: Cephalometrics for you and me. Am J Orthod Dentofacial Orthop 39:729–755, 1953.
10. Burstone CJ: The integumental profile. Am J Orthod 44:1–25, 1958.
11. Burstone CJ: Integumental contour and extension patterns. Angle Orthod 29:93–104, 1959.
12. Ricketts RM: Perspectives in clinical application of cephalometrics. Angle Orthod 51:115–150, 1981.
13. Ricketts RM: Planning treatment on the basis of the facial pattern and an estimate of its growth. Angle Orthod 43:105–119, 1957.
14. Ricketts RM: The influence of orthodontic treatment on facial growth and development. Angle Orthod 30:103–133, 1960.
15. Burstone CJ: Lip posture and its significance to treatment planning. Am J Orthod 53:262–284, 1967.
16. Wolford LM: Surgical-orthodontic correction of dentofacial and craniofacial deformities. Syllabus, Baylor College of Dentistry, Dallas, TX, 1990.
17. Bell WH, and Jacobs JD: Tridimensional planning for surgical/orthodontic treatment of mandibular excess. Am J Orthod 80:263–288, 1981.
18. Epker BN, and Fish LC: Evaluation and treatment planned. In *Dentofacial Deformities,* edited by BN Epker and LC Fish. St. Louis: C.V. Mosby Co.; 1986, p. 18.
19. Bass NM: The aesthetic analysis of the face. Eur J Orthod 13:343–350, 1991.

Chapter 5

Anteroposterior Skeletal Assessment

The anteroposterior position of the jaws is assessed based on measurements that use the true horizontal (TH) as the reference line[1] (Fig. B5.1). See Chapter 3 in this part for a glossary of abbreviations used here.

Size of the Mandible (GoGn) Relative to the Anterior Cranial Base (SNa)

A ratio of GoGn:SN = 1 indicates a well-balanced mandibular body relative to the cranial base (Fig. B5.2). A differential of 0 to 5 mm (SNa > GoGn) would be expected for the prepubertal period and the opposite (SNa > GoGn) for the postpubertal period. The size of the anterior cranial base, unless severely deformed due to a genetic disorder/malformation, may be considered constant or of normal size in all cases. Therefore, the maxilla and mandible have to be in good anteroposterior relation to the "normal" anterior cranial base length.

The importance of this measurement lies in the fact that a very retrognathic profile may be due to a short mandibular body (that affects the anteroposterior plane), which may require surgical intervention, depending on the deformity and the age of the patient.

Maxillomandibular Ratio (PNS–ANS:ArGn)

According to the Michigan growth atlas,[2] the length of the mandible, defined from articulare (Ar) to gnathion (Gn), is almost exactly double of the maxillary length, defined from the posterior and anterior nasal spine (PNS–ANS), for all age groups and for both males and females. The actual length is not as important as is the maxillomandibular ratio, PNS–ANS:ArGn (similar to the maxillomandibular differential[3]), that provides the relationship of the two jaws relative to each other (Fig. B5.2). A ratio of 1:2 indicates that the actual lengths of the maxilla and mandible are in good balance with each other. This information, along with the relationship of the body of the mandible to the cranial base, relate the cranial base, maxilla, and mandible with each other.

Assessment of the Position of the Jaws Using Linear and Angular Measurements

Proffit and White[4] have proposed using a perpendicular from the nasion with the TH in assessing the maxillary and mandibular anteroposterior relationship with linear measurements. Three suggested linear measurements from points A, B, and pogonion (Pg) to nasion perpendicular to TH relate the position of the maxilla, mandible, and chin, respectively. A-point should be 1 mm in front of the Na-perpendicular, whereas B-point and Pg should be 3 mm and 1 mm behind the line, respectively (Fig. B5.3).

	Measurement	**Patient**
SN:GoGn	1 : 1	
PNS ANS: ArGn	1 : 2	
A:NperpTH	+1 mm	
B:NperpTH	−3 mm	
P:NperpTH	−1 mm	
"True Wits" (ab)	4 ± 2 mm	
Chin Length (bp)	2 mm ± 2 mm	
NaA-TH	90° ± 3°	
NaB-TH	87° ± 3°	
NaP-TH	89° ± 3°	
ANB	3° ± 2°	
BNPg	−2° ± 2°	

B5.1

Figure B5.1 The 12 cephalometric measurements used in the anteroposterior assessment of the jaws.

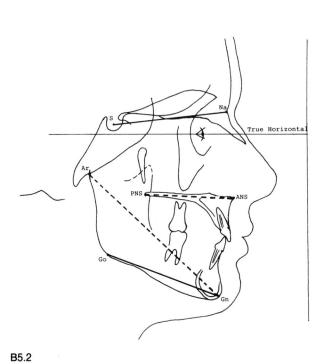

B5.2

Figure B5.2 The cranial base mandibular differential *(solid lines)* and the maxillomandibular ratio *(dotted lines)* of the jaws.

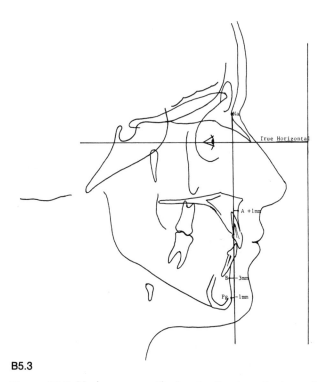

B5.3

Figure B5.3 Nasion perpendicular to the true horizontal. Note the relationships of points A, B, and P to this line.

Due to the importance of accurate assessment of the anteroposterior position of both the maxilla and the mandible relative to each other and the cranial base, angular measurements are also calculated between the TH and NaA, NaB, and NaP. These are 90 degrees ± 3 degrees, 87 degrees and 89 degrees ± 3 degrees, respectively[5] (Fig. B5.4).

Assessment of the Relative Anteroposterior Position of the Maxilla and the Mandible — the True Horizontal Wits and the ANB Angle

If points A and B are projected on the TH through perpendicular lines, points A and B are defined, respectively.[1] The AB distance is defined as the *true horizontal* Wits (Fig. B5.5) versus the original *Wits on the occlusal plane.* The TH Wits provides a better and more clear relationship of the anteroposterior position of the jaws relative to each other than does the original Wits, which can sometimes be affected by the inclination of the occlusal plane or by the inclinations of the Frankfort horizontal[6–12] (Fig. B5.6). The Wits appraisal does not necessarily focus attention on changes actually occurring in the sagittal relation between the mandible and the maxilla.[6,7] Rather, because of changes in the angulation of the occlusal plane, the true sagittal changes are likely to be disguised.[11,12] A correlation between angle ANB and Wits would not be expected because they each involve an exclusive point or plane, which is not necessarily biologically related. The mean ± SD for this measurement is 4 ± 2 mm.

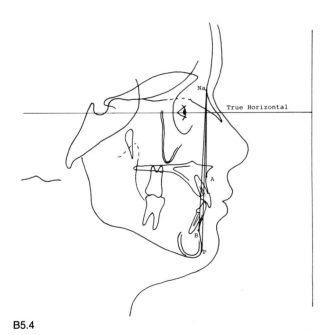

B5.4

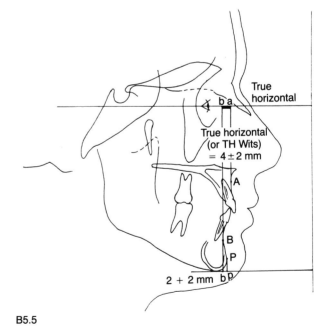

B5.5

Figure B5.4 Angular measurements that assess the anteroposterior position of the jaws from points A, B, and P. Values above the mean indicate prognathism, whereas values less than the mean (especially more than 1 standard deviation) indicate retrognathia.

Figure B5.5 The "true horizontal Wits" and the chin length measurements.

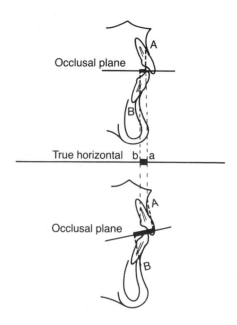

Occlusal plane

True horizontal   b   a

Occlusal plane

B5.6

Figure B5.6 The value of the Wits can be affected by the inclination of the occlusal plane.

In addition to the TH Wits linear measurement, an angular measurement, the ANB angle, is also used to assess the anteroposterior position of the jaws. The ANB angle is a very popular measurement; its use has been well documented in the literature.[1-12] The mean ± SD is 3 degrees ± 2 degrees (see Fig. B5.4).

Anteroposterior Assessment of the Chin — the Chin Length and the BNP Angle

A line parallel to the TH is drawn tangent to the mandible at menton (Me). Projections of B-point and Pg define the *chin length* (BP). The mean ± SD for this measurement is 2 ± 2 mm[1] (see Fig. B5.5). An angular measurement, the BNP angle, assesses the prominence of the chin relative to the body of the mandible (see Fig. B5.4). The mean ± SD for the BNP angle is − 2 degrees ± 2 degrees.

By applying the aforementioned measurements, the clinician will develop an appreciation of the position of the jaws in the anteroposterior plane (Fig. B5.7 through B5.12) and will then be ready for the evaluation of the skeletal substrate in the vertical plane.

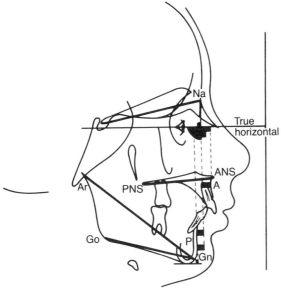

B5.7

Figure B5.7 Ten-year-old patient who, according to the 12 cephalometric measurements of anteroposterior skeletal assessment, demonstrates a slightly small mandible (the differential with the cranial base is 7 mm and the maxillomandibular ratio greater than 1:2, approximately 1.1:2). There is a significant discrepancy of the true horizontal Wits and the ANB measurements, due partly to the size of the mandible but mostly to the procumbency of the maxillary substrate. These observations are in accordance with the clinical impression of a retrognathic profile.

	Measurement	**Patient**
SNaGoGn	1:1	7 mm differential (SN > GoGn)
PNS ANS: ArGn	1:2	5 mm shorter body
A:NaperpTH	+1 mm	+11 mm
B:NaperpTH	−3 mm	−5 mm
P:NaperpTH	−1 mm	−4 mm
"True Wits" (ab)	4 ± 2 mm	11 mm
Chin Length (bp)	2 mm ± 2 mm	1 mm
NaA-TH	90° ± 3°	97°
NaB-TH	87° ± 3°	87°
NaP-TH	89° ± 3°	88°
ANB	3° ± 2°	10°
BNPg	−2° ± 2°	−1°

B5.8

Figure B5.8 The 12 cephalometric measurements of the patient in Figure B5.7.

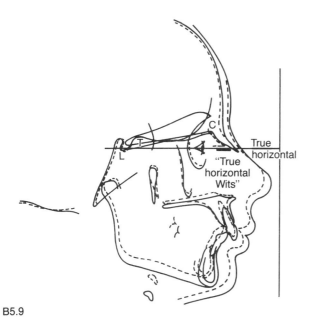

B5.9

Figure B5.9 A follow-up of this same patient after 5 years clearly shows that the true horizontal Wits has remained the same.

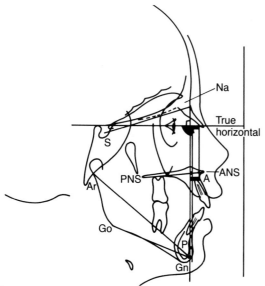

B5.10

Figure B5.10 This 11-year-old patient has a cranial base differential and maxillomandibular ratio within normal limits. The cephalometric measurements reveal a slight procumbency of both maxillary and mandibular skeletal bases relative to the cranial base. The true horizontal Wits reveals that the two jaws are in good anteroposterior relationship to each other, even though the ANB angle is slightly increased.

	Measurement	**Patient**
SNa:GoGn	1 : 1	Differential is 4 mm (within normal limits)
PNS ANS: ArGn	1 : 2	Approximately 1 : 2
A:NaperpTH	+1 mm	+7 mm
B:NaperpTH	−3 mm	+1 mm
P:NaperpTH	−1 mm	+2 mm
"True Wits" (ab)	4 ± 2 mm	6 mm
Chin Length (bp)	2 mm ± 2 mm	1 mm
NaA-TH	90° ± 3°	97°
NaB-TH	87° ± 3°	90
NaP-TH	89° ± 3°	91°
ANB	3° ± 2°	7°
BNPg	−2° ± 2°	−1°

B5.11

Figure B5.11 The 12 cephalometric measurements of the patient in Figure B5.10.

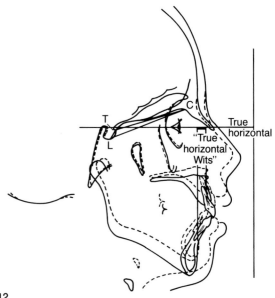

B5.12

Figure B5.12 Five years later, at the age of 16, the same skeletal relationships are still evident.

References

1. Viazis AD: Anteroposterior assessment of the maxilla and the mandible based on the true horizontal. J Clin Orthod 26:673–680, 1992.
2. Riolo ML, Moyers RE, McNamara JA, and Hunter WS: *An Atlas of Craniofacial Growth: Cephalometric Standards.* Ann Arbor, MI: University School Growth Study, the University of Michigan. Monograph Number 2, Craniofacial Growth Series, Center for Human Growth and Development, 1972.
3. McNamara LA, Jr.: A method of cephalometric evaluation. Am J Orthod 86:449–469, 1984.
4. Proffit WR, and White R: *Surgical Orthodontic Treatment.* St. Louis: C.V. Mosby Co.; 1990, pp. 109–111, 117–124.
5. Viazis AD: A cephalometric analysis based on natural head position. J Clin Orthod 25:172–182, 1991.
6. Oktay H: A comparison of ANB, WITS, AF–BF, and APDI measurements. Am J Orthod Dentofacial Orthop 99:122–128, 1991.
7. Sherman SL, Woods M, and Nanda RS: The longitudinal effects of growth on the Wits appraisal. Am J Orthod Dentofacial Orthop 93:429–436, 1988.
8. Wallen T, and Bloomquist D: The clinical examination: Is it more important than cephalometric analysis in surgical orthodontics? International Journal of Adult Orthodontics and Orthognathic Surgery 1:179, 1986.
9. Ellis E, III, and McNamara JA, Jr.: Cephalometric reference planes—Sella nasion vs. Frankfort horizontal. International Journal of Adult Orthodontics and Orthognathic Surgery 3:31, 1988.
10. McNamara JA, Jr., and Ellis E, III: Cephalometric analysis of untreated adults with ideal facial and occlusal relationships. International Journal of Adult Orthodontics and Orthognathic Surgery 3:221, 1988.
11. Jarvinen S: The relation of the Wits appraisal to the ANB angle: Statistical appraisal. Am J Orthod Dentofacial Orthop 94:432–435, 1988.
12. Rushton R, Cohen AM, and Linney AD: The relationship and reproducibility of angle ANB and the Wits appraisal. Br J Orthod 18:225–231, 1991.

Chapter 6

Vertical Skeletal Assessment

The influence of mandibular growth rotation in the development of deep or open bites before, during, or after orthodontic intervention has been the center of extensive investigations over the past 40 years.[1-17] A number of diagnostic modalities have been introduced to provide the clinician with the ability to "predict" abnormal rotational patterns that may appear as part of the growth and development of the patient's facial skeleton, especially of the mandible.[4-6,8-10,14-17] It has been shown that there is no measurement or set of measurements that can be used successfully to predict growth rotation, even by experienced clinicians.[10] Conversely, the orthodontist may use some cephalometric parameters to assess the individual patient. The following 10 cephalometric measurements may aid the clinician in appreciating a patient's facial vertical growth.[18] A fair number of these measurements indicate a rotational pattern tendency that will increase the relative prediction ability of the clinician when evaluating the unique features of each individual case (Figs. B6.1 and B6.2). See Chapter 3 in this part for a glossary of abbreviations used here.

Width of the Symphysis Parallel to the True Horizontal from Pogonion (P TH)

The greater this measurement is, the more of a forward growth rotation (a deep bite tendency in most cases) is to be expected (see Part C, Chapter 1, *Growth Considerations*). A narrow symphysis corresponds to a backward growth rotation (an open-bite tendency).[14-16] The mean ± SD is 16.5 mm ± 3 mm.

Angle of the Symphysis (BP–MeTH)

This is defined by the line connecting B-point and pogonion (P) as it crosses a line parallel to the true horizontal (TH) at menton (Me). The mean ± SD is 75 degrees ± 5 degrees. If the symphysis is inclined backward, that is, if the angle of the symphysis is acute, this is an indication of a forward growth rotational pattern.[9,14-16] If it is inclined forward (angle is obtuse), there will be backward rotation.[9,14-16]

Mandibular Plane Angle (GoMe–TH)

One of the most widely used cephalometric measurements, this angle may sometimes mask the true growth tendencies of the mandible due to extensive remodeling changes occurring at the angle of the mandible and the symphysis. High values indicate a backward growth rotator, and low ones indicate a horizontal growth pattern. The mean ± SD is 27 degrees ± 5 degrees. The angle will decrease approximately 2 degrees ± 2 degrees from childhood to adulthood.

Measurement	Mean ± SD/ Ratios	Patient
1. Symphysis Width (PgTH)	16.5 mm ± 3 mm	
2. Symphysis Angle (BPg-MeTH)	75° ± 5°	
3. Mandibular Plane Angle (GoMe-TH)	27° ± 5°	
4. Sum of Posterior Angles (SNa - SAr - ArGo - GoMe)	396° ± 4°	
5. Gonial Angle (ArGo-GoMe)	130° ± 7°	
6. Gonial Angle Ratio (ArGoNa:NaGoMe)	75%	
7. Post.Cranial Base to Ramus Height Ratio (SAr:ArGo)	75%	
8. Posterior/Anterior Facial Height Ratio (SGo:NaMe)	65%	
9. Posterior/Anterior Maxillary Height Ratio (EPNS:NaANS)	90%	
10. Lower to Total Facial Height Ratio (ANSMe:NaMe)	60%	

B6.1

Figure B6.1 The 10 cephalometric measurements used to assess the vertical relationship of the jaws.

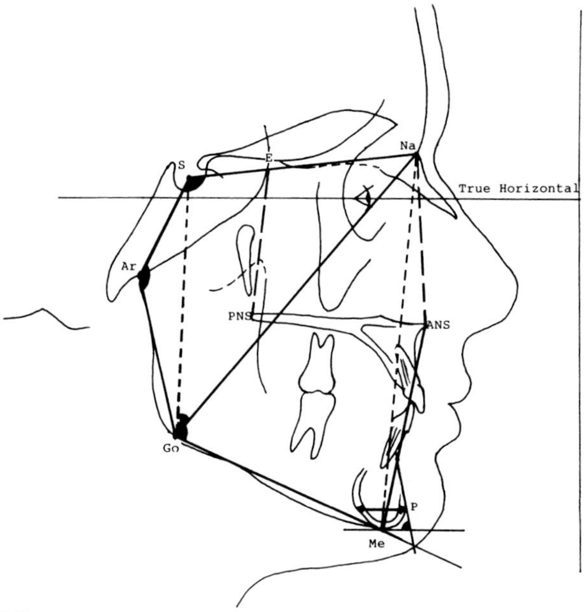

B6.2

Figure B6.2 The 10 measurements of vertical assessment drawn on a single tracing.

Sum of Posterior Angles

The mean value of the sum of the cranial flexure angle SNa–SAr (saddle angle), articular angle (SAr–ArGo), and gonial angle (ArGo–GoMe) is 396 degrees ± 4 degrees.[3,17] High values indicate a vertical growth pattern (clockwise, opening, or backward rotation), whereas low ones show a horizontal growth pattern (counterclockwise, closing, or forward growth rotation). The mean ± SD of the individual angles is: SNa–SAr, 123 degrees ± 5 degrees; SAr–ArGo, 143 degrees ± 6 degrees; ArGo–GoMe; 130 degrees ± 7 degrees. The saddle and the articular angle increase approximately 1 degree each from ages 12 to 20 years, but the sum remains the same because the gonial angle will decrease by 2 degrees during this period.[3,17]

Gonial Angle (ArGoMe)

As described by Björk[17] and Jarabak and Fizzell,[3] with a mean of 130 degrees ± 7 degrees, an increased gonial angle indicates a backward growth rotator, and a decreased one indicates a forward growth rotator.

Gonial Angle Ratio

A line from gonion to nasion divides the gonial angle into upper (ArGoNa) and lower (NaGoMe). If the ratio of the upper to the lower angle is more than 75% (high upper angle), we have an increased horizontal growth rotation.[3] The opposite (high lower angle) indicates a vertical growth pattern.

Posterior Cranial Base to Ramus Height Ratio (SAr:ArGo)

The length of the posterior cranial base needs to be measured and compared to the mean for the individual sex and age group. Providing that the length of Ar is within normal limits, a ratio value of more than 75% would indicate a short ramus height, thus contributing to a clockwise rotation skeletal pattern. A short posterior cranial base is also indicative of a backward growth rotator.

Posterior/Anterior Face Height Ratio (SGo:NaMe)

Values higher than 65% favor a forward growth pattern, whereas a ratio of less than 65% indicates a backward growth rotator.

Posterior/Anterior Maxillary Height Ratio (EPNS:Na ANS)

Values higher than 90% indicate an upward rotation of the anterior maxilla and a downward movement of its posterior component, thus contributing to an open bite. Values lower than 90% may indicate a rotational pattern that contributes to a deep bite.

Lower to Total Anterior Facial Height Ratio (ANSMe:NaMe)

Values higher than 60% or a long lower face height are indicative of a backward growth rotator. Low ratio values suggest a forward growth rotator.

The distinction between open- and deep-bite tendencies, especially in borderline cases, is very important, not only for the initial diagnosis, but also for the planning of the treatment mechanics of choice. A deep mandibular antegonial notch is indicative of a diminished mandibular growth potential and a vertically directed mandibular growth pattern.[19] High-angle cases generally may be more prone to mechanical extrusion of posterior teeth during orthodontic treatment, primarily because the high mandibular plane angle is associated with less muscle strength.

The vertical assessment of the jaws aids the clinician in recognizing open-bite tendency patterns that may be detrimental to a successfully treated case (Figs. B6.3 through B6.8).

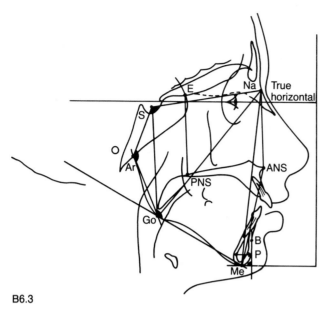

B6.3

Figure B6.3 A 12-year-old boy who presented clinically with a 1-mm open-bite relationship. It is apparent that a successful treatment outcome for this individual would depend greatly on the open-bite tendency that he may exhibit, especially during his pubertal growth spurt.

Measurement	Mean ± SD/ Ratios	Patient
1. Symphysis Width (PgTH)	16.5 mm ± 3 mm	7 mm*
2. Symphysis Angle (BPg-MeTH)	75° ± 5°	90*
3. Mandibular Plane Angle (GoMe-TH)	27° ± 5°	29°
4. Sum of Posterior Angles (SNa - SAr - ArGo - GoMe)	396° ± 4°	399
5. Gonial Angle (ArGo-GoMe)	130° ± 7°	141*
6. Gonial Angle Ratio (ArGoNa:NaGoMe)	75%	80%
7. Post.Cranial Base to Ramus Height Ratio (SAr:ArGo)	75%	81%*
8. Posterior/Anterior Facial Height Ratio (SGo:NaMe)	65%	62%*
9. Posterior/Anterior Maxillary Height Ratio (EPNS:NaANS)	90%	100%*
10. Lower to Total Facial Height Ratio (ANSMe:NaMe)	60%	56%

B6.4

Figure B6.4 Same patient as in Figure B6.3. Six of the 10 measurements (*) are beyond 1 standard deviation from the mean, indicating a backward growth pattern, *i.e.,* a strong open-bite tendency. Not all of the measurements show us this tendency. The clinician may use his or her judgment and clinical expertise to balance the information presented by the individual case.

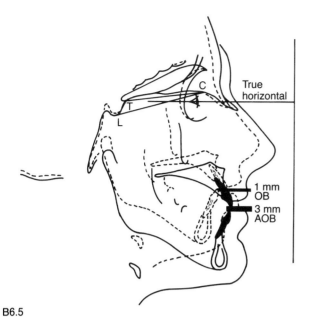

B6.5

Figure B6.5 Three years later, the patient in Figure B6.3 had expressed a significant vertical growth, which increased his open bite by 4 mm. A surgical approach was the treatment of choice.

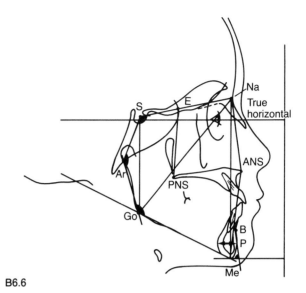

B6.6

Figure B6.6 This 10-year-old boy presents with 1-mm open-bite relationship.

Measurement	Mean ± SD/ Ratios	Patient
1. Symphysis Width (PgTH)	16.5 mm ± 3 mm	15 mm
2. Symphysis Angle (Bg-MeTH)	75° ± 5°	85°*
3. Mandibular Plane Angle (GoMe-TH)	27° ± 5°	21.5°**
4. Sum of Posterior Angles (SNa - SAr - ArGo - GoMe)	396° ± 4°	396°
5. Gonial Angle (ArGo-GoMe)	130° ± 7°	132
6. Gonial Angle Ratio (ArGoNa:NaGoMe)	75%	76%
7. Post.Cranial Base to Ramus Height Ratio (SAr:ArGo)	75%	87.5%*
8. Posterior/Anterior Facial Height Ratio (SGo:NaMe)	65%	60%*
9. Posterior/Anterior Maxillary Height Ratio (EPNS:NaANS)	90%	91%
10. Lower to Total Facial Height Ratio (ANSMe:NaMe)	60%	55%**

B6.7

Figure B6.7 The same patient as in Figure B6.6. The cephalometric evaluation shows that three (*) of the measurements indicate backward growth (open-bite tendency), whereas two (**) indicate forward growth (deep-bite tendency). The rest of the measurements are right on or around the mean values. It was decided that this patient would continue to grow in the same manner (the open bite would not get worse) and orthodontic mechanotherapy would try to limit any extrusive side effects as much as possible.

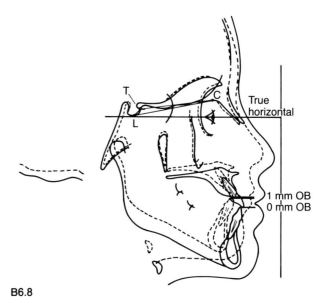

B6.8

Figure B6.8 Five years later, the patient has a similar relationship, with an overbite of 0 mm. Clinical judgment and realistic evaluation of the numbers from the cephalometric evaluation allowed for a thorough understanding of the individual patient's growth tendencies in the vertical plane.

References

1. Schudy FF: The rotation of the mandible resulting from growth: Its implications in orthodontic treatment. Angle Orthod 35:36–50, 1965.
2. Odegaard J: Growth of the mandible studied with the aid of metal implant. Am J Orthod 57:145–157, 1970.
3. Jarabak JR, and Fizzell JA: *Technique and Treatment with Light Wire Edgewise Appliances,* 2nd ed. St. Louis: C.V. Mosby Co., 1972.
4. Lavergne J, and Gasson N: A metal implant study of mandibular rotation. Angle Orthod 46:144–150, 1976.
5. Isaacson R, Zapfel R, Worms T, and Erdman A: Effects of rotational jaw growth on the occlusion and profile. Am J Orthod 72:276–286, 1977.
6. Isaacson R, Zapfel R, Worms F, Bevis R, and Speidel T: Some effects of mandibular growth on the dental occlusion and profile. Angle Orthod 47:97–106, 1977.
7. Lavergne J, and Gasson N: Analysis and classification of the rotational growth pattern without implants. Br J Orthod 9:51–56, 1982.
8. Lavergne J: Morphogenetic classification of malocclusion as a basis for growth prediction and treatment planning. Br J Orthod 9:132–145, 1982.
9. Skieller V, Björk A, and Linde-Hansen T: Prediction of mandibular growth rotation evaluated from a longitudinal implant sample. Am J Orthod 86:359–370, 1984.
10. Baumrind S, Korn EL, and West EE: Prediction of mandibular rotation: An empirical test of clinician performance. Am J Orthod 86:371–385, 1984.
11. Björk A: The face in profile: An anthropological x-ray investigation on Swedish children and conscripts. Svensk Tandlakare Tidskrift 40 (Suppl) (5B), 1947.
12. Ricketts RM: Planning treatment on the basis of the facial pattern and an estimate of its growth. Angle Orthod 27:14–37, 1957.
13. Ricketts RM: The influence of orthodontic treatment on facial growth and development. Angle Orthod 30:103–133, 1960.
14. Björk A: Variations in the growth patterns of the human mandible: Longitudinal radiographic study by the implant method. J Dent 42:400–411, 1963.
15. Björk A: Prediction of mandibular growth rotation. Am J Orthod 55:585–599, 1969.
16. Björk A, and Skieller V: Facial development and tooth eruption: An implant study at the age of puberty. Am J Orthod 62:339–383, 1972.
17. Björk A: The face in profile: An anthropological x-ray investigation on Swedish children and conscripts. Svensk Tandlakare Tidskrift 40 (Suppl), 1947.
18. Viazis AD: Assessment of open and deep bite tendencies using the true horizontal. J Clin Orthod 26:338–343, 1992.
19. Singer CP, Mamandras AH, and Hunter WS: The depth of the mandibular antegonial notch as an indicator of mandibular growth potential. Am J Orthod Dentofacial Orthop 91:117–124, 1987.

Chapter 7

Cephalometric Dental Evaluation

The inclination of the dentition relative to the skeletal substrate is provided with the following measurements[1] (Fig. B7.1). See Chapter 3 in this part for a glossary of abbreviations used here.

Inclination of the Functional Occlusal Plane (Occlusal Plane Angle)

The angle between TH and the functional occlusal plane (OP) is derived from the lower molar and bicuspid cusp tips and locates the teeth in occlusion relative to the rest of the face. As with the mandibular plane, high values indicate a backward and low values a forward growth rotation. The mean ± SD is 8 degrees ± 2 degrees.

Inclination of the Upper Incisor to the Maxillary Plane (Upper Incisor Angle)

This is the angle formed from the long axis of the upper incisor (U1) and the ANS/PNS line. The mean ± SD is 110 degrees ± 5 degrees.

Inclination of the Lower Incisor to the Mandibular Plane (Lower Incisor Angle)

The long axis of the lower incisor (L1) and the GoGn plane form this angle. The mean ± SD is 92 degrees ± 5 degrees (GoMe can be used as well).

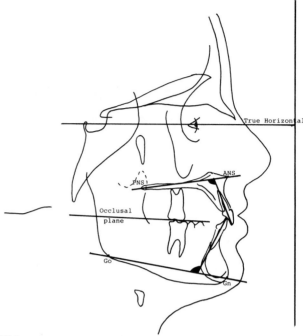

B7.1

Figure B7.1 The inclination of the dentition is determined from the occlusal plane angle and the relation of the incisors to their skeletal substrate.

Reference

1. Viazis AD: A cephalometric analysis based on natural head position. J Clin Orthod 25:172–181, 1991.

Chapter 8

Posteroanterior Cephalometrics

As emphasized by Proffit and White,[1] the primary indication for obtaining a posteroanterior cephalometric film is the presence of facial asymmetry. A tracing is made and vertical planes are used to illustrate transverse asymmetries.[1] Lines are drawn through the angles of the mandible and the outer borders of the maxillary tuberosity (Figs. B8.1 and B8.2). Vertical asymmetry can be observed readily by drawing transverse occlusal planes (molar to molar) at various vertical levels and observing their vertical orientation.[1] If a significant skeletal asymmetry is detected, orthognathic surgery may be incorporated in the treatment plan. A more thorough evaluation would then be needed.[2,3]

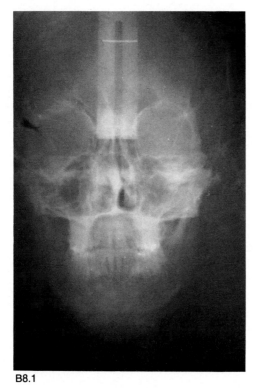

B8.1

Figure B8.1 A posteroanterior cephalometric radiograph.

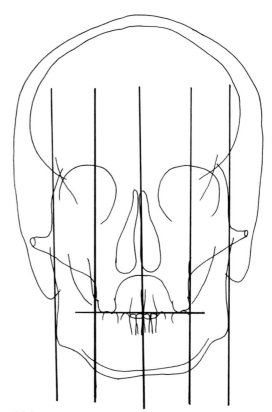

B8.2

Figure B8.2 Vertical and horizontal lines are a good first impression of the existence of facial asymmetry.

References

1. Proffit WR, and White RP, Jr.: *Surgical Orthodontic Treatment.* St. Louis, MO: Mosby Year Book; 1991, p. 127.
2. El-Mangoury NH, Shaheen SI, and Mostafa YA: Landmark identification in computerized posteroanterior cephalometrics. Am J Orthod Dentofacial Orthop 91:57–61, 1987.
3. Grummons DC, and Kappeyne van de Coppello MA: A frontal asymmetry analysis. J Clin Orthod 21:448–465, 1987.

Growth

Growth Considerations

Craniofacial growth is a complex phenomenon and its understanding requires an in-depth study of the changes that occur from infancy to adulthood.[1-12] The clinician should be aware of a few basic principles of maxillary and mandibular growth.[1-12]

The maxilla and the mandible grow in both a downward and forward direction relative to the cranial base (Fig. C1.1). At the peak of the juvenile growth spurt (7 to 9 years of age), the maxilla grows 1 mm/yr and the mandible 3 mm/yr, whereas during the prepubertal period (10 to 12 years of age) there will be a reduced rate of growth (maxilla, 0.25 mm/yr; mandible, 1.5 mm/yr), only to reach maximum growth levels during puberty (12 to 14 years of age) (maxilla, 1.5 mm/yr; mandible, 4.5 mm/yr).[8-11] The lower facial height (ANS–Me) increases approximately 1 mm/yr, and the pogonion (Pg) comes forward about 1 mm/yr.

In general, from 4 to 20 years of age, there will be on average 10 mm of pure alveolar growth (Fig. C1.2).[8-12] Overall, mandibular growth is approximately twice that of overall maxillary growth.[7] The average direction of maxillary sutural growth has been found to be 45 degrees to 51 degrees in relation to the nasion–sella line from 8.5 to 14.5 years of age.[8-11] Mechanisms responsible for the maxillary growth displacement may be different in the earlier and later periods of maxillary growth, as the direction of sutural growth changes to almost horizontal at the age of 14.5 years. This corresponds to the finding that the mean vertical maxillary displacement has terminated by the age of 15 years, whereas the horizontal displacement continues until 18 years of age in boys and until 16 years of age in girls. The angle of maxillary prognathism (NA–TH) remains almost constant during growth because the forward displacement of the maxilla is accompanied by a forward displacement of the nasion point due to periosteal apposition. If the maxillary growth in boys is assumed to have terminated by age 18 years and in girls by age 16 years, this corresponds to an average annual lowering of 0.7 mm. Furthermore, increase in facial height (vertical growth) continues at a much reduced rate throughout early adulthood both in men and women. The mean increase for total face height (nasion to menton) during adulthood is almost 3 mm, but in individual cases it may be in the order of 10 mm (1 cm)![12] All of the aforementioned guidelines should be taken into consideration when evaluating the cephalometric measurements of the individual patient relative to the presented average values.

The position of the condylar surfaces relative to the articular fossae probably does not change appreciably with growth. The lowering of the maxillary complex displaces the anterior, tooth-bearing part of the mandible, whereas condylar growth and lowering of the articular fossae displace its posterior part.[2,12] If the amounts of lowering of the anterior and posterior parts are not equal, the mandibular displacement will contain a component of rotation.[2]

When the direction of condylar growth is upward and forward in relation to the mandibular base, the lowering of the posterior part of the mandible usually exceeds that of the anterior part. The resulting type of mandibular rotation is termed *forward growth rotation*[1,2,8-11] (counterclockwise rotation). If, during the forward growth rota-

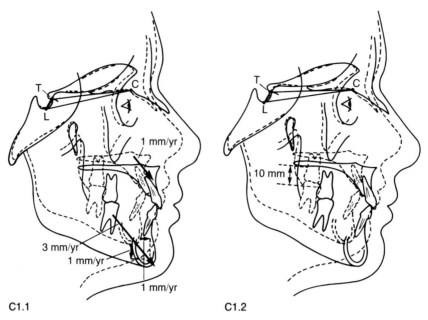

C1.1   C1.2

Figure C1.1 Growth of the jaws in a downward and forward direction.

Figure C1.2 Alveolar growth from childhood to adulthood.

tion, there is occlusal contact in the incisal region, the eruption of the posterior teeth normally serves to maintain occlusal contact in the posterior part of the dental arches. If there is no occlusal contact in the incisal part of the dental arches, the forward growth rotation occurs as a rolling movement around a point in the bicuspid region of the dental arches. The incisal segment of the lower dental arch is thereby carried inside the incisal segment of the upper dental arch, leading to the development of *skeletal deep bite*[1,2,8-11] (Figs. C1.3 and C1.4). Depending on the severity of these cases, adjunctive orthodontic/surgical treatment may be needed.[13,14]

If the lowering of the anterior and posterior parts of the mandible is identical, there will be no component of rotation and the mandibular displacement with growth will be a pure translation.

In subjects with a predominantly backward direction of the condylar growth or with only a small amount of condylar growth, the lowering of the posterior part of the mandible can be smaller than that of its anterior part. Mandibular displacement in such instances will contain a component of backward rotation and the mandible will seem to roll backward around a point in the molar region. This is termed *backward growth rotation*[2,8-11] (clockwise rotation). In such cases, occlusal contact in the anterior segment of the dental arches can be maintained by increased eruption of the front teeth. If the teeth are not able to compensate by supra-eruption, a *skeletal open bite* develops (see Figs. C1.20 to C1.22). Again, an orthognathic surgical approach should be considered for the severe cases.[13,14]

It should be emphasized that facial changes also occur in adulthood. Males tend to have a counterclockwise rotation of the mandible, whereas the mandibles of females seem to rotate clockwise. This may have a bearing on the long-term stability of treated cases; a treated class II female might be more prone to relapse toward a class II situation, and a treated class III male might be more prone to relapse to class III. In addition, as some individuals age, the mandible might appear less protrusive owing to a number of factors: the maxillary incisors are continually uprighting during adulthood, and with the continued growth of the nose and chin, the repositioning of the lips, and the vertical increase, one could easily envision that the adult face would appear less protrusive over time.[6] This might make us more conservative in our diagnosis of bimaxillary protrusion.[6]

Every clinician who practices contemporary orthodontics should be able to recognize and diagnose cases with skeletal problems that should not be treated by orthodontic means alone, but with an adjunctive orthognathic procedure. These problems may involve the anteroposterior dimension, mandibular retrognathia (Figs. C1.3 through C1.11), mandibular prognathism (Figs. C1.12 through C1.18), or the vertical dimension (Figs. C1.19 through C1.24) with the clinical appearance of a skeletal open bite. Sometimes, they may involve skeletal discrepancies in both dimensions (Figs. C1.25 through C1.29). Problems in the transverse dimension should be detected as well (Fig. C1.30). The ability to evaluate and recognize these cases should be in the realm of every practitioner.

The description of the treatment of these cases is beyond the scope of this text. The clinician who becomes involved in the treatment of such cases must first spend a considerable amount of time studying the state-of-the-art literature on the subject of comprehensive surgical/orthodontic treatment.[13,14] A thorough understanding of the numerous orthognathic procedures available (and their advantages and drawbacks) is an absolute must for the successful management of these cases; failure, sometimes beyond repair, is otherwise guaranteed.

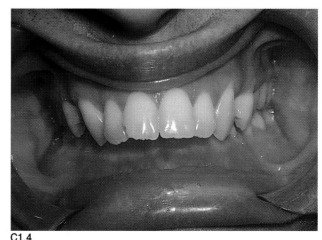

C1.4

Figure C1.4 Same patient as in Figure C1.3. The anterior view of his occlusion reveals a very deep bite (the lower incisors cannot even be seen!). His overjet was 12 mm, and he had a full class II molar relationship.

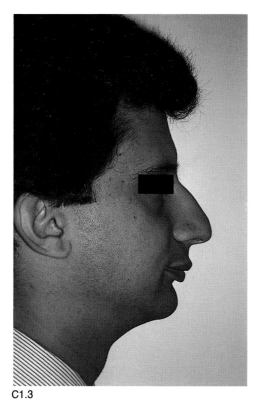

C1.3

Figure C1.3 Adult patient with the clinical impression of a retrognathic mandible. Note the deep labiomental fold.

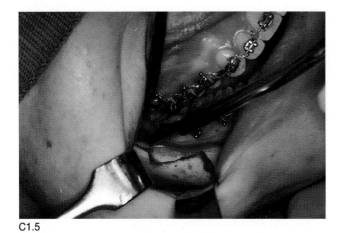

C1.5

Figure C1.5 A mandibular advancement orthognathic procedure is the surgery performed on patients with mandibular retrognathia.

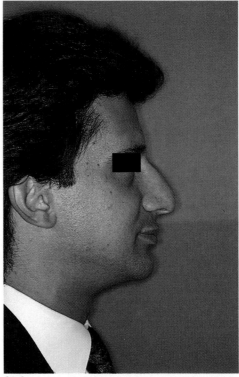

C1.6

Figure C1.6 The same patient as in Figure C1.3 after orthodontic treatment and surgery. Note the improvement in the patient's profile.

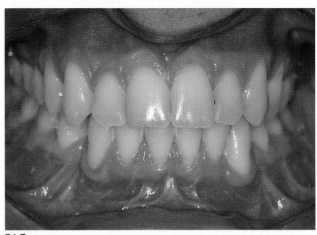

C1.7

Figure C1.7 The dentition after surgery in the patient seen in Figure C1.3.

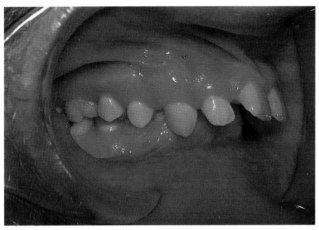

C1.8

Figure C1.8 Buccal view of a patient with mandibular retrognathia. Note the 15 mm overjet. The molar relationship is a full (100%) class II. The bite is very deep (more than 150% OB!).

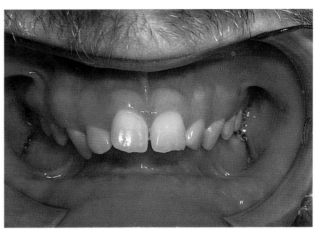

C1.9

Figure C1.9 Anterior view of the same patient as in Figure C1.8.

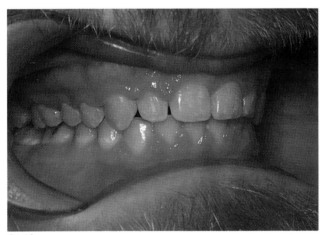

C1.10

Figure C1.10 Buccal view of the patient in Figure C1.8 after orthodontic treatment followed by orthognathic surgery (mandibular advancement). Note the class I cuspid and molar relationship.

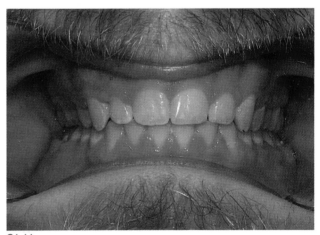

C1.11

Figure C1.11 Anterior view of the patient in Figure C1.10. Note the dramatic improvement in the overbite relationship.

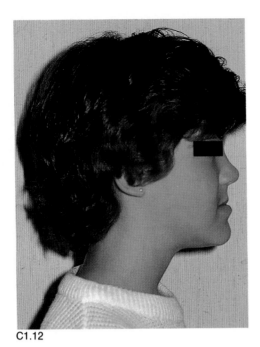

C1.12

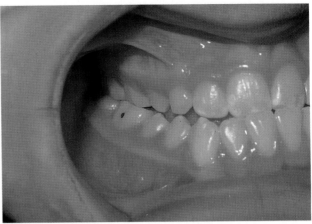

C1.13

Figure C1.13 Same patient as in Figure C1.12. Right buccal view of the occlusion. Note the retroclined lower incisors and the end-to-end multiple crossbites.

Figure C1.12 A 10-year-old girl with evident mandibular prognathism.

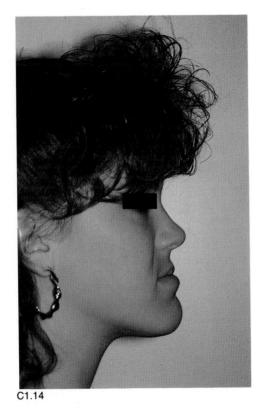

C1.14

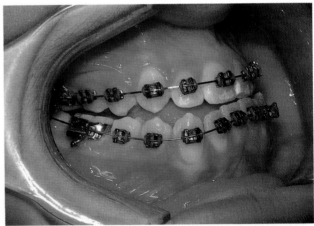

C1.15

Figure C1.15 Same patient as in Figure C1.14. Fixed orthodontic appliances in preparation for surgery.

Figure C1.14 Same patient as in Figure C1.12 after puberty and cessation of mandibular growth. Note the prognathic profile.

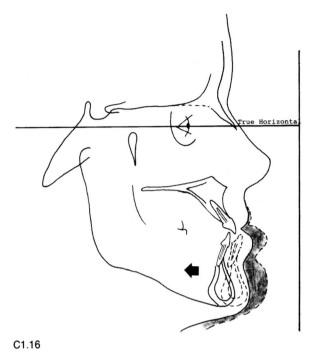

C1.16

Figure C1.16 Same patient as in Figure C1.14. In a mandibular setback procedure, the mandible is brought back until a positive overjet is achieved.

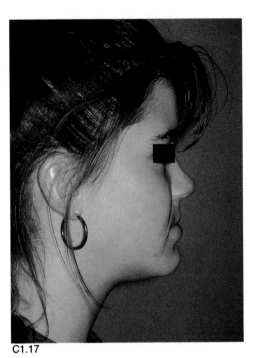

C1.17

Figure C1.17 Patient shown in Figure C1.14 after surgery.

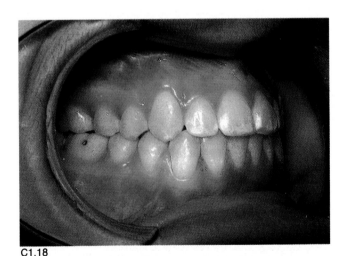

C1.18

Figure C1.18 Same patient as in Figure C1.17. Right buccal view of the occlusion after surgery. Note the improvement in the occlusion. The cuspid teeth are in a solid class I relationship.

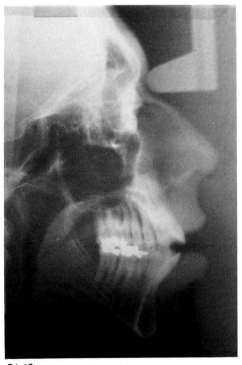

C1.19

Figure C1.19 Cephalometric radiograph of a patient with a significant vertical problem.

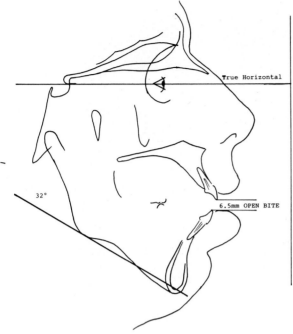

C1.20

Figure C1.20 Same patient as in Figure C1.19. The cephalometric tracing reveals a 6.5-mm open bite, high mandibular plane angle (32°), and a very long lower face.

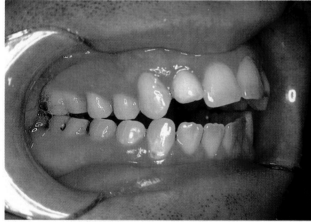

C1.21

Figure C1.21 Right buccal view of the same patient as in Figure C1.19. Note the extent of the open bite all the way to the posterior teeth.

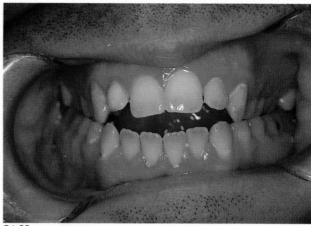

C1.22

Figure C1.22 Anterior view of the same patient as in Figure C1.19. Note the "rainbow" appearance of the skeletal open bite.

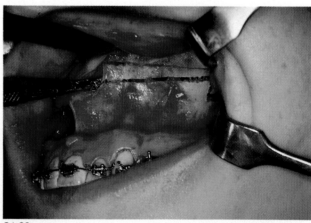

C1.23

Figure C1.23 In cases with such a significant vertical problem, a LeFort I osteotomy is performed above the maxilla.

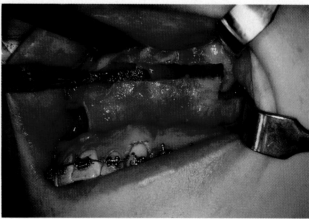

C1.24

Figure C1.24 A segment of bone is removed and the whole maxilla is repositioned superiorly. In most instances, the mandible autorotates and aids in the closing of the open bite.

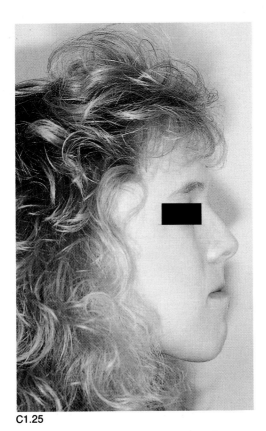

C1.25

Figure C1.25 Patient with mandibular prognathism (antero-posterior problem) and a very long lower face (vertical problem).

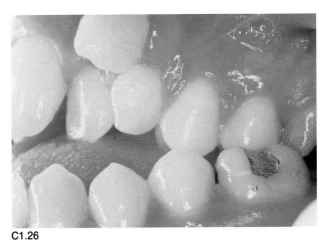

C1.26

Figure C1.26 Same patient as in Figure C1.25. Right buccal view of the occlusion. Note that the open bite extends posteriorly to the molar area.

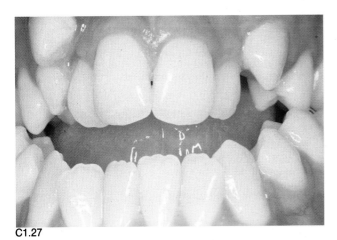

C1.27

Figure C1.27 Anterior view of the same patient as in Figure C1.25. This case requires a double-jaw orthognathic approach (three-piece maxillary LeFort I osteotomy and a mandibular procedure).

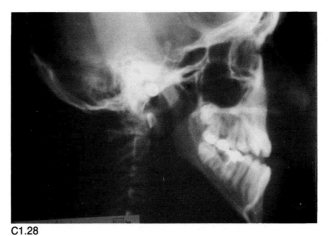

C1.28

Figure C1.28 Cephalometric radiograph of the patient in Figure C1.25.

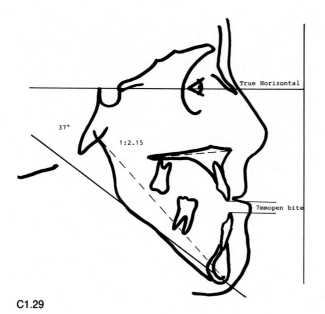

C1.29

Figure C1.29 The cephalometric tracing and analysis reveals a very high mandibular plane (37°), a large mandible relative to the size of the maxilla (ratio, 1:2.15), and a 7-mm open bite. Such a case is almost impossible to treat with orthodontic means alone at any age.

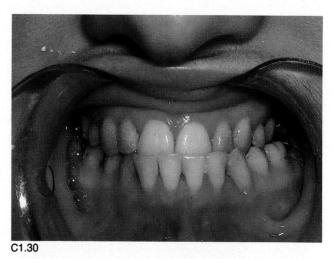

C1.30

Figure C1.30 Skeletal asymmetry of the jaws as a result of mandibular prognathism. A mandibular orthognathic procedure is the treatment of choice.

References

1. Skieller V, Björk A, and Linde-Hausen T: Prediction of mandibular growth rotation evaluated from a longitudinal implant sample. Am J Orthod 86:359–370, 1984.
2. Solow B: The dentoalveolar compensatory mechanism: Background and clinical implication. Br J Orthod 7:145–161, 1980.
3. Nielsen IL: Vertical malocclusions: Etiology, development, diagnosis and some aspects of treatment. Angle Orthod 61:247–260, 1991.
4. Korn EL, and Baumrind S: Transverse development of the human jaws between the ages 8.5 and 15.5 years, studied longitudinally with use of implants. J Dent Res 69:1298–1306, 1990.
5. Iseri H, and Solow B: Growth displacement of the maxilla in girls studied by the implant method. Eur J Orthod 12:389–398, 1990.
6. Behrents R: Adult craniofacial growth. J Clin Orthod 20:842–847, 1986.
7. Love RJ, Murray TM, and Mamandras AH: Facial growth in males 16 to 20 years of age. Am J Orthod Dentofacial Orthop 97:200–206, 1990.
8. Björk A: Variations in the growth patterns of the human mandible: Longitudinal radiographic study by the implant method. J Dent 42:400–411, 1963.
9. Björk A: Prediction of mandibular growth rotation. Am J Orthod 55:585–599, 1969.
10. Björk A, and Skieller V: Facial development and tooth eruption: An implant study at the age of puberty. Am J Orthod 62:339–383, 1972.
11. Björk A: The face in profile: An anthropological x-ray investigation on Swedish children and conscripts. Svensk Tandlakare Tidskrift 40 (Suppl) (5B), 1947.
12. Enlow DH: *Facial Growth.* Philadelphia: W.B. Saunders Co., 1990.
13. Proffit WR, and White RP, Jr.: *Surgical-Orthodontic Treatment.* St. Louis, MO: C.V. Mosby Co., 1991.
14. Bell WH: *Modern Practice in Orthognathic and Reconstructive Surgery,* vols. 1–3. Philadelphia: W.B. Saunders Co., 1992.

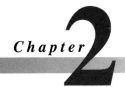
Growth Superimposition/ Evaluation

It has been well documented that the anterior wall of the sella turcica and the cribriform plate remain unchanged after the fifth year of life.[1-4] This means that no growth or remodeling changes affect these areas of the cranial base by the time the first permanent tooth erupts in the oral cavity, which is most likely the earliest time an orthodontic consultation or intervention may be needed. Growth changes of the facial skeleton can be carefully evaluated by superimposing cephalometric radiographs on these stable structures. Yet the various existing superimposition techniques do not concentrate on using this portion of the cranial substrate.[5-16] All of the other areas presently used are subject to growth changes.[17] Even the most popular superimposition technique—superimposition on the SN line by registering on S (sella)—expresses growth more anteriorly than it actually occurs.[9-12] A reason for avoiding the use of the aforementioned stable areas has been the difficulty in accurate location of the cribriform plate and the small dimension of the anterior wall of the sella turcica.

The following superimposition approach offers a sound and practical way of incorporating these structures in the evaluation of facial growth.[17] Three points are used to define the triangle (Fig. C2.1):

1. *T-point:* The most superior point of the anterior wall of the sella turcica at the junction with tuberculum sella. It can be quickly located on the radiograph and does not change with growth, as does the sella (S).
2. *C-point:* The most anterior point of the cribriform plate at the junction with the nasal bone. Even though the cribriform plate is not easily detectable, the C-point is always very clear on the cephalometric radiograph at the most posterior tip of the nasal bone.
3. *L-point:* The most inferior (lower) point of the sella turcica. This point also defines the most posterior point of the anterior wall of the sella turcica.

The triangle incorporates in its area the whole anterior wall of the sella turcica and extends over a large area that includes all of the anterior and part of the middle cranial base. The three points selected are at the greatest distance from each other within stable structures. This provides the clinician with a large marking area. By registering on the T-point and superimposing on the anterior wall of the sella turcica and the stable TC line (cranial base line), a solid formation is provided through the shape of the triangle in both the anteroposterior and the vertical planes for a practical and dependable evaluation of facial growth. The purpose of the triangle is to provide the clinician with a quick, solid, visual orientation of the most stable areas of the cranial base.

It is preferable to obtain a cephalometric radiograph of all growing patients at the age of 9 or 10 years or at the initial visit at the office. Just before orthodontic treatment is to begin and at least 6 months after the initial radiograph, a second cephalometric radiograph will give the clinician the ability to compare the two and evaluate facial growth. When superimposing the two triangles as described above, the two lower sides of the triangles may not necessarily fit right on top of each other,

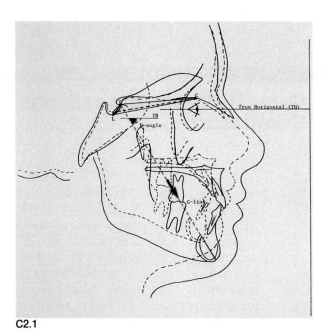

C2.1

Figure C2.1 The cranial base triangle (TLC), the G (growth) line, and D (directional) angle.

especially because of the L-point (due to slight remodeling changes in the area) (see Fig. C2.1). Focus should be placed, in the order of registering, on (1) the T-point and superimposing on (2) the inner structure of the triangle (anterior wall of the sella turcica) and (3) the TC line. This recommended methodology simplifies the procedure of the "best-fit" approach while recognizing the limits of realistic expectations of a superimposition technique.

A line connecting the T-point with gnathion (Gn) is defined as the G-line, which may be used as a growth line (see Fig. C2.1). The advantage of the G-line over the other ones that use sella is attributed to the stable position of the T-point versus the unstable S (sella point) due to growth and remodeling. In addition, the T-point is an anatomic landmark, whereas the sella is a constructed one (as the middle of sella turcica).

The mean ± SD of the angle formed between the G-line and the true horizontal (D-angle) is 58 degrees ± 4 degrees[17] (see Fig. C2.1). Growth is downward and forward along this line (D-angle stable with growth). Backward rotation of the G-line (by registering at the T-point) with growth indicates vertical growth (D-angle increases) (Fig. C2.2). Anterior rotation of the G-line with growth indicates a forward horizontal growth pattern (D-angle decreases) (Fig. C2.3).

The angle between the TC line (stable cranial base line) and the *true vertical* (TV) may be established on the first tracing of a patient (Fig. C2.4). Any additional radiographs of this patient taken to evaluate either growth changes or treatment effects may be oriented so that the *TC–TH angle* remains constant. In this way, the patient is treated to his or her initial natural head position (NHP), established in the beginning of treatment, irrespective of postural, behavioral, or surgical effects. In other words, the patient is treated to a constant NHP based solely on the line of vision, which is established when the pupil is in the middle of the eye and the individual is looking straight ahead.

In understanding the importance of craniofacial growth and its role in the development of an individual's malocclusion, one needs only to comprehend the role of dental compensation to the skeletal growth pattern.

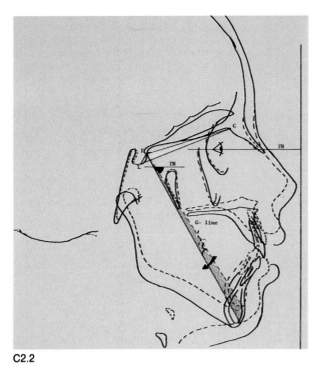

C2.2

Figure C2.2 Backward or clockwise rotation and the development of an open bite.

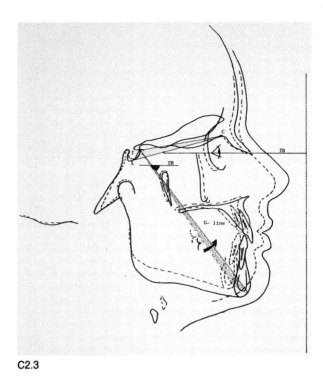

C2.3

Figure C2.3 Forward or counterclockwise rotation and the development of a deep bite.

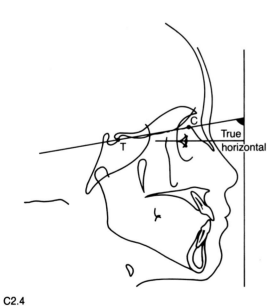

C2.4

Figure C2.4 The angle between TC and TV can be used to orient any future cephalometric radiographs of the same patient.

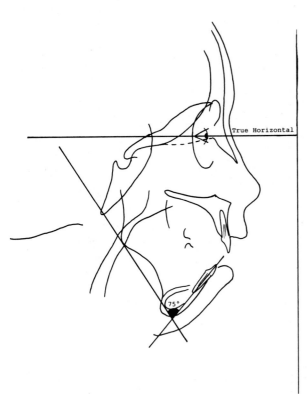

C2.5

Figure C2.5 Dental compensation in open bites: the anterior teeth tip lingually and supererupt. Here, the lower incisor to the mandibular plane angle is 75° (normal, 92° ± 5°).

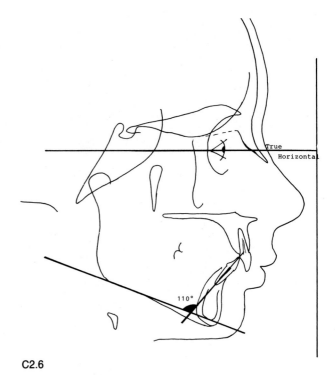

C2.6

Figure C2.6 Dental compensation in deep-bite cases. The lower incisors have flared (110°) in an effort to reduce the overbite (normal, 92° ± 5°).

Malocclusions stem from the inability of teeth to compensate for an abnormal skeletal pattern.[18] If we were to look at severe skeletal open-bite cases, we would notice that the anterior dentition (incisors) is retroclined (tipped lingually) and has supererupted in the majority of these cases[18] (Fig. C2.5). This is nature's attempt to compensate for the abnormal skeletal growth pattern that has created the open bite (backward rotation) with dental movement that decreases the extent of the open bite over the years. The opposite would take place in a deep-bite patient. The teeth would flare labially in an effort to decrease the deep overbite relationship[18] (Fig. C2.6). Of course, this is not clearly visible in all cases, because other factors play a role in the overall appearance of the dentition (muscles, soft tissue, tongue–lip equilibrium, tongue function, parafunctional habits, etc.).

The aforementioned differences in nature's dental compensations involve the vertical plane. If we were to look at skeletal development problems in the anteroposterior dimension, we would notice a similar compensatory pattern. In a class III mandibular prognathism patient, as the negative overjet (underjet) develops, the upper incisors tip labially and the lower incisors tip lingually in an effort to keep as normal an overjet relationship as possible. It is as if the teeth are trying to "hold on" while the mandible grows excessively anteriorly (Fig. C2.7).

The diagnosis of such problems may become more complicated when we have abnormal skeletal development in both dimensions, vertically and anteroposteriorly, such as the class III, open-bite patient presented previously (see Figs. C1.25 through C1.29). A thorough cephalometric evaluation along with proper superimposition of serial radiographs will help in locating the extent of the problem in both dimensions.

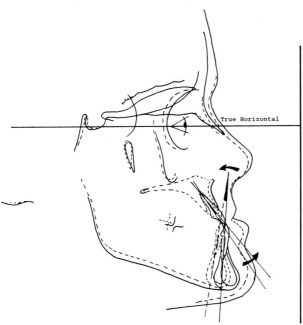

True Horizontal

C2.7

Figure C2.7 As the mandible continues to grow anteriorly, the mandibular teeth gradually tip lingually, whereas the maxillary teeth tip labially (the *arrows* show the direction of tipping). Note the angles formed from the long axes of the teeth (these axes would remain parallel if no dental compensation occurred).

An example of dental compensation is given in the situation of two patients who may have the same skeletal open-bite tendency, but one has a normal open bite/overjet of 2 mm and the other an open bite. The teeth of the first patient compensated by supereruption of the anteriors, whereas they did not for the second patient. In the past, when orthognathic surgery had not yet developed to its current level, clinicians would correct such malocclusions by completing nature's work; *i.e.,* extrude the teeth (in the case of an open bite) to close the bite.

Another example of the role of dental compensations involves the decision of extraction versus nonextraction on two individuals who have the exact same crowding and dental appearance, but one has an open-bite tendency (backward rotation) and the other a deep bite (forward rotation). Nature tends to compensate in open-bite cases by supererupting the anterior teeth and tipping them lingually. Nature compensates a deep bite by flaring the anteriors labially. We would rather extract teeth to resolve the crowding in an open-bite case, because this treatment modality would allow us to tip the rest of the teeth lingually (working along with nature's attempt to compensate) to close the bite. Extractions in a deep-bite case should be avoided if possible, because the remaining teeth would move lingually and make the bite deeper. Therefore, nonextraction approaches should be investigated for deep-bite cases.

Finally, if we were to consider two patients with identical malocclusion but totally different growth patterns, we would attempt to treat them in two different ways because it is not the malalignment of teeth that directs our treatment planning, but the individual growth patterns (Figs. C2.8 through C2.10).

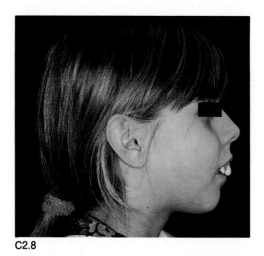

C2.8

Figure C2.8 This 10-year-old girl demonstrates severe dental projection of the upper anterior teeth. Note her long lower face height (Sn to Me′).

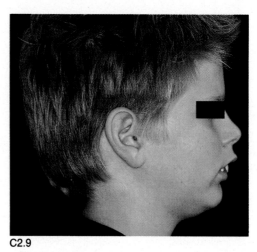

C2.9

Figure C2.9 This 10-year-old boy demonstrates a dental problem similar to that of the girl shown in Figure C2.8. Note his short lower face height (Sn to Me′). Also note the deep labiomental fold, indicative of a deep-bite, class II malocclusion.

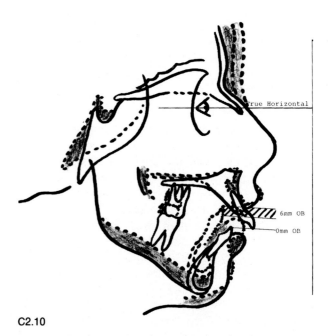

C2.10

Figure C2.10 Arbitrary superimposition of the cephalometric radiographs of the two patients presented in Figures C2.8 and C2.9. Although a very crude method of evaluating the growth of different individuals of the same age, one can notice the difference in their growth patterns. The girl with the long lower face has 0 mm overbite and is a backward growth rotator (vertical grower). The boy is a forward growth rotator and has a deep bite of 6 mm. Although these patients have the same dental problem (severe projection of the upper incisors and a Class II malocclusion), the treatment approach will be different according to their individual growth patterns.

References

1. Melsen B: The cranial base. The postnatal development of the cranial base studied histologically on human autopsy material. Acta Odontol Scand 32(Suppl):62, 1974.
2. Roche AF, and Lewis AB: Late growth changes in the cranial base. In *Development of the Basicranium,* edited by JF Bosma. Bethesda: DHEW Publications; 1976, pp 221–239.
3. Björk A, and Skieller V: Normal and abnormal growth of the mandible. A synthesis of longitudinal cephalometric implant studies over a period of 25 years. Eur J Orthod 5:1–46, 1983.
4. Buschang PH, LaPalme L, Tanguay R, and Demirjian A: The technical reliability of superimposition on cranial base and mandibular structures. Eur J Orthod 8:152–156, 1986.
5. de Coster L: The familial line, studies by a new line of reference. Trans Eur Orthod Soc 28:50–55, 1952.
6. Brodie G: Late growth changes in the human face. Angle Orthod 23:147–157, 1953.
7. Björk A: Cranial base development. Am J Orthod 41:198–255, 1955.
8. Coben SE: The integration of facial skeletal variants. Am J Orthod 41:407–434, 1955.
9. Ricketts RM: A foundation of cephalometric communication. Am J Orthod 46:330–357, 1960.
10. Ricketts RM: Cephalometric analysis and synthesis. Am J Orthod 31:141–156, 1961.
11. Ricketts RM: The value of cephalometrics and computerized technology. Angle Orthod 42:179–199, 1972.
12. Ricketts RM: Perspectives in clinical application of cephalometrics. Angle Orthod 51:115–150, 1981.
13. Björk A: Variations in the growth pattern of the human mandible: Longitudinal radiographic study by the implant method. J Dent Res 42:400–411, 1963.
14. Solow B, and Tallgren A: Natural head position in standing subjects. Acta Odontol Scand 29:591–607, 1971.
15. Coben SE: Basion horizontal coordinate tracing film. J Clin Orthod 13:598–605, 1979.
16. Frankel R: The applicability of the occipital reference base in cephalometrics. Am J Orthod 77:379–395, 1980.
17. Viazis AD: The cranial base triangle. J Clin Orthod 25:565–570, 1991.
18. Björk A, and Skiller V: Facial development and tooth eruption. An implant study at the age of puberty. Am J Orthod 62:331–383, 1972.

Chapter 3

Hand–Wrist Radiograph Evaluation

The course of orthodontic treatment often depends on the intensity of facial growth; thus, the knowledge of the growth velocity variations of the jaws is of importance in clinical orthodontics.[1,2] The clinician would like to know the onset of the growing patient's pubertal growth spurt so that he or she may intervene with maximum results in the minimum time frame. The physical maturity shown in a hand–wrist radiograph of the individual child can be visually compared with that of normal children of the same age and gender using Greulich and Pyle's *Atlas,*[3] where a number of hand–wrist radiographs are presented.[1,2] Consequently, the practitioner may evaluate the stage of development of the patient by matching the individual radiograph to one in the *Atlas.* Conversely, one may assess a hand–wrist radiograph without the *Atlas,* based on the following guidelines:[1,2]

1. When the width of the epiphysis of the second proximal phalanx (PP2) is equal to that of its diaphysis (PP2=), we are close to, but certainly before the onset of puberty.
2. When the width of the epiphysis of the third middle phalanx (MP3) is equal to that of its diaphysis (MP3=) and the sesamoid (s) bone has begun to ossify and can be seen on the radiograph, we are right at the onset of puberty or slightly past its onset (Fig. C3.1). One must remember that in one fifth of patients, the sesamoid is visible 2 years before maximum growth is reached.[1,2] This is why the information obtained from MP3 is very critical.
3. Capping of MP3 (where the epiphysis covers completely the diaphysis) occurs almost invariably simultaneously with the maximum of 1 year after the peak growth.[1,2]
4. The most intense period of growth may be expected between ossification of the sesamoid and onset of the capping stage.

Menarche in girls occurs well after the pubertal growth peak.[4] Dental development is of little value as a criterion of puberty.[4] The mean sesamoid bone appearance precedes mean peak mandibular velocity (puberty) by 0.72 year in males and 1.09 years in females.[5] One should note that in one quarter of males and one fifth of females, the adductor sesamoid appears after puberty.[5]

One may start his or her observation of the patient's hand–wrist radiograph by looking at the adductor sesamoid of the thumb.[6] If it is not ossified, we then look at the width of the epiphysis of the middle phalanx of the third finger (MP3). If this is equal to or less than the width of the diaphysis of MP3, then we know the patient has not yet reached puberty. If the sesamoid is ossified and we can see capping of MP3 (*i.e.,* the epiphysis is wider than the diaphysis and starts to cap it), then we know the patient has pretty much just reached puberty. Within 2 years after this, fusion of MP3 will occur, and this is an indicator that there is very little growth left. Finally, if we see fusion of the radius, we can be sure that growth for this patient has been completed.

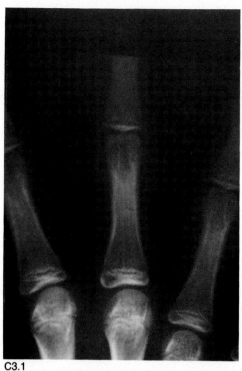

C3.1

Figure C3.1 This radiograph of the third finger shows that capping of MP3 is just beginning.

References

1. Helm S, Siersbael-Nelson S, Skieller V, and Björk A: Skeletal maturation of the hand in relation to maximum pubertal growth in body height. Tandlaegebladet 6:1223–1234, 1971.
2. Björk A, and Helm S: Prediction of the age of maximum pubertal growth in body height. Angle Orthod 37:134–143, 1967.
3. Greulich WW, and Pyle SI: *Radiographic Atlas of Skeletal Development of the Hand and Wrist,* 2nd ed. Stanford, CA: Stanford University Press, 1959.
4. Enlow DH: *Facial Growth.* Philadelphia: W.B. Saunders Co., 1990.
5. Pileski RCA, Woodside DG, and James GA: Relationship of the ulnar sesamoid bone and maximum mandibular growth velocity. Angle Orthod 43:162–170, 1973.
6. Fishman LS: Radiographic evaluation of skeletal maturation: A clinically oriented method based on hand–wrist films. Angle Orthod 52:88–111, 1982.

Chapter 4

Nasal Growth

The growth of the nose has been the focus of many investigations over the past 30 years, due to the important role that nasal development plays in orthodontic treatment planning.[1-12] Class I subjects tend to have straighter noses, class III subjects reveal a concave configuration of the nose along the dorsum, and class II individuals exhibit a more pronounced elevation of the nasal bridge (greater dorsal hump), leading to the increased convexity observed in the class II patient. Most investigators state that nasal growth for girls continues until the age of 16 years.[1,9] In addition, very small increments of nasal growth have been reported between the ages of 18 to 22 years, and as late as 26 to 29 years of age.[10,11]

The tip of the nose progressively attains a more forward and downward position with age (due to forward growth of the nasal, septal cartilages) and the forward growth of the nose is greater in proportion than that of other soft tissues of the face.[2,3] Nasal growth increases at a rate of about 25% greater than of the maxilla.[4] This contributes significantly to the increased convexity of the soft-tissue profile with age. In a recent study, it was concluded that patients with marked horizontal maxillary growth have more horizontal growth of the nose than those patients with vertical growth of the maxilla (who have more vertical nasal development).[12]

Developmentally, the greatest change occurs in the anteroposterior prominence of the nasal tip in both sexes, and because the forward positioning of the nose is greater than that of the soft-tissue chin, it appears that the lips are receding within the facial profile.[2,5] Having failed to explain the possibility of excessive nasal growth potential, the clinician finds it difficult to convince the parents or the patient that the unesthetic profile is due to the excessive nose and not to orthodontic mechanotherapy that resulted in retrusive lip position[12] (Figs. C4.1 through C4.3).

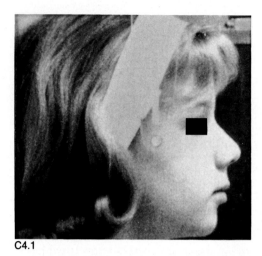

C4.1

Figure C4.1 Profile of a patient at age 12 years, before orthodontic treatment.

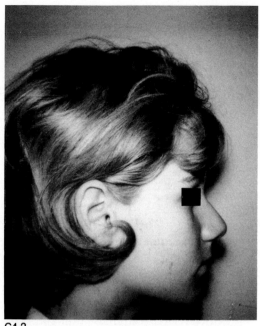

C4.2

Figure C4.2 Same patient as in Figure C4.1, at age 14 years, after orthodontic treatment. The nasal length appears to have remained the same.

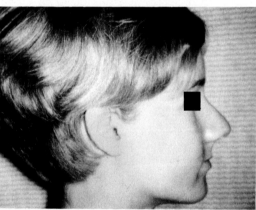

C4.3

Figure C4.3 Same patient as in Figure C4.2, 6 years later, at age 20 years. Note the excessive late nasal growth that resulted in the "false" appearance of retruded lips (attributed by the patient to the orthodontic treatment).

References

1. Posen TM: A longitudinal study of the growth of the nose. Am J Orthod 53:746–756, 1967.
2. Subtenly JD: A longitudinal study of soft tissue facial structures and their profile characteristics defined in relation to underlying skeletal structures. Am J Orthod 45:481–507, 1959.
3. Subtenly JD: The soft tissue profile, growth and treatment changes. Angle Orthod 31:105–122, 1961.
4. Proffit WR: *Contemporary Orthodontics.* St. Louis, MO: C.V. Mosby Co., 1986.
5. Rudee DA: Proportional profile changes concurrent with orthodontic therapy. Am J Orthod 50:421, 1964.
6. Chaconas SJ: A statistical evaluation of nasal growth. Am J Orthod 56:403–414, 1969.
7. Clements BS: Nasal imbalance and the orthodontic patient. Am J Orthod 55:244–264, 329–352, 477–497, 1969.
8. Burstone CJ: The integumental profile. Am J Orthod 44:1–25, 1958.
9. Meng HP, Goorhuls J, Kapila S, and Narida RS: Growth changes in the nasal profile from 7 to 18 years of age. Am J Orthod 94:917–926, 1988.
10. Sarnas KV, and Solow B: Early adult changes in the skeletal and soft tissue profile. Eur J Orthod 2:1–12, 1980.
11. Fosberg CM: Facial morphology and aging: Or longitudinal cephalometric investigation of young adults. Eur J Orthod 7:15–23, 1979.
12. Buschang PH, Viazis AD, DelaCruz R, and Oakes C: Horizontal growth of the soft-tissue nose relative to maxillary growth. J Clin Orthod 26:111–118, 1992.

Orthodontic Mechanotherapy

Chapter 1

Biomechanics of Tooth Movement

Tooth Movement Simplified

If we take a pencil, and place it flat on a desk, and try to move it with a finger by contacting it in its middle, we will notice that the pencil rolls and moves parallel to itself (Figs. D1.1 and D1.2). If we try to move it from its sharpened edge, we will see that it moves, but it also rotates slightly (Figs. D1.3 and D1.4).

Now if we imagine the *tooth* as the pencil, the *orthodontic forces* as our finger, the middle of the pencil as the *center of resistance of the tooth,* and the sharpened edge of the pencil as the *crown of the tooth,* and if we define as *bodily movement* the parallel motion of an object to itself and *tipping* as the movement of the object as it rotates and spins around itself, then we may appreciate the following when it comes to tooth movement in orthodontics[1-3]:

Because the center of resistance of the tooth is four tenths away from its apex, *i.e.,* within the alveolar bone, it would be impossible for us to apply a direct force on the tooth in order to make it move parallel to itself (Figs. D1.5 and D1.6). Thus, our only option is to attempt to move teeth by applying a force on the crown, which, according to the aforementioned correlation with the pencil, will cause the tooth to tip. This happens because there is a Moment = Force × Distance that rotates the tooth (Figs. D1.7 and D1.8). In order to move a tooth bodily, we need to apply a countermoment equal to and in the opposite direction of the one that is created by the orthodontic force. This can be done only with rectangular wires.[1-3]

Let us imagine the upper incisors as we try to retract into the available space that we have obtained from the extraction of the first bicuspids (Fig. D1.9). The bracket that is bonded onto the crown of the tooth has an opening in it, called the slot, where the archwire is placed. An elastic chain can be used to pull the brackets together and thus apply the necessary force to move the tooth. As soon as the force is applied, the tooth tends to tip, as explained previously. When that happens, the edges of the rectangular wire grab hold of the bracket slot and thus apply a couple (equal and opposite forces), which tends to spin the tooth in the opposite direction than the moment from the force is attempting to tip it (Fig. D1.10). In other words, the rectangular wire has created a countermoment. If the moment and countermoment are equal, they will cancel each other out.[1,3] This means that the tooth *will move bodily* (translation, parallel movement) from the action of the force from the elastic chain and solely from it.

The same principles apply if we were to look at a tooth from its occlusal surface, with an orthodontic bracket bonded on to its buccal surface[1-3] (Fig. D1.11). This time, the tooth will tend to spin around its long axis if the main archwire is not securely wire tied with a ligature in the bracket slot. In this dimension we do not have much control, whether we use a round or rectangular wire, unless we use a deltoid bracket.

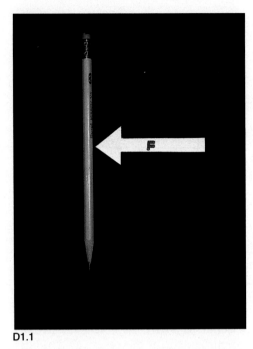

D1.1

Figure D1.1 A force (from our finger) is applied in the middle of the pencil at point A.

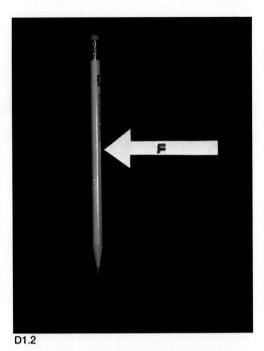

D1.2

Figure D1.2 Notice that the pencil moves parallel to itself to point B.

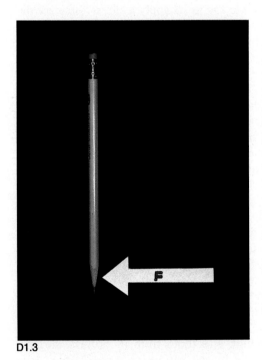

D1.3

Figure D1.3 Try to move the pencil from one of its ends.

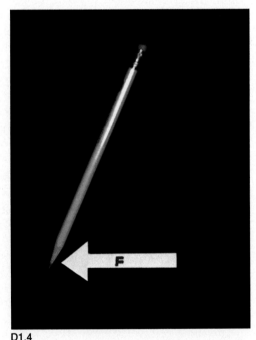

D1.4

Figure D1.4 It rotates as it moves from point A to B.

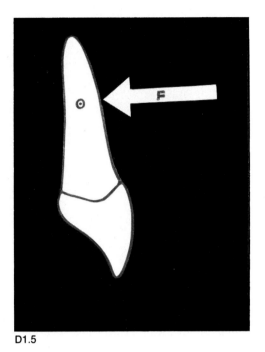

D1.5

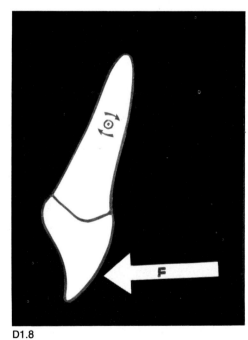

D1.6

Figures D1.5 and D1.6 It is impossible to apply a direct force at the center of resistance of a tooth (and thus move it bodily), because it is in the alveolar bone.

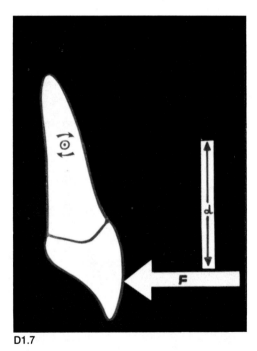

D1.7

D1.8

Figures D1.7 and D1.8 As we attempt to move the tooth by applying a force (F) on its crown, a moment (M) rotates the tooth as it moves; (d) is the distance of the point of application of the force from the center of resistance of the tooth.

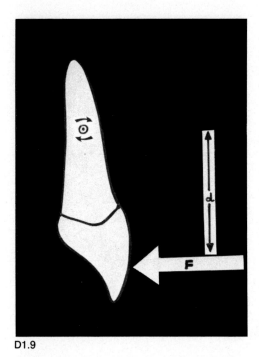

D1.9

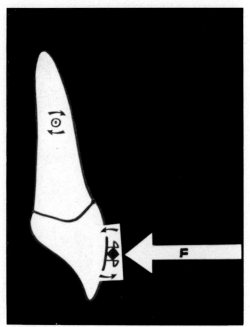

D1.10

Figures D1.9 and D1.10 As we try to move the upper incisor posteriorly by applying a force on it from point A to point B, the tooth moves bodily if the countermoment applied from the rectangular archwire is equal to the moment that tends to tip the tooth.

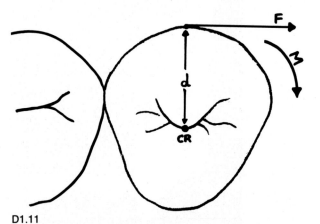

D1.11

Figure D1.11 As this bicuspid tooth is pulled from an orthodontic elastic wire chain to close the extraction space mesial to it, the tooth tends to rotate from the moment (M) that is created. CR is the center of resistance of the tooth.

Bracket Prescriptions

Contemporary orthodontic mechanotherapy[4-9] leads to treatment results that are based on the six keys to normal occlusion[6]: (1) a class I molar relationship (as described previously); (2) crown angulation (tip)—the gingival portion of the crown of teeth is distal to the incisal portion in most individuals; (3) crown inclination (torque)—anterior crowns have an anterior inclination, whereas posterior crowns have a lingual inclination; (4) absence of rotations; (5) absence of spaces; and (6) the plane of occlusion should vary from generally flat to a slight curve of Spee. In order to achieve these results, we need to understand the relationships and positions of teeth in the arches.

If one were to closely observe an ideal dental arch, it would immediately become apparent that the position of each tooth in the alveolus is defined by three parameters[4-6]: (1) the "in–out" position (Fig. D1.12), (2) the crown angulation to "tip" (Fig. D1.13), and (3) the crown inclination or "torque" (Fig. D1.14). These three parameters define the three-dimensional position of each tooth in its space. In the past, all orthodontic brackets were the same for all teeth, with the same slot. The clinicians had to incorporate into the main archwire three bends for each tooth, in order to maneuver each tooth in its ideal position: (1) the "in–out" or first-order bend, (2) the "tip" or second-order bend, and (3) the "torque" or third-order bend. Modern fixed appliances have all these bends built into their slots, thus making each bracket specific for each tooth. Providing that the bracket is positioned ideally on the tooth surface (in the middle of the crown, along the long axis, and parallel to the incisal edge), these preadjusted prescription appliances theoretically have the capability to finish the treatment with no bends in the archwires whatsoever! Obviously, this is like saying that everyone's feet should fit in the same size shoe. No matter how perfect bracket placement is with preadjusted appliances, compensating bends will always be needed at the end of treatment for final detailing and finishing of the occlusion.

A suggested prescription is given[4-8] (Fig. D1.15):

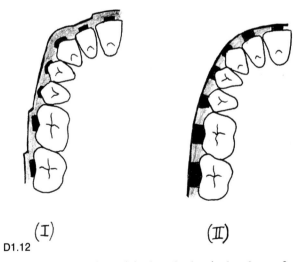

(I)   (II)

D1.12

Figure D1.12 In the original orthodontic brackets of one standard size and prescription *(I)*, the clinician had to place in-and-out bends in the wire to compensate for the difference in the buccolingual thickness of teeth. In the modern, preadjusted appliances *(II)*, different thickness in the brackets compensates for that of the teeth so that the clinician may use a straight wire without bends (the bracket thickness has been exaggerated for purposes of illustration).

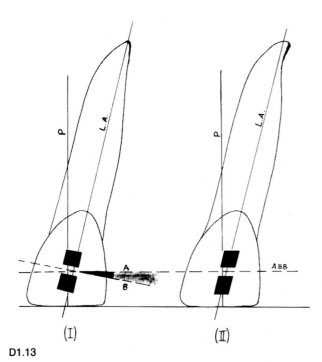

D1.13

Figure D1.13 The difference in the angulation of the teeth (tip) in the past forced the clinician to compensate with an up-and-down bend *(I)*. In contemporary, preadjusted appliances, this is not necessary because the tip is built into the bracket. If A is perpendicular to P (P forms 90° with incisal edge) and B is perpendicular to the base of the bracket slot, then the angle formed between the two represents the compensating bend that needs to be placed with the standard appliances *(I)*. A and B coincide in *II*.

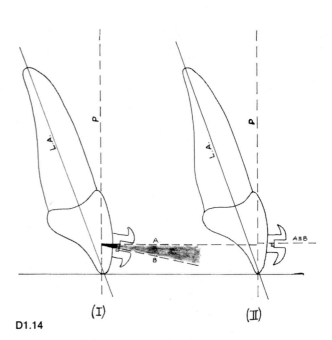

D1.14

Figure D1.14 The torque or inclination of teeth in the bone is again compensated for by the preadjusted appliance *(II)*. Note that the angle formed between the perpendicular (B) to the base of the slot and the perpendicular to line P, (A), coincide (A = B) for the preadjusted appliances *(II)*, whereas the two perpendiculars *B* and *A* form an angle in the standard brackets *(I)*.

BRACKET PRESCRIPTIONS

V		A		R		S		W		H		R	
Torque	Angulation	Torque	Angulation	Torque	Angulation	Torque	Angulation	Torque	Angulation	Torque	Angulation	Torque	Angulation
20	5	7	5	12	5	12	5	14	5	22	5	17	+3
10	10	3	9	8	9	8	9	7	8	14	8	11	+10
5	15	-7	11	-2	13	2	11	-3	10	7	10	5	+7
-5	0	-7	2	-7	0	-7	0	-7	0	-7	0	0	0
-5	0	-7	2	-7	0	-7	0	-7	0	-7	0	0	0
-10	0	-9	5	-14	0	-14	0	-10	0	-10	0	0	0
-10	0	-9	5	-14	0	-14	-5			-10	0	0	0
-5	0	-1	2	-1	2	2	2	-5	2	-1	0	0	0
-5	0	-1	2	-1	2	2	2	-5	2	-1	0	0	0
-5	5	-11	5	-11	7	0	7	-7	6	7	5	+2	+2
-15	0	-17	2	-17	-1	-17	-1	-11	0	-11	0	-6	0
-20	0	-22	2	-22	-1	-22	-1	-17	0	-17	0	-14	0
-30	-5	-30	2	-30	-1	-30	-1	-22	-6	-27	-5	-24	-5
-30	-5	-35	2	-30	-1	-25	-1	-27	-6	-27	-5	-34	-5

D1.15

Figure D1.15 Bracket prescriptions. V—Viazis; A—Andrews; first R—Roth; S—Swain; W—"Wick" Alexander; H—Hilgers; second R—Ricketts.

Upper Central Incisor

First-order bend (in–out): Standard
Second-order bend (tip): 5 degrees
Third-order bend (torque): 20 degrees

A specific thickness is given to the upper incisor bracket of a regular size. The 5-degree angulation is similar to the one proposed by Andrews' classic work.[6] It is also widely used in other prescriptions. The 20-degree torque is definitely greater than the torque proposed by Andrews,[6] Roth,[5] and Alexander,[7] and close to the 22 degrees suggested by Hilgers.[8] Because sliding mechanics are used, it would be quite easy to "dump" the anterior teeth lingually during retraction and space closure (Figs. D1.16 through D1.18). Accentuated torque would reduce this and, it is hoped, by the end of treatment the teeth would be in the area of 10 degrees of torque, similar to that proposed by Andrews for the ideal occlusion (7 degrees). In addition, it is easier to alleviate the torque effect by undersized rectangular wires than to add torque in the wire. Because 0.001 inch of play (tolerance) relates to approximately 4 degrees of torque lost, space closure with a .016- × .022-inch^2 stainless steel wire would theoretically have 8 degrees of torque effect lost, if desired. Accentuated lingual root torque of the upper central incisors is needed in the majority of cases during sliding mechanotherapy, and this prescription offers this advantage.

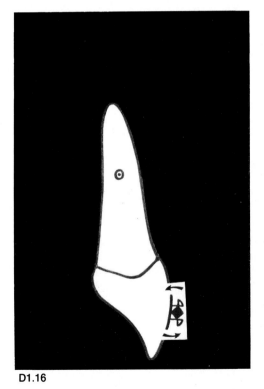

D1.16

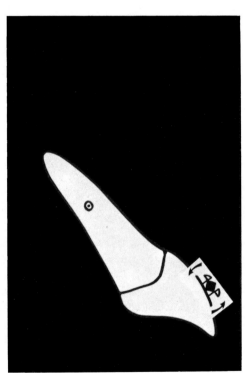

D1.17

Figures D1.16 and D1.17 The effect of additional torque in the bracket (note the twisted rectangular archwire in the bracket slot) rotates the tooth from A to B.

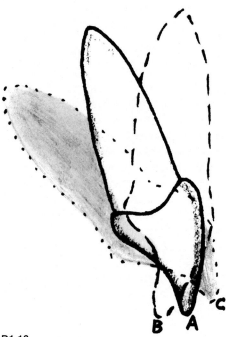

D1.18

Figure D1.18 If A is the correct inclination of the upper incisor teeth in the bone and B is the position they would assume if they tipped lingually during space closure if the countermoment provided by the wire is not enough, then C should be increased torque that is incorporated into the preadjusted appliance so that the tooth may end up in position A after space closure.

Upper Lateral Incisor

First-order bend (in–out): More thickness
Second-order bend (tip): 10 degrees
Third-order bend (torque): 10 degrees

More bracket thickness is needed to compensate for the buccal–lingual relationship of the lateral incisor compared to the central incisor. The 10-degree angulation is slightly greater than that suggested by Andrews[6] and Roth[5] (9 degrees) or Alexander[7] and Hilgers[8] (8 degrees), but similar to that recommended by Ricketts[8] (10 degrees). This additional angulation is needed to prevent close proximity of the central and lateral incisor roots, especially during space closure. The 10-degree torque is again greater than that in other prescriptions for the same reasons addressed for the central incisor bracket.

Upper Cuspid

First-order bend (in–out): Thinner than central incisor
Second-order bend (tip): 15 degrees
Third-order bend (torque): 5 degrees

The bracket thickness on the cuspid has to be thinner than the regular size of the upper central incisor due to the bulkiness of the cuspid. The 15 degrees of tip are similar to that proposed by Roth[5] (13 degrees). It positions the root of the tooth more distally, thus enhancing bodily movement and reducing the tipping effect of sliding mechanics. A 5-degree torque is necessary because, as supported by Hilgers,[8] there is a mechanical tendency to detorque the upper cuspids as they are retracted in extraction cases, and there is always the possibility of impacting the root on the dense cortical labial plate on space closure. In nonextraction cases, where a slight expansion occurs in all cases and the tooth is tipped outward anyway, the effect of the torque can be minimized by placing an undersized finishing wire (*i.e.,* a 0.016- × 0.022-inch² wire in the 0.018 slot system).

High lingual torque on the upper cuspid is also advocated in the prescriptions by Hilgers[8] and Ricketts[8] in order to maintain the integrity of the labial surface contours between the cuspid and the lateral by keeping their torque differential to a minimum. In addition, a more vertical inclination of the upper cuspids alleviates the detrimental effects of the "narrow cuspid" look, which is also detrimental to functional jaw movements and the periodontal health of the tissues overlying prominent roots. Thus, a nice, broad "Hollywood" type smile is created with a gentle rise in excursions and stability through reduction of excessive lateral forces.

Upper Bicuspids

First-order bend (in–out): Similar to the cuspid
Second-order bend (tip): 0 degrees
Third-order bend (torque): −5 degrees

The first-order compensation is the same as the cuspid one because of their similar prominence. The 0-degree tip agrees with the overcorrected position suggested in most prescriptions. The −5-degree torque placed on the bicuspids, although it encourages "dropping down" of the lingual cusps, does so just enough to ensure good intercuspation of the bicuspid teeth with their counterparts of the opposing arch. This comes as the result of numerous observations of finished cases that appeared fine from the buccal side but from the lingual side lacked the nice, solid occlusion of an ideally finished case. Undersized wires can be used in open-bite tendency cases.

Upper Molars

First-order bend (in–out): Very thin mesially/very thick distally (20 degrees)
Second-order bend (tip): 0 degrees
Third-order bend (torque): −10 degrees

As suggested by Hilgers,[8] a 15-degree distal rotation of this tooth ensures the shortest arch length occupied by the first molar tooth, which is 5 degrees more than Andrews'[6] recommendation. Thus, the bracket should be very thin around the mesiobuccal cusp and very thick on the distobuccal cusp. A 20-degree distal overrotation is especially helpful in the overcorrection of class II, division 1 cases, and it counteracts the movements placed on the molar teeth from the side effects of sliding mechanotherapy with elastic chains. The 0-degree angulation is similar to other prescriptions. The −10-degree torque allows a good intercuspal occlusion, especially of the lingual cusps. Incorporation of the second molar teeth is advisable only if absolutely necessary.

Lower Incisors

First-order bend (in–out): Thick
Second-order bend (tip): 0 degrees
Third-order bend (torque): −5 degrees

Thick brackets on the lower incisors compensate for their lingual relationship relative to the upper anteriors. The 0-degree tip positions these teeth in an upright position while the −5-degree torque, similar to that suggested by Alexander,[7] has been shown to hold the mandibular incisors in their original position, thus ensuring maximum retention stability.

Lower Cuspid

First-order bend (in–out): Thinner than regular
Second-order bend (tip): 5 degrees
Third-order bend (torque): −5 degrees

A thin bracket is necessary to compensate for the prominence of this tooth. The 5-degree tip is similar to that proposed by Andrews,[6] Alexander,[7] and Hilgers.[8] The −5-degree torque gives the lower cuspid a more labial version than in other prescriptions in order to articulate with the upper cuspid, as defined by this prescription, and offer the proper canine guidance during excursive movements. In addition, by having similar torque to the incisors, the cuspid tooth is positioned slightly lingual to the incisors (being at the corner of the arch). This supports the lower anterior dentition and enhances post-retention stability.

Lower First Bicuspid

First-order bend (in–out): As thin as the lower cuspid
Second-order bend (tip): 0 degrees
Third-order bend (torque): −15 degrees

A thin bracket is required due to the similarity of this tooth to the cuspid. The 0-degree tip is again similar to that suggested by the prescriptions of Alexander,[7] Hilgers,[8] and Ricketts.[8] The −15-degree torque provides a slightly greater elevation of the lingual cusp than that suggested by Andrews[6] (17 degrees) in order to provide a solid occlusion with the opposing dentition.

Lower Second Bicuspid

First-order bend (in–out): Same as the lower first bicuspid
Second-order bend (tip): 0 degrees
Third-order bend (torque): −20 degrees

All compensations for this tooth are made for the same reasons as for the lower first bicuspid.

Lower Molars

First-order bend (in–out): Mesially very thin/distally very thick
Second-order bend (tip): −5 degrees
Third-order bend (torque): −30 degrees

For the same reasons described for the maxillary molars, an overcorrection of the first-order compensation of 10 degrees is needed to counteract the mesial rotation imposed on the molars by the elastic chains of sliding mechanotherapy. The −5-degree tip maximizes the lower molar resistance to mesial tipping from the sliding mechanics and offers "tip-back" effect by placing the roots mesially, thus contributing to anchorage control during space closure. The −30-degree torque allows for good intercuspation of the lingual cusps without allowing unnecessary extrusion.

References

1. Smith RJ, and Burstone CJ: Mechanics of tooth movement. Am J Orthod 85:294–307, 1984.
2. Staggers JA, and Germane N: Clinical considerations in the use of retraction mechanics. J Clin Orthod 25:364–369, 1991.
3. Proffit WR: *Contemporary Orthodontics.* St. Louis, MO: C.V. Mosby Co., 1986.
4. Swain BF: Straight wire design strategies: Five-year evaluation of the Roth modification of the Andrews straight wire appliance, Chapter 18, pp. 279–298, in Graber LW: *Orthodontics—State of the Art, Essence of the Science.* St. Louis, MO: C.V. Mosby Co., 1986.
5. Roth RH: Treatment mechanics for the straight wire appliance, Chapter 11, pp. 665–716, in Graber TM, and Swain BF: *Orthodontics—Current Principles and Techniques.* St. Louis, MO: C.V. Mosby Co., 1985.
6. Andrews LF: *Straight Wire—Concept and Appliances.* San Diego: L.A. Wells Co., 1989.
7. Alexander RG: *The Alexander Discipline.* Glendora, CA: Ormco Co., 1986.
8. Hilgers JJ: Begin with the end in mind: Bioprogressive simplified. J Clin Orthod 9:618–627, 10:716–734, 11:794–804, 12:857–870, 1987.
9. McLaughlin RP, and Bennet TC: The transition from standard edgewise to preadjusted appliance systems. J Clin Orthod 23:142–153, 1989.

Chapter 2

Orthodontic Metal Fixed Appliances

Orthodontic fixed appliances are used to apply corrective forces to malaligned teeth.[1-4] These appliances generally include brackets, which are bonded onto the facial surface of the crown of the teeth, and a main archwire, which is inserted in the bracket (slot portion). The wire is allowed to slide through the brackets during tooth movement and guides tooth movement while applying a certain force to the bracket (and thus the tooth) if it is active (Fig. D2.1). Additional forces may be applied to the teeth by elastics (rubber bands) and/or elastomeric chain modules, especially during the closing of spaces (Fig. D2.2).

Conventional brackets have (1) a base, which has a mesh configuration that allows for adequate bond strength to the tooth surface; (2) a slot, which receives the wire; and (3) wings or hooks, on which elastics, elastomeric modules, ligatures, and coil springs, etc., can be attached (Fig. D2.3).

The twin-type brackets are basically made of two vertically oriented parallel bars that are spaced apart with a slot cut in each bar to receive the main archwire (Fig. D2.3). The single-type brackets are made of one vertical bar, with a smaller size slot than the twin brackets, and "wings" that are activated to contact the main archwire for rotational control, as needed (Fig. D2.4). The major disadvantage of the twin brackets is the narrow interbracket distance (between adjacent teeth), thus resulting in a small span of wire between the brackets, which reduces the flexibility of the arch-wire. Conversely, the rotational wings of the single brackets are too big; rotations are not easily corrected and teeth may tip into the extraction side more easily during space closure.

The deltoid bracket provides a narrow slot of the same dimensions of a single-wing bracket and delivers the same interbracket distance (see Figs. D2.3 and D2.4). It offers excellent rotational control due to the horizontal segment of the bracket and the triangular manner with which the O rings or the ligature wires encompass the bracket. It is smaller than the twin brackets and superior to the single bracket's rotational wings, which cause problems with the patient's oral hygiene. It is easy to orient onto the tooth surface (the vertical bar is along the long axis of the tooth and the horizontal parallel to its incisal edge). Sliding mechanics are greatly facilitated through the rotational and tip control that the horizontal bar offers during space closure. It greatly reduces friction during space closure due to the elevated slot.

The size of any bracket slot can be either 0.018-inch or 0.022-inch. Because we strive for as low a force as possible in orthodontic mechanotherapy, it is preferable to use the 0.018-inch slot system, because it takes a smaller size wire to fill its slot and thus lighter forces are exerted on the teeth. Brackets are bonded on all teeth except the first molars (Figs. D2.5 and D2.6). Metal bands are cemented onto these teeth. Bands provide better bond strength on these teeth, especially if a headgear appliance is used.

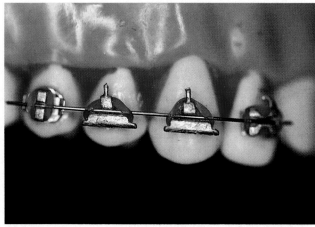

D2.1

Figure D2.1 Various contemporary orthodontic brackets (from left to right): single wing bracket (Ormco, CA), deltoid brackets (GAC, NY), and twin bracket (Unitek/3M, MN).

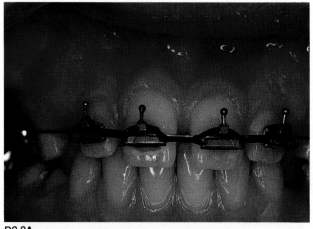

D2.2A

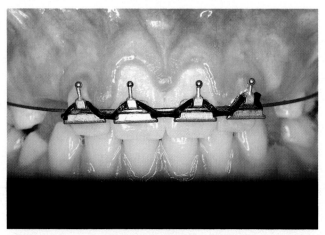

D2.2B

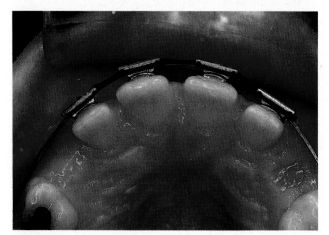

D2.2C

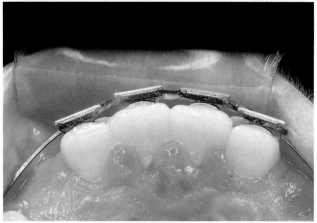

D2.2D

Figure D2.2. A–D. An elastomeric chain is applying a force on the teeth as it pulls all the brackets together. Note the rotational control of the deltoid bracket. Within one month, the anterior spaces were closed.

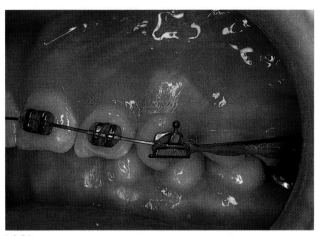

D2.3**A**

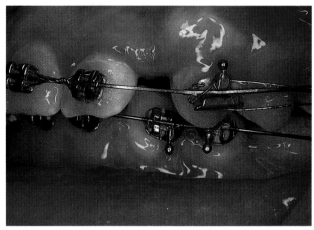

D2.3**B**

Figure D2.3. A, B. Close-up view of the deltoid (on the upper cuspid) and twin brackets (on the incisors). Note the hook on the deltoid bracket for the placement of auxiliary elastics. Within two months, cuspid retraction was completed (bodily movement and complete rotational control due to the horizontal bar of the deltoid bracket).

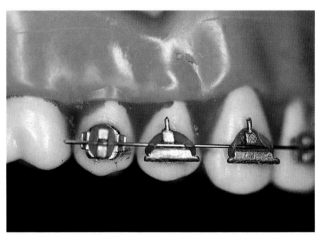

D2.4

Figure D2.4 Close-up view of the single wing (left) and the deltoid (right) brackets. Note the much bulkier single wing bracket. Also note the "stretch" of the "O" ring on the deltoid bracket, which aids in rotational control.

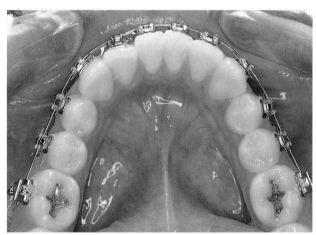

D2.5

Figure D2.5 The slot of the single wing bracket is too narrow and offers no rotational control. Note the rotated left lateral incisor despite correct bracket placement. Also note that brackets (instead of bands) can be bonded on the molar teeth when no headgear is to be used.

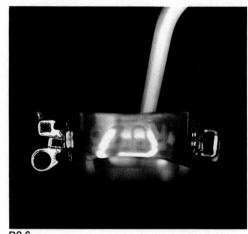

D2.6

Figure D2.6 An orthodontic band. Note the triple tubes. The upper one is for insertion of auxiliary wires (used in some techniques); the middle one receives the main archwire; the lower and bigger one receives the inner bow of a headgear. On the lingual side, the sheath receives the TPA or TCA appliances (see further).

References

1. Graber LW: *Orthodontics—State of the Art, Essence of the Science.* St. Louis, MO: C.V. Mosby Co., 1986.
2. Graber TM, and Swain BF: *Orthodontics—Current Principles and Techniques.* St. Louis, MO: C.V. Mosby Co., 1985.
3. Andrews LF: *Straight Wire—Concept and Appliances.* San Diego: L.A. Wells Co., 1989.
4. McLaughlin RP, and Bennet TC: The transition from standard edgewise to preadjusted appliance systems. J Clin Orthod 23:142–153, 1989.

Chapter 3

Esthetic Brackets

Recent advances in the field of esthetic fixed appliances have resulted in the development of fixed appliances made of polycrystalline or single-crystal aluminum oxide (99.5%), called ceramic brackets[1-24] (Figs. D3.1 and D3.2). The most apparent difference between polycrystalline and single-crystal brackets is in their optical clarity.[1] Polycrystalline brackets tend to be more translucent,[1] whereas both single-crystal and polycrystalline appliances resist staining and discoloration.[1] Almost all of the currently available ceramic brackets are made of polycrystalline material.[1-17] The physical properties of aluminum oxide that interest the practicing clinician are tensile strength, fracture toughness, material hardness, and friction.[1,4-8,20]

The tensile strength of ceramics is not a simple bulk material property, as it is for stainless steel;[2,15] it is very dependent on the condition of the surface of the ceramic. A shallow scratch on the surface of a ceramic will drastically reduce the load required for fracture, whereas the same scratch on a metal surface will have little, if any, effect on fracture under load.[2,15] In addition, the elongation for stainless steel is approximately 20% when it finally fails.[2] The elongation for the ceramic at failure is less than 1%, making these appliances more brittle[2] (Fig. D3.3).

The fracture toughness of material is the total energy loading required to cause its failure.[2] The fracture toughness values for ceramics are 20 to 40 times lower than those of stainless steel. It is, therefore, much easier to fracture a ceramic bracket than a metal one.

Thus, it is important for the orthodontist to inspect ceramic brackets for cracks at each patient visit.[2] Care should be taken during treatment not to scratch bracket surfaces with the instruments or overstress when ligating or activating a wire.[2,7] The patient should be cautioned against chewing on hard substances.[7] Pieces of bracket could be ingested or inhaled inadvertently if the fracture occurs in the mouth during function.[7] The problem of bracket fracture may also occur when placing or removing rectangular archwires, which almost completely fill the slot.[7] Placement of additional torque in the archwires may cause either tie-wing or slot microfractures on insertion.[7] The fracture resistance of the ceramic brackets appears to be adequate for clinical use in the range of 8 to 10 degrees of torque.[19]

In general, ceramic brackets produce more friction than metal brackets. In reference to the presence of friction between the ceramic bracket and the archwires, one study emphasized that it decreases with increased archwire sizes[20] because light wires are pressed not only against the edges of the bracket but along the anterior slot as well. A more recent study[21] showed that there is a decreased rate of tooth movement with ceramic brackets that ranges from 30% to 50% when compared to metal brackets, and that the amount of tooth movement decreased with an increase in wire size. In general, slot surfaces and edges of the ceramic brackets were more porous and rougher than those of the metal bracket,[21] and wire surfaces are obviously scratched by the ceramic brackets, whereas only slight scratches are observed on the wires used with metal brackets.

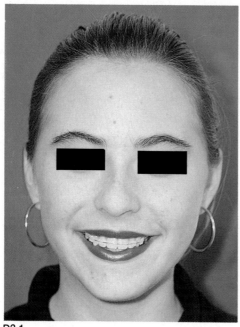

D3.1

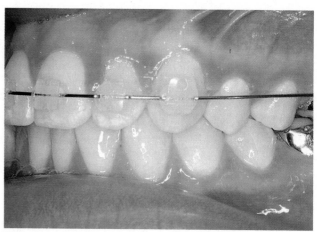

D3.2

Figures D3.1 and D3.2 Ceramic brackets offer patients an esthetic smile while undergoing orthodontic treatment.

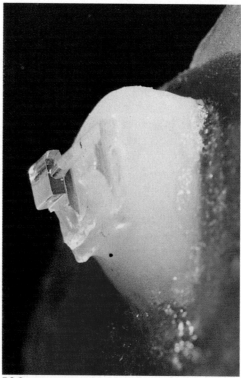

D3.3

Figure D3.3 A fractured, single-crystal ceramic bracket (Starfire, "A" Company, CA), caused by the brittle nature of the material. (Reproduced from Viazis AD, Cavanaugh G, and Bevis RR: Bond strength of ceramic brackets under shear stress: An in vitro report. Am J Orthod Dentofacial Orthop 98:214–221, 1990. With permission of Mosby-Year Book, Inc.)

As a result of this, efficiency of tooth movement is significantly reduced by ceramic brackets when compared to metal brackets. Refinement of ceramic brackets, slot edges, and surfaces in particular should one day produce more efficient and desired tooth movement. Stainless steel is the smoothest wire, followed by Sentalloy (GAC).[24] At present, these wires are the most suitable for use with ceramic brackets in sliding mechanics.

A very important physical property of ceramic brackets is the extremely high hardness values of aluminum oxide.[5] The hardness of ceramic brackets is almost nine times that of stainless steel brackets or enamel.[5,6] Serious consideration should be given to the possibility of enamel contact with an opposing ceramic bracket and the detrimental effects it may have on the integrity of the enamel.[5,6]

Ceramic brackets cause significantly greater enamel abrasion than stainless steel brackets[6] (Figs. D3.4 and D3.5). We should realize that the constraints faced by prosthodontists in not opposing natural enamel with porcelain apply equally to the field of orthodontics.[5] It would be rather simple to state that as long as the brackets are kept out of occlusion, this undesirable side effect is not to be expected.[5] Unfortunately, during the course of orthodontic treatment one cannot be sure of avoiding this problem, especially in extraction cases in which tooth retraction is initiated.[5]

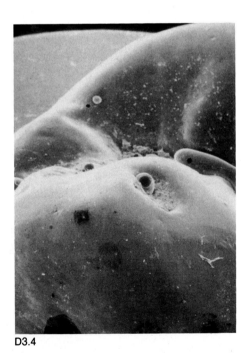

D3.4

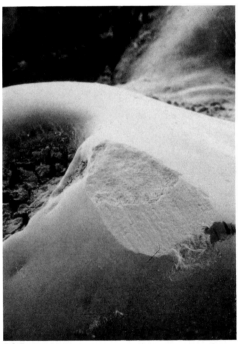

D3.5

Figures D3.4 and D3.5 Scanning electron micrographs showing abrasion of a bicuspid cusp tip before and after contact with an opposing ceramic bracket. Note the cat scratch-like surface. Half of the abraded area has been delaminated, revealing the intact enamel prisms underneath. (Reproduced from Viazis AD, DeLong R, Bevis RR, et al: Enamel surface abrasion from ceramic orthodontic brackets: A special case report. Am J Orthod Dentofacial Orthop 96:514–518, 1989. With permission of Mosby-Year Book, Inc.)

Avoid placing ceramic brackets in deep-bite cases.[5] Ceramic brackets used on the mandibular teeth should be kept out of occlusion at all times during treatment.[5,6] Routine check of this matter is advised at every visit.[5,6] Crossbites should first be corrected before the application of ceramic brackets.[5] Use of ceramic brackets on the anterior maxillary teeth is possibly the best way to benefit from the esthetics of porcelain while avoiding potentially deleterious enamel wear of occluding teeth.[5] It is not an exaggeration to correlate this type of abrasion to a saw blade applied against a hard surface area.[5] Severe enamel abrasion from ceramic brackets might occur during a single meal, sometimes within a few seconds.[5,6] Clinically, damage occurs immediately on tooth contact with these appliances.[5,6] (Figs. D3.6 and D3.7). Enamel wear may occur from metal appliances as well, but this would be gradual (weeks or months) and not as aggressive.[6] The use of elastomeric rings with covers for the occlusal part of the ceramic brackets may be a way to avoid this problem.

According to the literature, the incidence of enamel damage on debonding of ceramic brackets ranges from 0% to 40% for clinically sound teeth and is as high as 50% for compromised teeth (enamel cracks, endodontic therapy, large restorations).[7,8] The incidence of bracket failure on debonding is in the range of 6% to 80%.[7,8] The design of the bracket, more specifically of the tie wing itself, affects the performance of the bracket during debonding.[7] The junction between the bracket body and the tie wing is relatively narrow and reduces the bulk of ceramic material supporting the tie

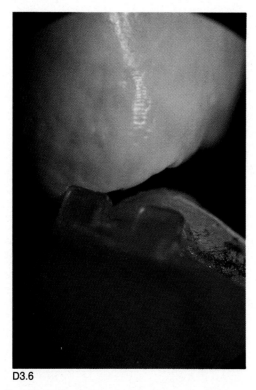

D3.6

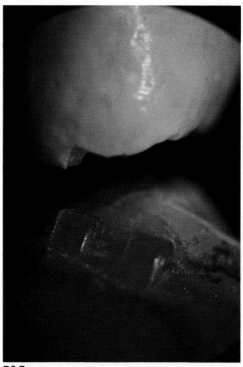

D3.7

Figure D3.6 Contact of a lower ceramic appliance with an opposing tooth. (Reproduced from Viazis AD, DeLong R, Bevis RR, et al: Enamel abrasion from ceramic orthodontic brackets under an artificial oral environment. Am J Orthod Dentofacial Orthop 98:103–109, 1990. With permission of Mosby-Year Book, Inc.)

Figure D3.7 Dramatic damage done to the opposing tooth in Figure D3.6 within seconds after contact with the ceramic appliance. (Reproduced from Viazis AD, DeLong R, Bevis, RR, et al: Enamel abrasion from ceramic orthodontic brackets under an artificial oral environment. Am J Orthod Dentofacial Orthop 98:103–109, 1990. With permission of Mosby-Year Book, Inc.)

wing extension.[7] Absence of adequate bulk, in addition to crack propagation, is contributory to bracket failure at the site of application of the debonding force.[7]

The mean shear bond strength of the silane chemical bond provided by some ceramic brackets is significantly higher than the mean shear bond strength of the grooved mechanical bond of various other ceramic appliances and the foil mesh base of the stainless steel brackets.[8]

Mechanical bonds, that is, metal foil mesh and grooved-base ceramic bracket bases, under shear stress fail primarily within the adhesive itself[8] (Fig. D3.8). This is called brittle failure of the adhesive from localized stress areas due to the bracket base design.[8] Chemical bonds, provided by silane-treated ceramic bracket bases, fail mostly at the adhesive–bracket interface.[8] This is defined as pure adhesive failure caused by wider stress distribution over the whole interface.[8]

The maximum value of shear bond strength reported in the literature exceeded 100 lb of force.[8] This occurred with the first-generation Transcend (Unitek/3M) bracket, which is no longer available and has been withdrawn from circulation[8,14,17] (Figs. D3.9 and D3.10). The high bond attributed to this bracket was due to a combination of micromechanical and chemical adhesion that was provided by the coupling effect of the silane layer of the bracket base, giving it a shiny, smooth surface area that increased the stress distribution during debonding.[17]

It must be noted that the new bracket base of the Transcend 2000 (Unitek/3M) appears to be much "safer" when compared to the original Transcend.[17] No tooth failures were noted in a study with the Transcend 2000.[17] Both Fascination (Dentaraum, Germany) and the original Transcend caused enamel failure in the same study, which is in accordance with the findings of previous investigations.[8,14,17] The new

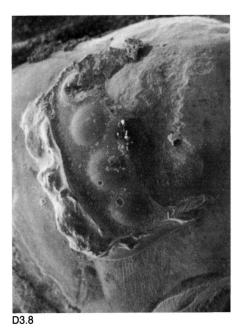

D3.8

Figure D3.8 Mechanical bonds fail safely within the adhesive upon debonding. This is a scanning electron micrograph of the residual adhesive on the tooth after debonding of an Allure (GAC) ceramic bracket. Note the imprints of the bracket base.

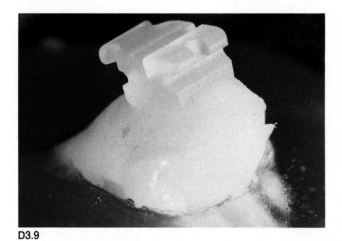

D3.9

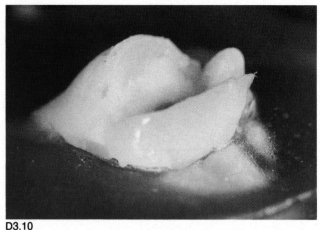

D3.10

Figure D3.9 First-generation Transcend (Unitek/3M) ceramic bracket bonded onto a bicuspid tooth. (Reproduced from Viazis AD, Cavanaugh G, and Bevis RR: Bond strength of ceramic brackets under shear stress: an in vitro report. Am J Orthod Dentofacial Orthop 98:214–221, 1990. With permission of Mosby-Year Book, Inc.)

Figure D3.10 Tooth failure upon debonding of the bracket shown in Figure D3.9. Debonding force levels of these brackets exceeded 100 lb. These appliances have been withdrawn from the market. (Reproduced from Viazis AD, Cavanaugh G, and Bevis RR: Bond strength of ceramic brackets under shear stress: an in vitro report. Am J Orthod Dentofacial Orthop 98:214–221, 1990. With permission of Mosby-Year Book, Inc.)

generation of the Starfire brackets also appeared to have been improved.[17] There were less cohesive bracket failures than previously reported.[8,14,17]

The Allure (GAC) brackets demonstrate safe debonding.[17] Their bond strength appears to be strong enough to bond to the enamel throughout the length of treatment without compromising the integrity of the tooth on debonding[8] (Fig. D3.8). As supported by various studies,[8,9] the Allure bracket is the ceramic bracket system of choice for both predictability and bond strength. For those clinicians still using the original Transcend or the Fascination brackets, a more flexible, lower, filled adhesive may be the answer to lower bond strength and prevention of enamel fractures.[17]

In the event that part of a bracket remains on the tooth on debonding, a high-speed diamond handpiece with ample water spray may be used to take the residual ceramic material off.[7,18] Sensitivity of the tooth may develop if the pulp is irritated by this procedure.[7]

The need for relatively strong forces to obtain bond failure may result in various degrees of patient discomfort.[7] In the clinical setting, such a force would be transmitted to teeth that are often mobile and sometimes sensitive to pressure at the end of the active phase of orthodontic treatment.[7] To minimize such an episode, the teeth should be well supported during bracket removal.[7] It has been suggested that the orthodontist have the patients bite firmly into a cotton roll to help stabilize these sensitive and relatively mobile teeth.[7]

It needs to be pointed out to the clinician that the likelihood of bracket failure can be minimized if the debonding instrument is fully seated to the base of the bracket and to the tooth surface[7] (Fig. D3.11). This firm seating allows the forces used for bracket removal to be transmitted through the strongest and bulkiest part of the bracket; namely, the bracket base. Failure to adhere to this requirement as a result of hastiness by the clinician or the presence of large amount of composite flash on the surface of the tooth and around the bracket periphery could result in a greater incidence of bracket failure.[7] Because bracket failure is usually quick and sudden, it could result in injury to the pericoronal soft tissue, the oral mucosa, the tooth, or the clinician if debracketing is performed carelessly.[7]

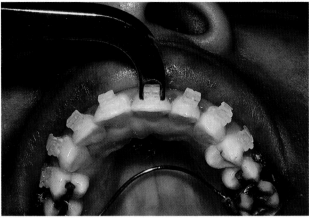

D3.11

Figure D3.11 Special instruments are recommended by various manufacturers to debond ceramic appliances. This instrument, by Unitek/3M, should be fully and firmly seated before the debonding force is applied.

Whole or fractured bracket particles can become dislodged into the field of operation and ingested or aspirated by the patient, creating a significant medical emergency.[7] Furthermore, the flying bracket particles subject both the patient and the clinician to possible eye injury if protective eyewear is not available or not worn by both individuals.[7] If the pliers designed for removal of brackets have a protective sheath that covers the working end of the instrument, the probability that bracket fragments will become dislodged in the patient's mouth or in the field of operation is decreased. The plier blades progressively lose their sharpness because of the interaction between the stainless steel blade and the much harder and more abrasive ceramic material. As the plier blades become dull, debonding efficiency is reduced.

It has been advocated that techniques used during debonding of conventional stainless steel brackets may be inappropriate for removal of ceramic brackets. Alternative debonding, such as ultrasonic and electrothermal debracketing, techniques that minimize the potential for bracket failure as well as the trauma to the enamel surface during debonding, have been investigated. These may be more time consuming, and the likelihood of pulpal damage needs to be thoroughly investigated. Prototype debracketing instruments are, at present, undergoing clinical trials.

A lot of the aforementioned problems will be avoided if the orthodontist performs a very careful clinical examination of the patient, with particular attention to compromised teeth, goes over a thorough informed consent and treatment agreement with the patient, emphasizes to the patient the advantages and disadvantages of ceramic brackets, adheres to the manufacturer's instructions, and is kept up to date with the information that becomes available in the literature.

References

1. Swartz ML: Ceramic brackets. J Clin Orthod 22:82–88, 1988.
2. Scott GE: Fracture toughness and surface cracks—The key to understanding ceramic brackets. Angle Orthod 1:3–8, 1988.
3. Odegaard T, and Segnes D: Shear bond strength of metal brackets compared with a new ceramic bracket. Am J Orthod Dentofacial Orthop 94:201–206, 1988.
4. Gwinnett AJ: A comparison of shear bond strengths of metal and ceramic brackets. Am J Orthod Dentofacial Orthop 93:346–348, 1988.

5. Viazis AD, DeLong R, Beris RR, Douglas WH, and Speidel TM: Enamel surface abrasion from ceramic orthodontic brackets: A special case report. Am J Orthod Dentofacial Orthop 96:514–518, 1989.
6. Viazis AD, DeLong R, Beris RR, Rudney TD, and Pintado MR: Enamel abrasion from ceramic orthodontic brackets under an artificial oral environment. Am J Orthod Dentofacial Orthop 98:103–109, 1990.
7. Bishara SE, and Trulove TS: Comparison of different debonding techniques for ceramic brackets: An in vitro study. Am J Orthod Dentofacial Orthop 98:263–273, 1990.
8. Viazis AD, Cavanaugh G, and Beris RR: Bond strength of ceramic brackets under shear stress: An in vitro report. Am J Orthod Dentofacial Orthop 98:214–221, 1990.
9. Britton JC, McInnes P, Weinberg R, Ledoux WR, and Retief DH: Shear bond strength of ceramic orthodontic brackets to enamel. Am J Orthod Dentofacial Orthop 98:348–353, 1990.
10. Angolkar PV, Kapila S, Duncanson MG, and Nanda RS: Evaluation of friction between ceramic brackets and orthodontic wires of four alloys. Am J Orthod Dentofacial Orthop 98:499–506, 1990.
11. Kusy RP, and Whitley JQ: Coefficients of friction for arch wires in stainless steel and polycrystalline alumina bracket slots. Part I: The dry state. Am J Orthod Dentofacial Orthop 98:300–312, 1990.
12. Pratten DH, Popli K, Germane N, and Gunsolley JC: Frictional resistance of ceramic and stainless steel orthodontic brackets. Am J Orthod Dentofacial Orthop 98:398–403, 1990.
13. Harris AMP, Joseph VP, and Rossoun E: Comparison of shear bond strength of orthodontic resins to ceramic and metal brackets. J Clin Orthod 24:725–728, 1990.
14. Eliades T, Viazis AD, and Eliades G: Bonding of ceramic brackets to enamel: Morphological and structural considerations. Am J Orthod Dentofacial Orthop 99:369–375, 1991.
15. Viazis AD: Direct bonding in orthodontics. Journal of Pedodontics 1:1–23, 1986.
16. Gwinnett AJ: A comparison of shear bond strengths of metal and ceramic brackets. Am J Orthod Dentofacial Orthop 93:346–348, 1988.
17. Eliades T, Viazis AD, and Lekka M: Failure mode analysis of ceramic brackets bonded to enamel. Am J Orthod Dentofacial Orthop (in press)
18. Vukovich ME, Wood DP, and Daley TD: Heat generated by grinding during removal of ceramic brackets. Am J Orthod Dentofacial Orthop 99:505–512, 1991.
19. Holt MH, Nanda RS, and Duncanson MG, Jr.: Fracture resistance of ceramic brackets during arch wire torsion. Am J Orthod Dentofacial Orthop 99:287–293, 1991.
20. Bednar JR, Gruendemau GW, and Sandrik JL: A comparative study of frictional forces between orthodontic brackets and archwires. Am J Orthod Dentofacial Orthop 100:513–522, 1991.
21. Tanne K, Matsubara S, Shibaguchi T, and Sakuda M: Wire friction from ceramic brackets during simulated canine retraction. Angle Orthod 61:285–290, 1991.
22. American Association of Orthodontists: Ceramic bracket survey, memorandum to members, April 7, 1989.
23. American Association of Orthodontists: Ceramic bracket survey results update, memorandum to members, December 1989.
24. Prososki RR, Bagby MD, and Erickson LC: Static frictional force and surface roughness of nickel-titanium arch wires. Am J Orthod Dentofacial Orthop 100:341–348, 1991.

Direct Bonding of Brackets/ Adhesive Systems

Since the introduction of the acid-etching technique by Buonocore,[1,2] which enhanced the adhesion of resins to enamel, rapid developments have led to the concept of direct bonding in orthodontics, where attachments are directly bonded to the enamel surface.[1-18] Naturally, the effectiveness of the bonded appliances in transferring the desired forces to the teeth is dependent on the bond strength to the tooth. This can be accomplished by an adhesive system that will bond the brackets directly to the tooth surface and maintain them throughout the duration of treatment (Figs. D4.1 through D4.20).

Orthodontic resins must ideally have adequate strength, be able to bond to both ceramic and metal brackets, remain stain-free and thus be esthetically pleasing, have variable setting times for multiple uses, and possess adequate hardness to facilitate debonding.[3] They are divided into two systems: the ultraviolet (UV)- and self-cured systems.[3]

The UV curing systems rely on externally supplied, long-wavelength, UV radiation to produce a free-radical–liberating compound, such as benzoin methylether, in the resin.[3,4] They are one-component systems and therefore are easier to use; the most important advantage is that of unlimited working time. In general, there is no statistically significant difference between the mean shear bond strength of light-cured and chemically cured adhesives (two pastes or no mix).[8] The fact that visible, light-cured resins are being used successfully would seem to indicate that, although their *in vitro* shear bond strength is clinically less than that of the chemically cured resin, visible, light-cured resins can be used clinically with good results.[9]

Both lightly filled and heavily filled resins predispose to plaque formation without significant qualitative differences between them.[5] There is a trend toward an increased bond strength with increased filler concentration.[6] The removal of highly filled composite cements on average causes more loss of enamel than removal of an unfilled adhesive.[10] A lower filler content decreases the abrasive resistance and simplifies polishing and finishing of the enamel surface after debonding.

Recently, glass ionomer cements were introduced in clinical orthodontics (Figs. D4.21 through D4.26). A great advantage of glass ionomer cements is their ability to act as reservoirs of fluoride ions, thus reducing the possibility of decalcification.[11-24] Fluoride ions are released in the immediate vicinity of the cement soon after placement, and this ion release continues at significant levels for at least 12 months.

Glass ionomer cements were found to adhere without etching; simple prophylaxis and drying of the enamel produced the strongest bond. Etching actually reduced bond strength, because glass ionomers form a direct chemical bond with the enamel, unlike the mechanical bond of composite resins. They also bond relatively better to the bracket than to the enamel; fractures tended to be cohesive failures, within the cement itself. The clinical implication is that little cement will be left on the tooth after debonding.

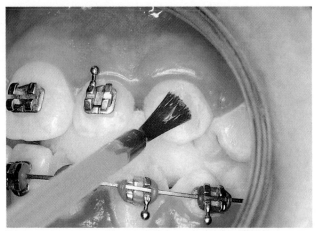

D4.1

Figure D4.1 After isolation with cheek retractors (for both arches) or cotton rolls (for single-tooth procedures), the teeth are pumiced and adequately rinsed, followed by acid etching with a disposable brush for 15 seconds.

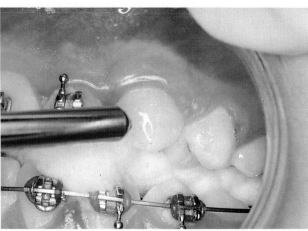

D4.2

Figure D4.2 Thorough rinsing and drying are absolutely necessary in order to obtain the chalky-white etched tooth surface that allows for a good bond. At this point, the tooth is ready to receive the bracket.

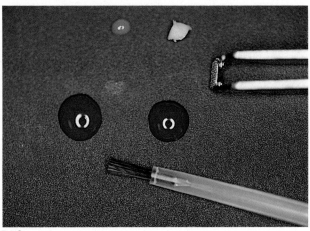

D4.3

Figure D4.3 Most adhesives come with two parts: a liquid form and a paste form.

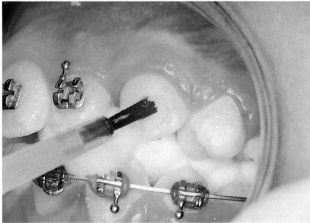

D4.4

Figure D4.4 The liquid part is applied onto the tooth surface with a brush by the clinician.

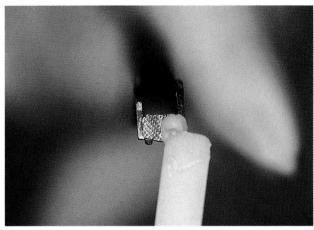

D4.5

Figure D4.5 The paste is placed onto the bracket base by the chairside assistant.

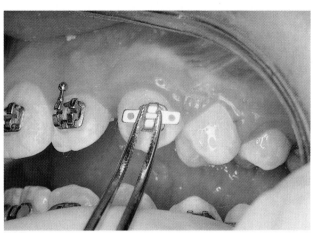

D4.6

Figure D4.6 The bracket is then placed on the center of the tooth with a special holding plier or even a pair of cotton pliers.

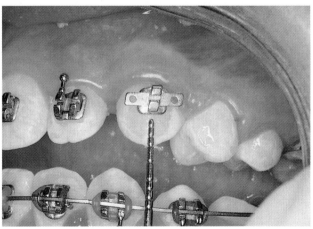

D4.7

Figure D4.7 The clinician then aligns the bracket along the long axis of the tooth at a specific distance from the incisal edge.

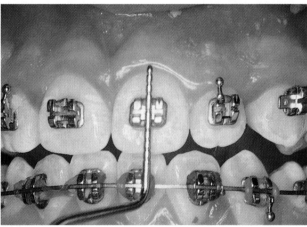

D4.8

Figure D4.8 This is more easily done for the twin and deltoid brackets with the perio probe, due to the convenient shape of these appliances.

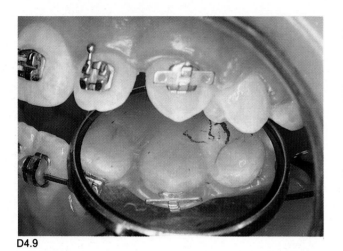

D4.9

Figure D4.9 At the end, as a final check, the bracket is checked with a mouth mirror to ensure that it is aligned properly.

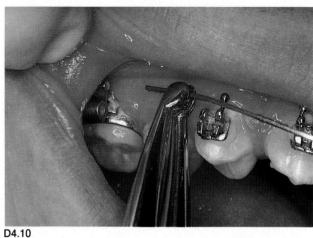

D4.10

Figure D4.10 Wire placement is done intraorally with the Howe pliers which allow a firm grip of the wire and easy placement in the molar tubes and the bracket slots.

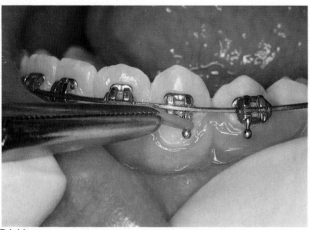

D4.11

Figures D4.11 through D4.15 The placement of the elasto-meric modules ("O" rings) over the bracket is done with a hemostat. The module is hooked around one wing and then, with the "baseball home-run" twisting motion, all four rings of the twin bracket are engaged.

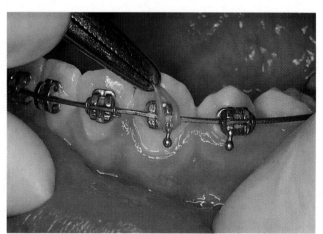

D4.12

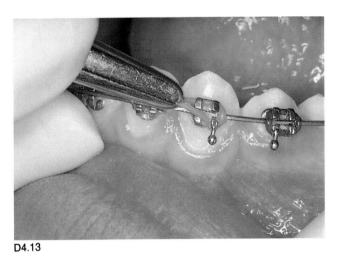

D4.13

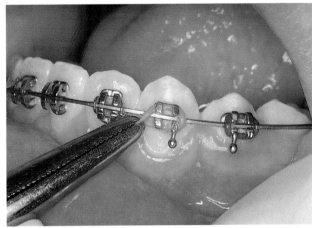

D4.14

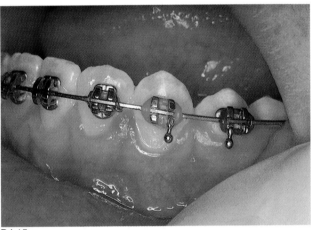

D4.15

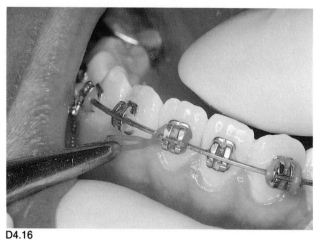

D4.16

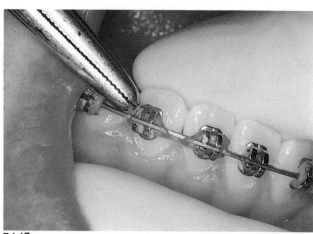

D4.17

Figures D4.16 and D4.17 For the hook-up of the elastic chains, the procedure is quite similar: on insertion of one of the loops, the chain is stretched and the rest is tied in a similar manner.

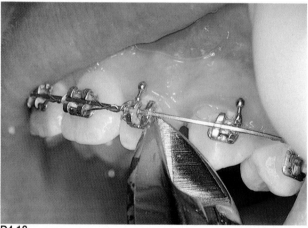

D4.18

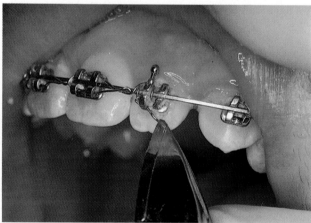

D4.19

Figure D4.18 To secure the archwire in the bracket slot tightly, a ligature wire-tie is used. It is placed beneath first the mesial wings of the bracket and then the distal ones while sliding along the main archwire. At this point, the two legs are crossed over, twisted by hand a few times, and then securely tightened with a hemostat. The excess ligature is cut off and the remaining 3-mm twisted part is placed beneath the main arch wire.

Figure D4.19 When removal of a ligature wire-tie is desired, a ligature-cutter plier may be used to cut the wire and, without letting go of it, the ligature tie is removed with the same plier.

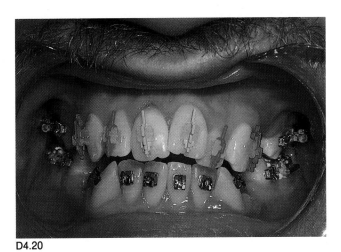

D4.20

Figure D4.20 Colored jigs aid the practitioner in the correct placement of the ceramic appliances. These jigs are removed after the adhesive has set.

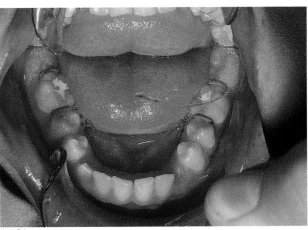

D4.21

Figure D4.21 One week before band fitting and cementing, separators are placed around the teeth that are to be banded.

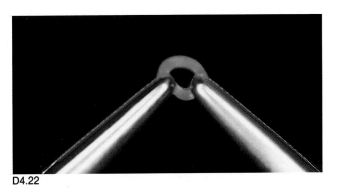

D4.22

Figure D4.22 The separator is held by two hemostats at a 90-degree angle.

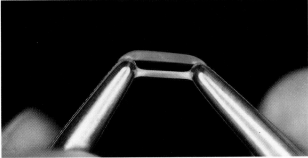

D4.23

Figure D4.23 The separator is stretched and then inserted between the teeth. Its thin, stretched section (the lower, partly white area) can easily slide through the tooth contacts.

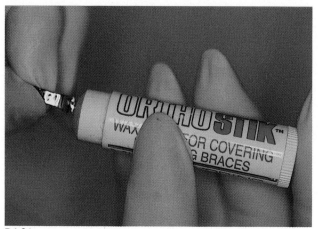

D4.24

Figure D4.24 The band's triple tubes are waxed so that adhesive will not enter the tubes.

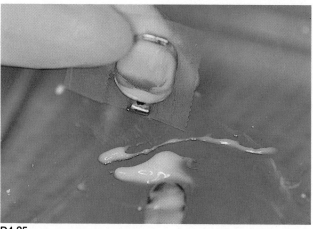

D4.25

Figure D4.25 A glass ionomer cement is used to bond teeth because the bond is stronger than that of zinc phosphate cements, especially if headgear is used at some point during treatment.

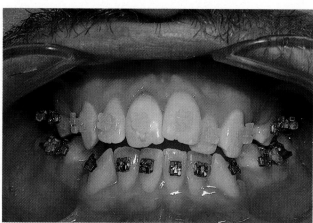

D4.26

Figure D4.26 Regardless of the bracket type used, brackets should all be placed in the middle of each tooth, at the same distances (x) from the incisal edge, with the exception of the cuspids, which should be 1 mm more gingivally (x + 1 mm), and molar teeth, which should be 1 mm more occlusally (x − 1 mm). This bracket placement ensures cuspid guidance at the end of treatment and minimizes the extrusion of the molar teeth, which may otherwise lead to interferences.

In a recent study, it was found that a glass ionomer cement, Ketac–Cem (Espe, Fabrik Pharmazutischer Preparate GMBH & Co., Germany), had a 12.4% failure rate when it was used to bond brackets on teeth of 40 consecutive patients.[11] More recent investigations showed that conventional composite adhesives leave a considerably higher bond strength than glass ionomer cements.[13,14] It is recommended that if glass ionomer cements are used for bonding of orthodontic brackets, the archwires not be placed until the next day, in order to have sufficient clinical strength.[11] In a recent study,[24] it was concluded that the mean shear bond strength of light-cured, fluoride-releasing glass ionomer is higher than that of the chemically cured ionomer.

A problem that may arise during treatment with direct-bonded appliances is corrosion. Corrosion appears as black and green stains around the corner of the brackets, some of which permanently mark the enamel, especially on anterior teeth.[15] It is primarily caused by the percolation of the salivary fluids, which are rich in electrolytes, at the junction of the resin–enamel or resin–mesh interface for a long period.[16] Contributory factors may be corrosion susceptibility of the alloy, the effect of welding or brazing on the structure, and galvanic action arising from contact with other alloys in the mouth.[16] It is advisable that the clinician remove the affected bracket and rebond.[15]

Visible, light-activated, fluoride-releasing orthodontic bonding systems are capable of adequately retaining brackets while aiding in the prevention of decalcification around bonded appliances.[18] Such bonding systems were found to provide bracket retention rates similar to those of conventional orthodontic bonding systems.[18] Acid etching the enamel before fluoride application increases fluoride uptake.[19] This type of post-etch fluoride treatment does not alter bond strength.[20] Use of fluoride-exchanging adhesive resulted in a reduction of early demineralization.[21] Findings indicate that the application of either 2% or 4% sodium fluoride (NaF) in a diluted orthophosphoric acid (H_3PO_4) solution does not significantly influence the tensile bond strength of the adhesive material to the enamel surface.[22] Equal susceptibility to white spot formation has been reported whether teeth are banded or bonded.[23] Fluoride-releasing base liners are not acceptable as orthodontic adhesives, but they may be placed around already-bonded brackets.[25]

It should be noted that an allergic reaction to the nickel element of the metal brackets has been reported.[17] It seems that there is a high initial release of metals but that the effect diminishes with time. There are fewer symptoms associated with oral exposure to nickel. Inter-individual differences must be considered.

In reference to bonding to gold teeth, roughing the surface before bonding is necessary to provide a successful bond. Acid etching should then be used to provide a clean gold surface and should be followed by bonding with highly filled resins.[26]

The technique used to bond orthodontic brackets to porcelain relies on a hydrolyzed silane coupling agent. If a nonhydrolyzed silane agent is used (Ormco porcelain primer, Ormco, CA), it needs to be applied onto the tooth without removal of the acid etchant. The phosphoric acid etchant activates the silane and hydrolyzes it. The process of hydrolyzing activates the silane and prepares it for chemical interaction with the porcelain surface. A second layer of nonhydrolyzed silane should follow. After a thorough rinse and air dry, the adhesive resin may be applied. When a hydrolyzed silane is used (Scotch prime, Unitek/3M), it should be applied only once for 2 minutes without acid etching and dried with warm air. To remove the brackets during debonding, a tensile pull with a "pinching and peeling" force should be applied.[26] The porcelain should not be touched with the finishing bur (No. FG 7909, Teledyne Densco Co.) that removes the residual composite from the tooth.[26] Insta-Glaze (Taub Products and Fusion Co.) can be used to polish the porcelain surface at the end of the procedure.[26]

Various adhesive systems currently exist in the market that allow for clinically successful bonds to porcelain teeth: System 1 (Ormco) with porcelain bonding primer, Enamelite 500 enamel coating/porcelain repair (Lee Pharmaceutical), Isopast with Silanit contact-resin (Vivadent), and Concise with Scotchprime (Unitek/3M). Generally speaking, debonding and clean up with scalers and pliers create surface defects such as craters, pits, and porcelain fracture as the resin is removed. Diamond polishing paste is better in restoring the surface than are polishing stones. Irreversible damage to porcelain may also occur. Because the bond strengths to glazed and deglazed porcelain are not significantly different, it may be desirable to bond to glazed porcelain to minimize surface damage.[27] Roughening of porcelain with silane treatment allows for clinically acceptable bond strengths of orthodontic brackets to porcelain.[28] Roughened surfaces and surfaces with microfractures can be satisfactorily finished and polished with either a series of graded ceramist's points (Shofu Dental Co.) or a diamond-impregnated polishing wheel (Meissinger, Jan Dental Co.), followed by a diamond polishing paste (Vident).[29]

References

1. Buonocore MG: A simple method of increasing the adhesion of acrylic filling materials to enamel surfaces. J Dent Res 34:849–853, 1955.
2. Viazis AD: Direct bonding of orthodontic brackets. J Pedodontics 11:1, 1986.
3. Maijer R: *Bonding Systems in Orthodontics. Biocompatibility of Dental Materials.* Vol. II. Boca Raton, FL: CRC Press, 1982, pp. 3:51–76.
4. Lee HL, Orlowski JA, and Rogers BJ: A comparison of ultraviolet-curing and self-curing polymers in preventive, restorative and orthodontic dentistry. Int Dent J 26:134–151, 1976.
5. Gwinnet AJ, and Ceen RF: Plaque distribution on bonded brackets. A scanning microscope study. Am J Orthod 75:667–678, 1979.
6. Ostertag AJ, Dhuru VB, Ferguson DJ, and Meyer RA: Shear, torsional, and tensile bond strengths of ceramic brackets using three adhesive filler concentrations. Am J Orthod Dentofacial Orthop 100:251–258, 1991.
7. Delport A, and Grobler SR: A laboratory evaluation of the tensile bond strength of some orthodontic bonding resins to enamel. Am J Orthod Dentofacial Orthop 93:137, 1988.
8. Viazis AD, Cavanaugh G, and Beris R: Bond strength of ceramic brackets under shear stress: An in-vitro report. Am J Orthod Dentofacial Orthop 98:214, 1990.
9. Greenlaw R, Way DC, and Galil KA: An in vitro evaluation of a visible light-cured resin as an alternative to conventional resin bonding resins. Am J Orthod Dentofacial Orthop 96:214–220, 1989.
10. Brown CR, and Way DC: Enamel loss during orthodontic bonding and subsequent loss during removal of filled and unfilled adhesives. Am J Orthod 74:663–671, 1978.
11. Cook PA: Direct bonding with glass ionomer cement. J Clin Orthod 24:509–511, 1990.
12. Rezk-Lega F, Ogaard B, and Arends J: An in-vivo study on the merits of two glass ionomers for the cementation of orthodontic bands. Am J Orthod Dentofacial Orthop 99:162–167, 1991.
13. Rezk-Lega F, and Ogaard B: Tensile bond force of glass ionomer cements in direct bonding of orthodontic brackets: An in vitro comparative study. Am J Orthod Dentofacial Orthop 100:357–361, 1991.
14. Bishara SE, Swift EJ, and Chan DCN: Evaluation of fluoride release from an orthodontic bonding system. Am J Orthod Dentofacial Orthop 100:106–109, 1991.
15. Gwinnet AJ: Corrosion of resin-bonded orthodontic brackets. Am J Orthod 82:441–446, 1982.
16. Maijer R, and Smith DC: Corrosion of orthodontic bracket bases. Am J Orthod 80:43–48, 1982.
17. Gjerdet NR, Erichsen ES, Remlo HE, and Evjen G: Nickel and iron in saliva of patients with fixed appliances. Acta Odontol Scand 49:73–78, 1991.
18. Sonis AL, and Snell W: An evaluation of a fluoride releasing visible light-activated bonding system for orthodontic bracket placement. Am J Orthod Dentofacial Orthop 95:306, 1989.
19. Kajander KC, Uhland R, Ophang RH, and Sather AH: Topical fluoride in orthodontic bonding. Angle Orthod 57:70–76, 1987.
20. Klockowski R, Davis EL, Joynt RB, Wieczkowski G, and McDonald A: Bond strength and durability of glass ionomer cements used as bonding agents in the placement of orthodontic brackets. Am J Orthod Dentofacial Orthop 96:60–64, 1989.
21. Underwood ML, Rawls HR, and Zimmerman BF: Clinical evaluation of a fluoride-exchanging resin as an orthodontic adhesive. Am J Orthod Dentofacial Orthop 96:93–99, 1989.
22. Bishara SE, Chan D, and Abadir EA: The effect on the bonding strength of orthodontic brackets of fluoride application after etching. Am J Orthod Dentofacial Orthop 95:259–260, 1989.
23. Geiger AM, Gorelick L, Gwinnett AJ, and Griswold PG: The effect of a fluoride program on white spot formation during orthodontic treatment. Am J Orthod Dentofacial Orthop 93:29–37, 1988.
24. Compton AM, Meyers CE, Jr., Hondrum SO, and Lorton L: Comparison of the shear bond strength of a light-cured glass ionomer and a chemically cured glass ionomer for use as an orthodontic bonding agent. Am J Orthod Dentofacial Orthop 101:138–144, 1992.
25. McCourt JW, Cooley RL, and Barnwell S: Bond strength of light-wire fluoride-releasing base-liners as orthodontic bracket adhesives. Am J Orthod Dentofacial Orthop 100:47–52, 1991.
26. Andreasen GF, and Stieg MA: Bonding and debonding brackets to porcelain and gold. Am J Orthod Dentofacial Orthop 93:341–345, 1988.

27. Eustaquio R, Garner LD, and Moore BK: Comparative tensile strengths of brackets bonded to porcelain with orthodontic adhesive and porcelain repair systems. Am J Orthod Dentofacial Orthop 94:421–425, 1988.
28. Smith GA, McInnes-Ledoux P, Ledoux WR, and Weinberg R: Orthodontic bonding to porcelain—Bond strength and refinishing. Am J Orthod Dentofacial Orthop 94:245–252, 1988.
29. Kao EC, Boltz KC, and Johnston WM: Direct bonding of orthodontic brackets to porcelain veneer laminates. Am J Orthod Dentofacial Orthop 94:458–468, 1988.

Chapter 5

Basic Orthodontic Instruments: Wire Bending

A few pliers are needed in the modern practice of orthodontics (Fig. D5.1). Here are some basic ones[1,2]:

The *bird beak* plier: (the most popular orthodontic plier) used to bend round wires.

The *square* plier: used to bend rectangular wires.

The *Howe* plier: the clinician's "hand" in the mouth; mostly used to place the archwire in the bracket slots.

The *three-prong* plier: used to bend larger size wires; *i.e.,* 0.030-inch round retainer wire and clasps.

The *hemostat*: used to place elastomeric modules, elastic chains, and ligature wires over the bracket wings.

The *wire cutter* plier: used to cut wires outside of the mouth.

The *distal-end cutter* plier: used to cut the archwire distal to the molar tube in the mouth.

The *band-sitter*: facilitates the smooth fit of the molar bands around these teeth.

The *bracket remover*: is the same for all metal appliances, but varies depending on the manufacturer for the ceramic brackets.

The *band remover*: has a soft end, which contacts the tooth surface, and a metal end, which dislodges the band from its position.

***Cotton pliers/bracket-holding pliers*:** used to place brackets onto the tooth surface.

A *3-mm periodontal probe*: aids in the accurate placement of the brackets onto the teeth.

Despite the existence of modern, preadjusted appliances, compensating bends are almost always needed to finish a case.[1,2]

"In–out" or First-Order Bends

These are done in the horizontal plane. One should remember that we always start with an archwire that lies flat on the table, and that it should still lie flat after the bend has been placed in it (Figs. D5.2 through D5.15). This is why "orientation" of the archwire is of vital importance: we should always hold the pliers (bird beak for round or square for rectangular wires) perpendicular to and the archwire parallel to the floor. This way, we are not introducing any unnecessary bends in the wire that we may not be able to take out later on.

"Up and Down" or "Tip" or Second-Order Bends

These are done just like the first-order bends, only in the vertical plane (Figs. D5.16 through D5.19).

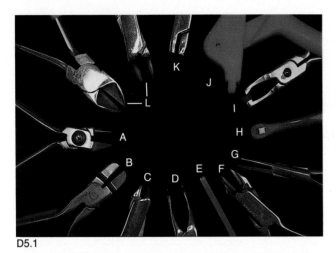

D5.1

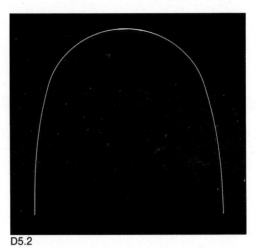

D5.2

Figure D5.1 Various instruments and pliers used in the modern practice of orthodontics: *(A)* bird beak pliers, *(B)* square pliers, *(C)* three-prong pliers, *(D)* Howe pliers, *(E)* torquing key, *(F)* torquing pliers, *(G)* hemostat, *(H)* band sitter, *(I)* band remover, *(J)* bond remover, *(K)* distal-end cutter pliers, *(L)* wire cutter plier.

Figure D5.2 Archwire preformed to the shape of the dental arch as it is available in the market.

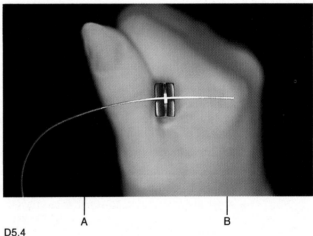

D5.3

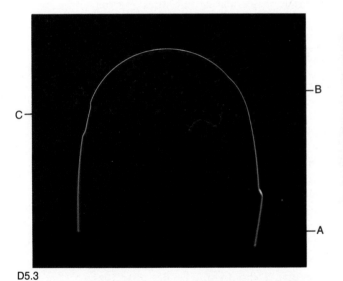

D5.4

Figure D5.3 First-order bends. *(A)* A *molar offset* is placed to move the mesiobuccal cusp of the molar slightly more buccally while at the same time smoothly curving its distal cusps lingually. The latter is accomplished because the end of the archwire points lingually ("toe-in"). This bend also helps to counteract the mesiolingual rotational movement exerted on the molar from the elastomeric chain modules during space closure. *(B)* A *cuspid offset* is placed to accentuate the position of the cuspid buccally, especially in a broad, full "Hollywood" smile. *(C)* An *inset* is the opposite of an offset. Its purpose is to move a tooth lingually.

Figure D5.4 Proper orientation during wire bending is very important. Always hold the pliers perpendicular to and the wire parallel to the floor. In a clinical situation, mark with an indelible pencil in the patient's mouth the point where to bend the wire. That is where the pliers should hold the wire. This is usually toward the mesial side of a tooth. For purposes of orientation while looking at the photograph, we will call *A* the segment of the wire on the left side of the pliers and *B* the segment on the right side.

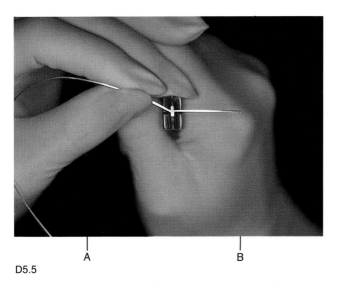

D5.5

Figure D5.5 To place an offset on *B*, start by bending *A* out with the thumb of the other hand. (It is the fingers that do the wire bending, *not* the pliers. The instruments are simply used to hold the wire.)

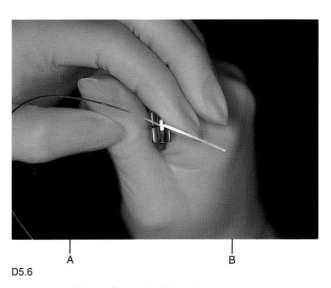

D5.6

Figure D5.6 Side B of the wire is bent inward.

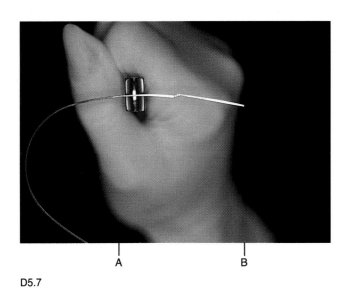

D5.7

Figure D5.7 The molar offset bent has been created.

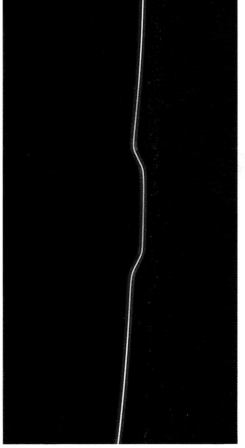

D5.8

Figure D5.8 To create an offset for an incisor or bicuspid (in the middle of the arch), all one needs to do is repeat the same procedure on the distal side of that specific tooth.

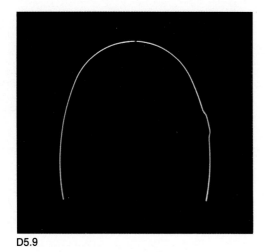

D5.9

Figure D5.9 A bicuspid offset.

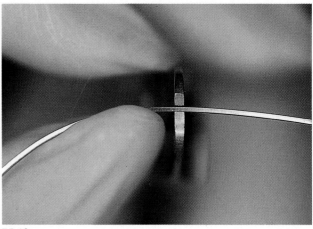

D5.10

Figure D5.10 The placement of a cuspid offset is done a little differently, due to the smooth curve that must be given to the archwire. Start by holding the wire at a point that corresponds mesial to the cuspid bracket.

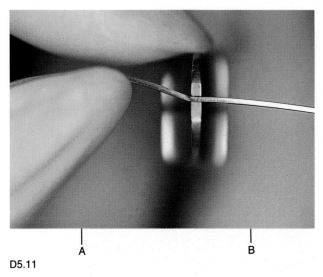

A   B

D5.11

Figure D5.11 The *A* segment is bent out, similar to the molar offset.

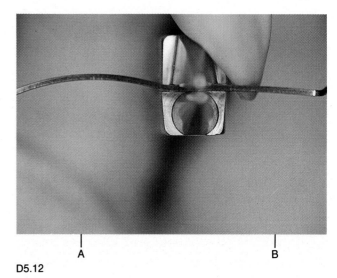

A   B

D5.12

Figure D5.12 Because square pliers have been used up to now (for bending rectangular wires), one needs to switch to bird beak pliers. Position the wire in the middle of the prongs of the pliers, distal to the point initially marked on the *B* segment.

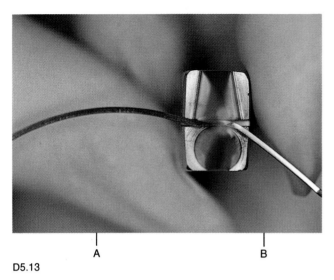

D5.13

A   B

Figure D5.13 Taking advantage of the roundness of the beak of the pliers, bend the *B* segment inward.

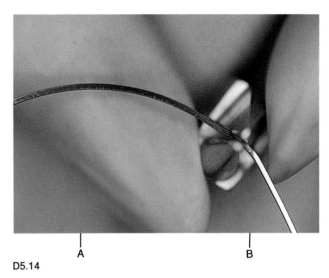

D5.14

A   B

Figure D5.14 The bird beak pliers are then repositioned slightly more distally on the *B* segment; again, exert light pressure to curve the wire around the beak of the pliers.

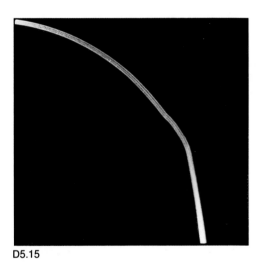

D5.15

Figure D5.15 The cuspid offset that was created. The offset should curve as smoothly as possible past the initial point of contact with the pliers.

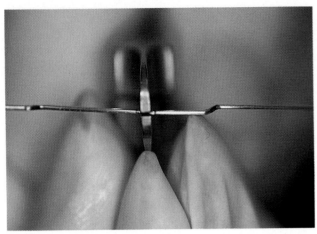

D5.16

Figure D5.16 The placement of a second-order bend is done just like the bicuspid offsets, but in the vertical plane. Shown is the first bend, which has already been placed on the mesial side. The square pliers are holding the archwire on the distal side of the bracket (as it would appear in the mouth).

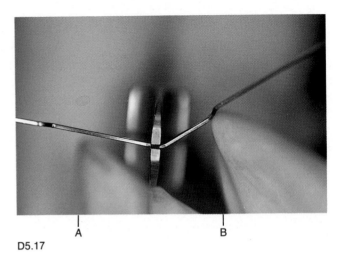

D5.17

Figure D5.17 In order to complete the second-order bend, the *B* segment is bent upward.

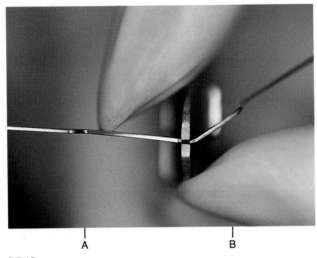

D5.18

Figure D5.18 The *A* segment is then bent downward.

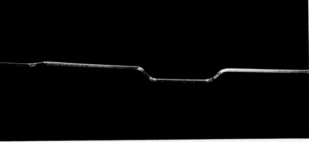

D5.19

Figure D5.19 The completed second-order bend. Usually, when placing such a bend, the tooth, as it is brought down, tends to roll in (lingually) as well. Therefore, it is a good idea to place a first-order bend (offset) as well to counteract this side effect.

"Torque" or Third-Order Bends

These are a little different from the other two. In order to apply "torque," we need to "twist" the wire so that the roots of the teeth may move either buccally or lingually (buccal root torque and lingual root torque, respectively). There are generally three types of "torque" bends (Figs. D5.20 through D5.32): (a) single-tooth torque, (b) anterior torque, and (c) posterior torque.

The following needs to be emphasized: even if a bend is necessary to compensate for bad bracket placement, it is much easier to reposition the brackets than to place unnecessary bends. Without anterior archwire bends, the wire slides through the bracket slots far more efficiently, allowing effective use of sliding mechanics for space closure. Although it is true that very little bending is needed during the first five stages of treatment, finishing requires some wire bending in almost every case. Because the appliance prescriptions are based on averages, they cannot possibly account for all the variations of tooth size and shape. This means that detailing bends will be needed in the finishing wires of some patients.

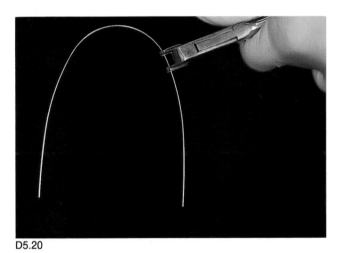

D5.20

Figure D5.20 The placement of torque or third-order bends is achieved with the help of the torquing (holding) pliers and torquing key. The pliers hold the wire as shown.

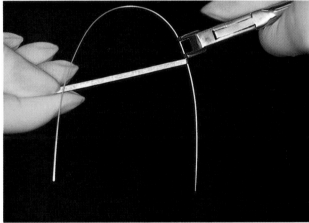

D5.21

Figure D5.21 In order to torque (twist) the wire distal to the holding pliers, the key is positioned next to the pliers, parallel to the pliers and the wire.

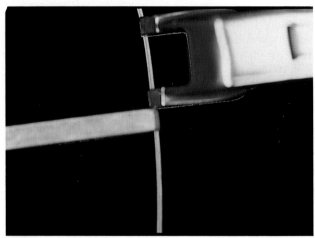

D5.22

Figure D5.22 A closer view shows the relationship of these auxiliary instruments. If torquing one tooth only, the torquing key would have to be placed between the two legs of the torquing pliers.

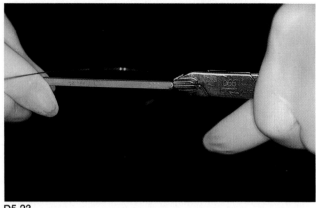

D5.23

Figure D5.23 Side view. Note that the pliers are parallel to the floor.

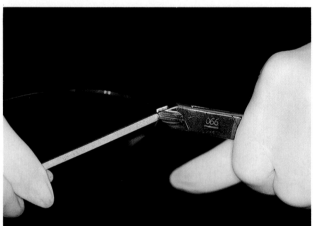

D5.24

Figure D5.24 If the archwire is of the upper arch and we wish to place lingual root torque on the upper right posterior teeth, then the key is moved inferiorly.

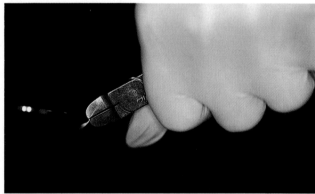

D5.25

Figure D5.25 If we now hold the posterior segment of the archwire with the square pliers, we notice that the pliers have moved upward posteriorly and are no longer parallel to the floor. When we place this archwire in the mouth and into the bracket slots, the roots of the upper right posterior teeth will move toward the same direction as the pliers did, *i.e.,* palatally (lingual root torque).

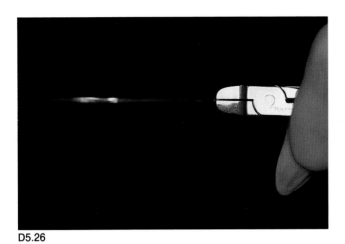

D5.26

Figure D5.26 The rest of the archwire has not been affected by the torque applied in the posterior segment. The pliers are still parallel to the floor.

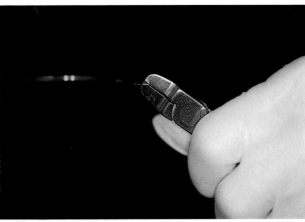

D5.27

Figure D5.27 Movement of the roots of the upper right posterior teeth toward the buccal cortical plate (buccal root torque) would require the opposite twisting activation of the wire. Similar logic can be applied for a mandibular wire.

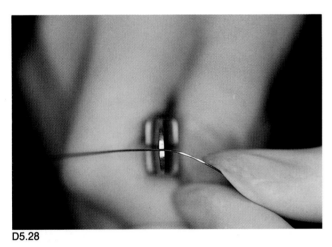

D5.28

Figure D5.28 Placement of anterior torque, usually from lateral incisor to lateral incisor but often from cuspid to cuspid, starts by gently bending the anterior part of the archwire.

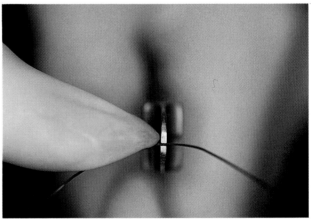

D5.29

Figure D5.29 The pliers are moved toward the midline as the fingers of the other hand continue to gently bend the wire. The same sequence is followed from the other side toward the midline.

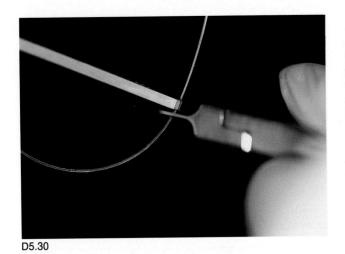

D5.30

Figure D5.30 With the help of the torquing key, any residual torque in the posterior segments of the archwire is taken out.

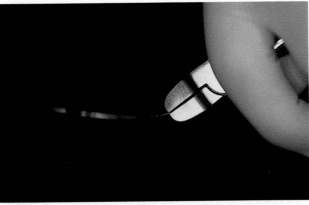

D5.31

Figure D5.31 As the orientation of the pliers relative to the torqued anterior part of the archwire shows, upon placement of this wire in the upper arch the roots of the anterior teeth will move toward the palatal cortical plate (lingual root torque).

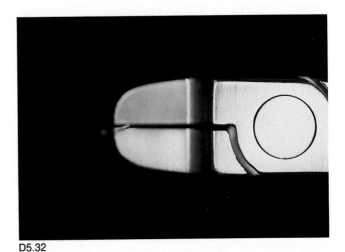

D5.32

Figure D5.32 The posterior archwire is flat.

The wires need to be handled with care in the patient's mouth (Fig. D5.33). In addition, apart from the main archwire, other auxiliary wires may be used when needed (Fig. D5.34). If we need to secure the wires tightly in the bracket slots, a ligature tie is preferred to the elastomeric modules (especially for the expression of torque) (Fig. D5.35).

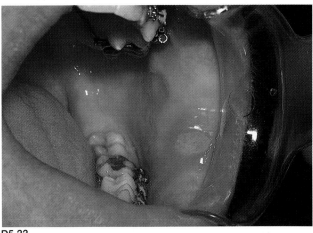

D5.33

Figure D5.33 It is very important that the main archwire is cut close to the most posterior molar band with the distal-end cutter pliers. Wires that "stick" the patient's soft tissue can create quite an ulceration between 3- to 4-week appointment periods.

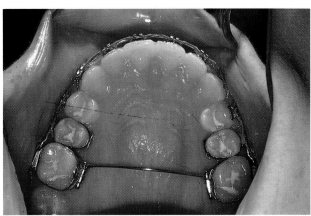

D5.34

Figure D5.34 The transpalatal arch (TPA) is available in different sizes and is easily inserted in the sheaths of the first molar bands with Howe pliers when headgear is used (to control the position of the molar teeth in the transverse dimension). For crossbite correction, an RME appliance is preferred for more stable results.

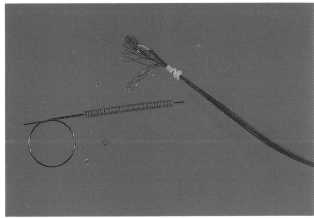

D5.35

Figure D5.35 The elastomeric modules and ligature wires used to tie the wires in the bracket slots.

References

1. Vanarsdall PL, Jr.: *Uprighting the Inclined Mandibular Molar in Preparation for Restorative Treatment.* Chicago: Quintessence Publishing Co., 1980.
2. Proffit WR: *Contemporary Orthodontics.* St. Louis, MO: C.V. Mosby Co., 1986.

Chapter 6

Orthodontic Wires

There are generally two types of orthodontic wires: round and rectangular.[1-10] Even though in the past most of these wires were made of stainless steel, the development of the nickel-titanium (NiTi) wires has led to the wide range of "elastic" wires that are available today.[1-10]

After the procedure of bonding the bracket onto the teeth has taken place, the steps in treatment that are followed during the 12- to 24-month treatment period are[1-10]:

Alignment
This is where the initial archwire will, over a period of a few months, bring the teeth into their correct "aligned" position in the dental arch. This is when rotations and crossbites are corrected.

Leveling
This is where the curve of Spee is leveled (in most instances) and all the teeth are brought into their normal vertical positions within the alveolus and in comparison to the adjacent teeth.

Space Closure
This is the third step of orthodontic treatment. Any remaining extraction spaces are closed during this phase with rectangular wires for the reasons that were discussed in the biomechanics section of this book. The rectangular wires provide the three-dimensional control of the teeth in the bone (tip/torque control), whereas elastomeric chain modules, rubber bands, and coil springs are used to pull the teeth together and close the spaces in the arch. One millimeter per month is, on average, the rate of space closure.

Finishing
This is the final phase of treatment, where bends are placed in the archwires to compensate for incorrect bracket position or peculiar tooth morphology. In an 0.018-inch slot system, a wire that completely fills the bracket slot and thus provides maximum torque control is the 0.018×0.025-inch^2 rectangular wire (finishing wire). Often, a 0.017×0.025-inch^2 or even an 0.016×0.022-inch^2 wire is used (they are not as stiff and are easier to insert in the bracket slot). It may be better to use the 0.016×0.022-inch^2 wire because it reduces the friction in the bracket slot, especially if finishing elastics are used to correct the midlines.

In the past, both alignment and leveling were done simultaneously with light, round stainless steel wires with monthly progression to a larger diameter wire. This sequence in the 0.018-inch slot system is 0.012-inch, followed by 0.014-inch, and then 0.016-inch diameter round wire (Fig. D6.1). The objective was to start with a very light wire, such as 0.012-inch wire, that would have the least stiffness (stiffness is a measure of the amount of force required to bend a wire a certain distance), so that it may be fully engaged in the bracket slot without deformation and thus start tooth movement with the least discomfort for the patient. If even lighter force levels were needed, braided stainless steel archwires were also used (Fig. D6.2). Usually, within a month or two, the teeth would have moved toward the correct arch form and the next size wire would be inserted in the brackets. One must remember that the stiffer the wire, the more force it takes to place it in the bracket; thus, the more force it will deliver and the more pain it will elicit. Space closure in the 0.018-inch slot system would begin with a 0.016×0.016-inch^2 rectangular stainless steel wire, followed by a 0.016×0.022-inch^2 size wire. The finishing archwire would be a 0.016×0.022-inch^2 wire or a 0.017×0.022-inch^2 wire.

The amount of force needed to move teeth is very low, approximately 0.025 g/cm^2, equal to the pressure in the capillaries. Higher force levels will cause "hyalinization" or "temporary necrosis" of the surrounding tissues, which will take about a 7- to 14-day period to reorganize. Pain will occur as well. The forces applied with the stainless steel wires are always heavier than needed, thus causing a delay period of 7 to 14 days of no tooth movement.

During this time, undermining resorption occurs (from within the bone) until it reaches the bone surface after 7 to 14 days, at which point the bone is resorbed and the tooth is moved abruptly. Hyalinization occurs again, and so on. This happens even with the lightest stainless steel wires (*i.e.,* 0.012 inch).

The recent introduction of the "elastic" wires has changed all this. Over the past few years, the use of NiTi wires has truly brought modern clinical orthodontics to another level. NiTi wires may deflect as much as six-fold compared to a stainless steel wire of the same size.[12] Research of the unique properties of this alloy over the past two decades,[1-7] along with the satisfactory results from its preliminary clinical application, has offered new horizons for research of biomechanics and challenging chapters in the practice of orthodontics. The superelastic NiTi wires can be displaced a considerable distance without developing excessive force. In addition, they can be reactivated (*i.e.,* manipulated to increase the force on a tooth after it has been partially moved into position) simply by releasing the elastomeric module holding it in the bracket slot, allowing it to spring back to its original shape (by pulling it out of the bracket), and then retying it.[9]

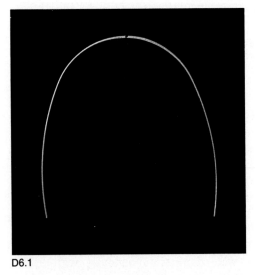

D6.1

Figure D6.1 A round stainless steel initial archwire (0.012 inch).

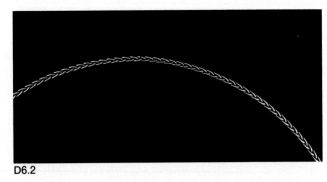

D6.2

Figure D6.2 A braided stainless steel initial archwire. This wire, before the introduction of the superelastic wires, exerted the lightest forces on the teeth.

The work by Andreasen and co-workers[1,2] led to the development of the Nitinol wire (Unitek). Although Nitinol has an excellent spring-back property, it does not possess shape memory or superelasticity because it has been manufactured by a work-hardening process.[6] Shape memory is a phenomenon occurring when the alloy is soft and readily amenable to change in shape at a low temperature but can easily be reformed to its original configuration when it is heated to a suitable transition temperature.[6] The superelastic property is demonstrated when the stress value remains fairly constant up to a certain point of wire deformation and, as the wire deformation rebounds, the stress value again remains fairly constant.[6] Miura et al.[6] claim that Japanese NiTi wire possesses all of the aforementioned properties and can therefore deliver a relatively constant force for a long period of time, which is considered a physiologically desirable force for tooth movement. Their research findings and clinical application of this round wire, under the trade name Sentalloy (GAC), showed that, due to the superelasticity of the archwire, tooth movement occurred effectively and patients did not exhibit any discomfort because the wire delivered a constant force for a long period during the deactivation of the wire.

In a more recent study,[7] it was found that the new superelastic NiTi rectangular wires, NeoSentalloy (GAC), can be used with extremely light force in the initial phase of treatment. Based on their three-point bending test and torque test on these wires, Miura et al. support findings that this new NiTi alloy shows extremely light continuous force, regardless of deflection, and that this superelastic force can be applied at low levels, regardless of wire size.

The rectangular NiTi wires have excellent clinical application, especially in the early phases of orthodontic treatment; *i.e.,* alignment and leveling. The greatest archwire flexibility and least patient discomfort in clinical trials appear to be provided with the NeoSentalloy (GAC) wires (Figs. D6.3 through D6.5). The rectangular NiTi wires can replace all of the stainless steel round wires, as well as some of the rectangular ones, but certainly not the finishing stainless steel wires that are necessary for fine detailing, arch coordination, and finishing bends (Figs. D6.6 through D6.21). A recommended treatment sequence with the 0.018-inch system would be a rectangular NiTi wire as initial archwire and 0.016×0.022-inch² stainless steel as finishing archwire. By using rectangular archwires from the onset of treatment, torque control

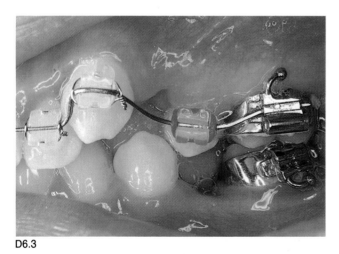

D6.3

Figure D6.3 The rectangular superelastic NeoSentalloy (GAC) archwire provides the greatest archwire flexibility available today, as well as control of torque from the onset of treatment.

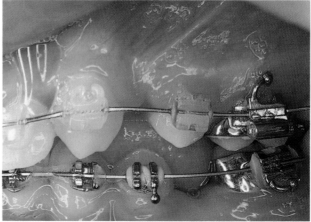

D6.4

Figure D6.4 The same patient as in Figure D6.3 after 1 month. Note that the cuspid has almost reached the occlusal plane (5 mm movement!). No patient discomfort was expressed.

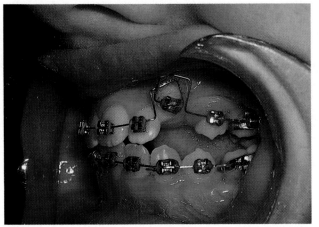

D6.5

Figure D6.5 A 0.014-inch stainless steel wire in a box configuration in a patient. This configuration allows for more wire to be incorporated between the adjacent brackets; otherwise the stainless steel wire would have been deformed had it been activated like the superelastic wire. In comparison, the efficacy in treatment is quite obvious with the NiTi wires.

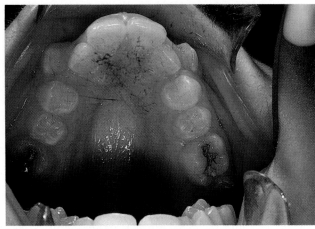

D6.6

Figures D6.6 through D6.9 A 12-year-old patient with a class I molar occlusion, orthognathic skeletal substrate, and severe upper and lower crowding (12 mm and 10 mm, respectively) requiring extraction of the upper first and lower second bicuspids. Note the overbite of 3 mm.

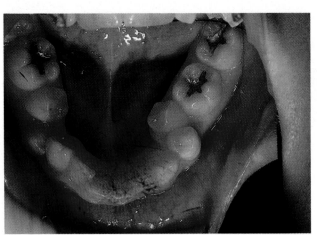

D6.7

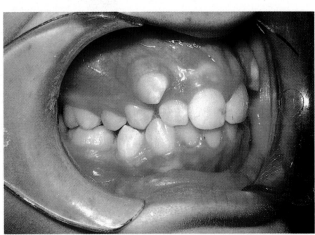

D6.8

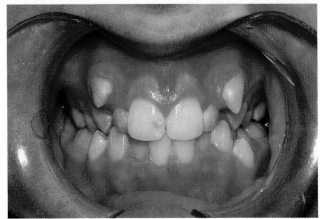

D6.9

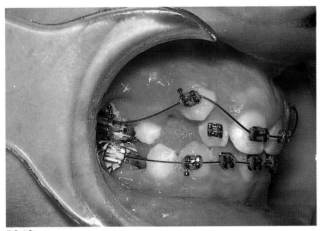

D6.10

Figure D6.10 A Sentalloy (GAC) round NiTi wire is placed as the initial archwire in the maxillary arch. A 0.012-inch, round, stainless steel wire is placed in the lower arch. The upper lateral incisors and bicuspids were not incorporated in this alignment phase in order to avoid unnecessary tipping of these teeth.

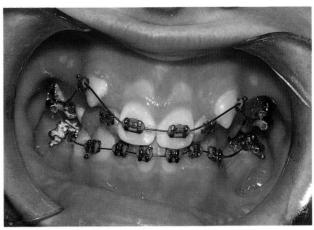

D6.11

Figure D6.11 Anterior view. Compare the vertical activation of more than 7 mm of the Sentalloy (GAC) round wire in the maxillary arch to the 0.5 mm of activation of the 0.012-inch stainless steel wire in the mandibular arch.

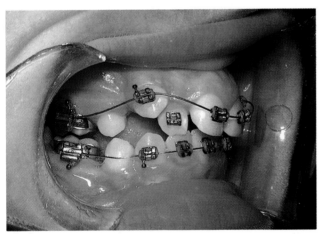

D6.12

Figure D6.12 After 1 month of treatment. The cuspid tooth has come down 3 mm. A 0.014-inch round wire is placed in the lower arch as the next step of stainless steel mechanotherapy.

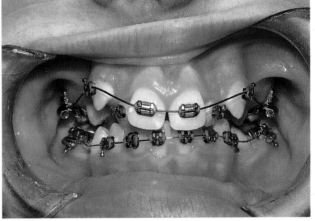

D6.13

Figure D6.13 Anterior wire. Note that there is a slight diastema that has opened between the central incisors as these teeth moved slightly mesially from the reaction to the cuspid movement.

is immediately obtained. This may have significant importance in posttreatment stability. In addition, cuspid retraction can be initiated from the onset of treatment (Figs. D6.22 through D6.27). By the time the cuspid teeth are in a solid class I relationship (about 5 months into treatment), alignment and leveling have been completed and the patient is ready to receive the stainless steel finishing coordinated archwires (0.016 × 0.022 inch), which will be the final archwires of therapy.

Finally, depending on the type of growth pattern being treated, the clinician should use the appropriate mechanotherapy sequence (Fig. D6.28).

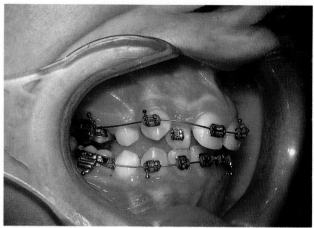

D6.14

Figure D6.14 After 2 months of treatment. The initial activation of the upper wire has brought the cuspids 5 mm more occlusally.

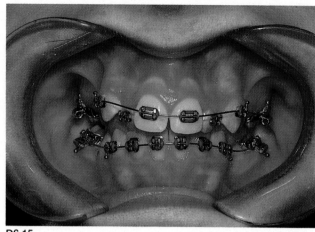

D6.15

Figure D6.15 Anterior view. Note that the diastema is closing as the cuspids are coming down and the incisors return to their original position.

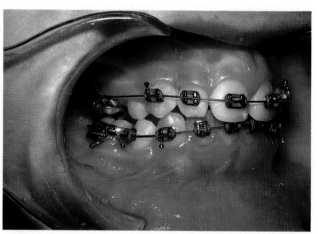

D6.16

Figure D6.16 After 3 months of treatment, the cuspid has reached the occlusal plane. A 0.016-inch round wire is the next size of stainless steel wire that is placed in the lower arch.

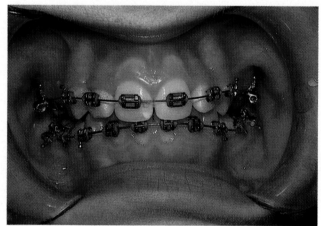

D6.17

Figure D6.17 Anterior view. The cuspid teeth have been brought into the arch without any side effects (the overbite is still 3 mm). The diastema has almost closed. Had the two central incisor teeth been wire tied together with a ligature tie, the diastema would not have been created.

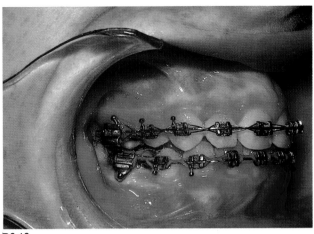

D6.18

Figure D6.18 Six months into treatment, 0.016×0.022-inch^2 stainless steel finishing wires are placed in both arches.

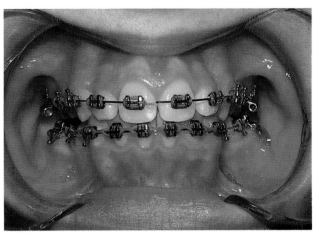

D6.19

Figure D6.19 Anterior view. Elastic chains help in closing of any remaining spaces in the lower arch.

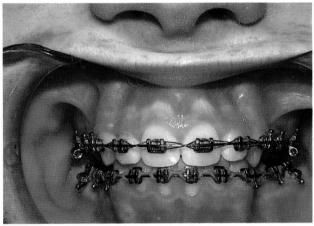

D6.20

Figure D6.20 Eight months into treatment, a figure-8 configuration of ligature wire (from the left first molar to the right one) consolidates and keeps the teeth in contact after space closure.

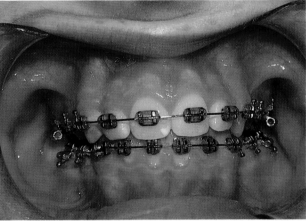

D6.21

Figure D6.21 Toward the end of treatment (10 months). This case will be finished in less than 1 year. A total of two wires were used in the upper arch: the initial superelastic wire and the finishing stainless steel.

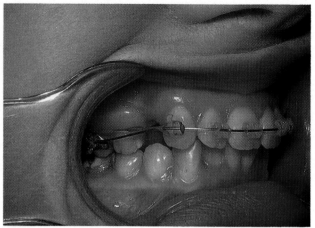

D6.22

Figure D6.22 Initiation of cuspid retraction using a rectangular, superelastic NeoSentalloy (GAC) wire immediately after bracket placement.

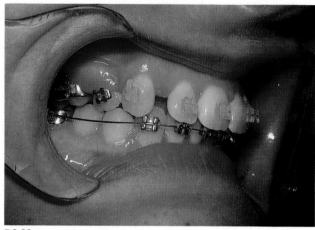

D6.23

Figure D6.23 Three months into treatment. The extraction space is closed. Space closure occurred rapidly due to the presence of osteoclastic activity brought about by the extraction of the bicuspid; 30% of this closure was the result of the tipping of the teeth.

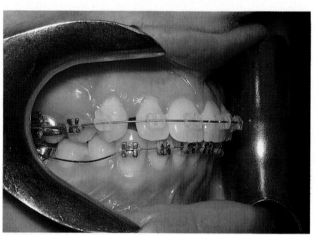

D6.24

Figure D6.24 Five months into treatment, the tipped teeth have uprighted into a solid class I occlusion simply by holding them tied together (with a ligature figure-8 pattern) as the prescription in the preadjusted appliance bracket system is given the time to "work-out" in relation to the wire.

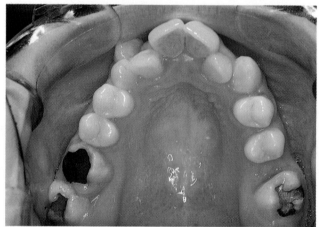

D6.25

Figure D6.25 This case shows a retained right primary cuspid, moderate crowding on the same side, and spacing on the opposite side from the previous extraction of the left first permanent molar. It was decided to extract the right first molar and alleviate the crowding.

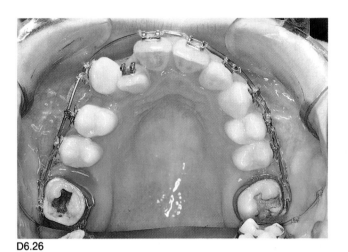

D6.26

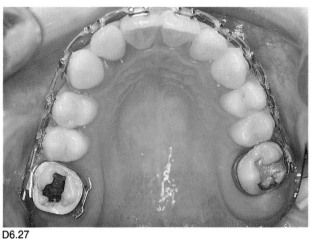

D6.27

Figure D6.26 A superelastic, rectangular NeoSentalloy (GAC) wire was placed and space closure was initiated immediately after bracket placement, 1 week after the extraction of the first molar (to take advantage of the presence of osteoclastic and osteoblastic activity in the extraction side). Within 3 months, the 10-mm extraction space had been reduced to only 3 mm. Also note how rapidly the right cuspid is moving into the space provided by the extraction of the retained primary tooth.

Figure D6.27 Five months into treatment. The superelastic wire allowed for quiet space closure and easy alignment of the cuspid tooth into the arch.

Open Bites	Deep Bites
1. Placement of upper anterior brackets more gingivally	Normal placement of upper anterior brackets
2. Banding of lower second molars late in treatment if needed	Banding of lower second molars early in treatment
3. Placement of molar bands or brackets more occlusally	Normal placement of posterior bands and brackets.
4. Preservation of the curve of Spee in the archwires	Placement of reverse curve of Spee in the lower arch and accentuated in the upper
5. Use of flexible rectangular archwires (NiTi's)	Use of stiff rectangular archwires (stainless steel)
6. Placement of lingual crown torque on the upper molars if needed	No additional torque necessary
7. Use of high pull headgear as needed	Use of low occipital headgear as needed
8. Use of bonded RME appliances for expansion as needed	Use of hygienic banded RME appliances for expansion as needed

D6.28

Figure D6.28 Open versus deep-bite orthodontic mechanotherapy.

References

1. Andreasen GF, and Hilleman TB: An evaluation of 55 cobalt substituted nitinol wire for use in orthodontics. J Am Dent Assoc 82:1373–1375, 1972.
2. Andreasen GF, and Morrow RD: Laboratory and clinical analyses of nitinol wire. Am J Orthod 73:142–151, 1978.
3. Lopez I, Goldberg J, and Burstone CJ: Bending characteristics of nitinol wire. Am J Orthod 75:569–575, 1979.
4. Watanabe K: Studies on new superelastic NiTi orthodontic wire, part 1. Japanese Journal of Dental Materials 1:47–57, 1982.
5. Burstone CJ, Qin B, and Morton JY: Chinese NiTi wire—a new orthodontic alloy. Am J Orthod 87:445–452, 1985.
6. Miura F, Mogi M, Ohura Y, and Hamanaka H: The superelastic property of the Japanese NiTi alloy wire for use in orthodontics. Am J Orthod 90:1–10, 1986.
7. Miura F, Mogi M, and Okamoto Y: New application of superelastic NiTi rectangular wire. J Clin Orthod 24:544–548, 1990.
8. Johnson E, and Lee RS: Relative stiffness of orthodontic wires. J Clin Orthod 23:353–363, 1989.
9. Proffit WR, and White RP: *Surgical–Orthodontic Treatment.* St. Louis, MO: C.V. Mosby Co., 1991.
10. Oakes C, and Hatcher JE: Determining physiologic archforms. J Clin Orthod 25:79–80, 1991.
11. Creekmore TD: The importance of interbracket width in orthodontic tooth movement. J Clin Orthod 10:530–534, 1976.
12. Kuzy RP, and Greenberg AR: Comparison of the elastic properties of nickel-titanium and beta titanium arch wires. Am J Orthod 81:199, 1982.
13. Proffit WR: *Contemporary Orthodontics.* St. Louis, MO: C.V. Mosby Co., 1986.

Chapter 7

Archforms

Determination of the correct archform is one of the most important aspects of orthodontic treatment.[1,2] The archform, especially in the mandible, cannot be permanently expanded by appliance therapy. The mandibular model with all permanent teeth present provides the best basis for construction of a correct or physiologic archform. Although preformed arches have been made using various geometric or computer-generated data, the fit to an individual mandibular model is highly variable.

It is recommended that the clinician place a sheet of tracing paper over the mandibular cast at the onset of treatment and mark with dots the most outer point of the buccal surfaces of all the teeth.[1] The points should then be connected to form the dental archform of treatment for the mandibular wires. The maxillary wires should always be coordinated with the mandibular ones (Fig. D7.1); otherwise various discrepancies may occur (Figs. D7.2 through D7.5).

In the event that there is excess buccal overjet on the right posterior dentition and an end-to-end (no overjet) on the left side, the upper archwire is skewed to the left side (Fig. D7.6). Occasionally, a reverse curve of Spee is added in the lower archwire during space closure with elastomeric chains (Fig. D7.7). In the upper arch, we can simply increase the curve. This prevents the teeth from tipping lingually, but it also tends to extrude the bicuspids and flare the anteriors.

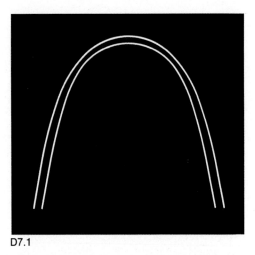

D7.1

Figure D7.1 Coordinated archwires must be used from the onset of treatment so that a normal buccolingual relationship (transverse dimension) can be achieved from the earlier stages of corrective orthodontic mechanotherapy.

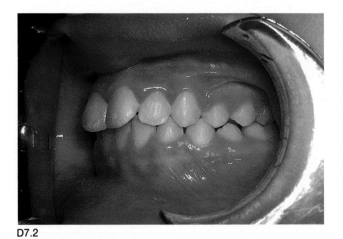

D7.2

Figure D7.2 Patient before treatment. Note the good buccal intercuspation of teeth.

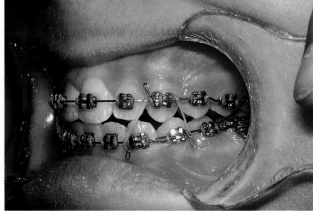

D7.3

Figure D7.3 Development of posterior open bite from incorrect bracket placement and arch incoordination. Same patient as in Figure D7.2.

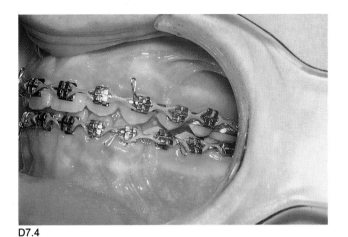

D7.4

Figure D7.4 Patient in fixed appliances during space closure.

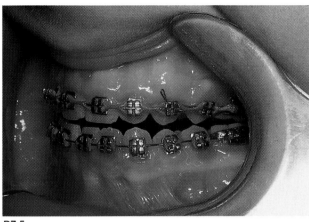

D7.5

Figure D7.5 Incorrect bracket placement, lack of coordination in the archwires, and lingual tipping of teeth during space closure led to the development of this open-bite situation. Same patient as in Figure D7.4.

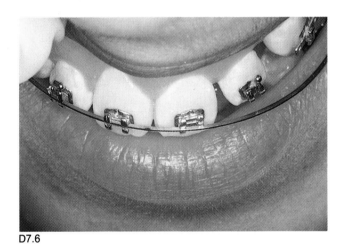

D7.6

Figure D7.6 Archwire "skewed" to the left.

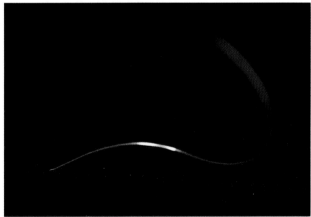

D7.7

Figure D7.7 Reverse curve of Spee in the lower archwire. This wire configuration is available for NiTi wires. Stainless steel archwires can be bent to this shape quite easily with the thumb.

References

1. Oakes C, and Hatcher JE: Determining physiologic archforms. J Clin Orthod 25:79–80, 1991.
2. Proffit WR, and White RP: *Surgical–Orthodontic Treatment.* St. Louis, MO: C.V. Mosby Co., 1991.

Chapter 8

Coil Springs

The most important characteristic of the Japanese NiTi alloy coil springs is the ability to exert a very long range of constant, light, continuous force over months for a single activation.[1-3] The new Sentalloy (GAC) coil springs have opened new horizons in the treatment of anteroposterior discrepancies,[2-3] *i.e.,* the correction of a full class II malocclusion into a class I occlusion with 4 to 7 mm of sequential distal movement of all maxillary teeth (Figs. D8.1 through D8.36). It is very important to note that this posterior movement is bodily in nature. According to the literature,[1,3] the superelastic coils should produce distal movement of posterior teeth at a rate of 1 to 1.5 mm/ month. Adjunctive headgear therapy, along with the juvenile and pubertal growth spurts, make the correction of Class II malocclusion in contemporary orthodontics an easy task to accomplish.

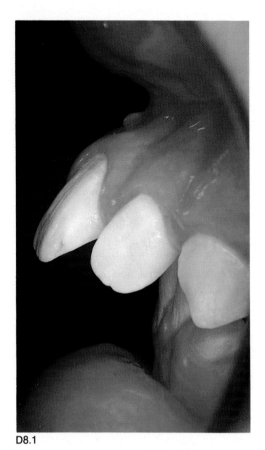

D8.1

Figure D8.1 Typical class II, division I with a 12-mm over-jet. In the past, cases such as this one were treated with headgear for at least 2 to 3 years (for correction of the 7-mm class II discrepancy into a class I occlusion) or with extraction of the upper first bicuspids. These cases can now be treated without extraction with the sequential use of the superelastic Sentalloy (GAC) coil springs.

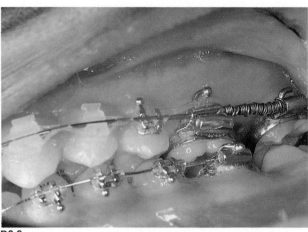

D8.2

Figure D8.2 A 100 g light section of the superelastic coil spring is compressed between the first and second molars, immediately after bracket and wire placement (from the first appointment of the patient's treatment). The initial wire is a superelastic rectangular wire. An elastomeric chain may also be placed from the onset of treatment from the first molar to the one on the opposite side in order to close any anterior spaces and retract the flared anteriors. This photograph is 2 months into treatment.

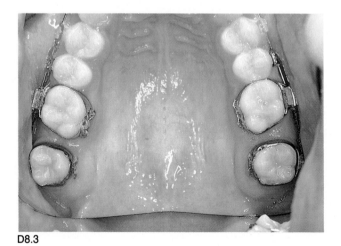

D8.3

Figure D8.3 Occlusal view. Note the significant second molar movement (2 to 3 mm) distally.

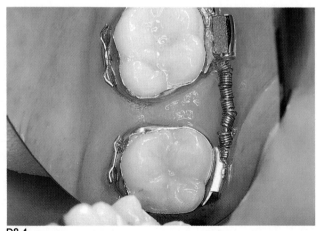

D8.4

Figure D8.4 Closer view. The typical mesial rotation of the class II molars is simultaneously corrected as the molars are moved distally.

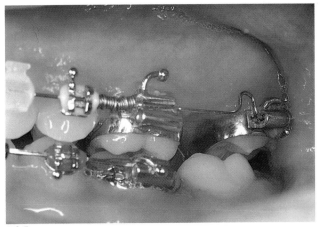

D8.5

Figure D8.5 After 4 months into treatment, the second molar has moved 6 mm distally in a 1- to 2-mm over-corrected position. A stop is placed in the archwire in front of the second molar to prevent its mesial movement during the distal movement of the first molar. The same coil spring is used again, but this time it is compressed between the second bicuspid and first molar. The archwire is now a 0.016 × 0.016 inch^2 stainless steel that allows placement of the stop in the archwire (the superelastic wires are difficult to bend).

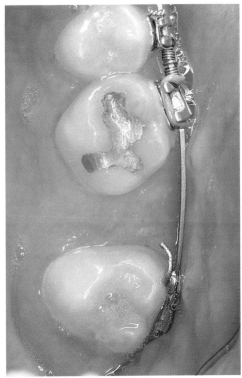

D8.6

Figure D8.6 This photograph, of another patient, shows the extent of distal movement of the molar that can be obtained (7 to 8 mm).

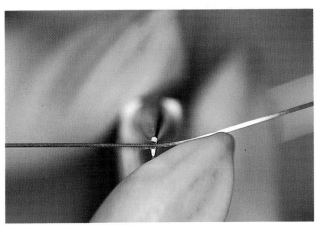

D8.7

Figure D8.7 The stop in front of the molar is fabricated around the round part of the birdbeak pliers.

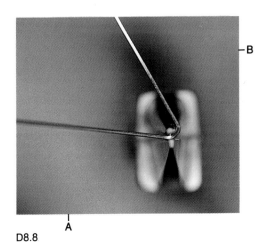

A

D8.8

Figure D8.8 The wire (segment B) is bent at a 45-degree angle to segment A.

B

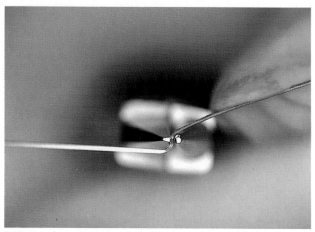

D8.9

Figure D8.9 Segment B is brought back down again.

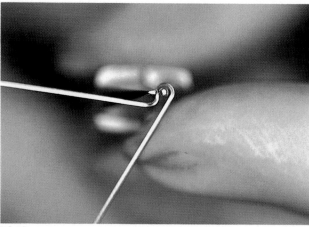

D8.10

Figure D8.10 The stop (in the form of a loop) is formed around the beak of the pliers.

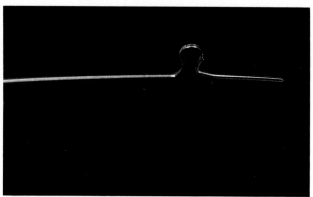

D8.11

Figure D8.11 The molar stop.

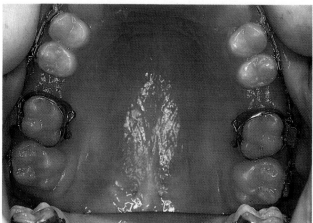

D8.12

Figure D8.12 After distal movement of the first molar teeth on a patient after 9 months of treatment.

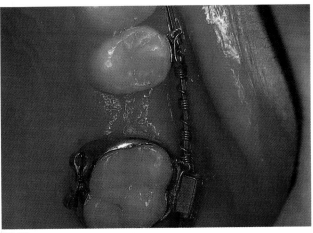

D8.13

Figure D8.13 Deactivated coil spring after significant distal molar movement.

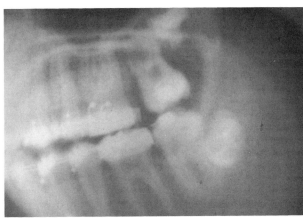

D8.14

Figure D8.14 Radiograph showing the second molar in its overcorrected position. Note the position of its roots in reference to their proximity to the first molar roots.

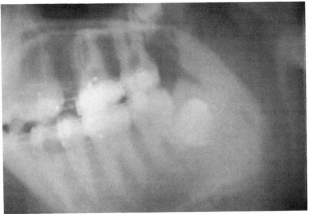

D8.15

Figure D8.15 Radiograph after the distal movement of the first molar is completed. Note that during this period, the second molar roots have uprighted (they are not in proximity with the first molar roots any longer). In essence, both molars have moved posteriorly bodily about 6 mm. This happens because, as the second molars are held in the overcorrected position (with the stop in the archwires), the roots upright on their own and with some aid from the moment created by the high-pull headgear appliance (see later), above the center of resistance of the molar teeth.

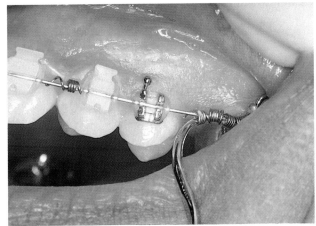

D8.16

Figure D8.16 The coil spring can be easily reactivated without taking out the main archwire, simply by compressing it distally with a scaler and adding the residual springs from the adjacent interbracket area. The clinician should try to avoid cutting the springs in a way that may impinge on the soft tissue. As soon as all posterior teeth and the cuspid have been sequentially brought back with the coil springs, the four incisor teeth can then be retracted with elastomeric chains.

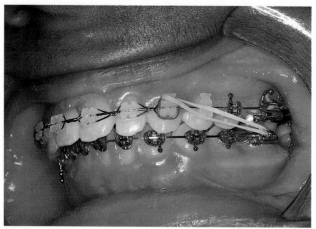

D8.17

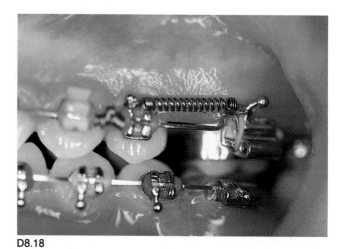

D8.18

Figure D8.17 During the movement of the second molar distally, there should not be any significant reaction from the coil spring anteriorly (*i.e.,* increased overjet). The three roots of the second molar move faster than the roots of all the rest of the teeth anterior to the second molar (three of the first molar, three of the bicuspids, three of the cuspid and incisor teeth; total: nine) because the root ratio is 3:9 or 1:3. When we attempt to move the first molar, the ratio increases to 3:6 or 1:2. It is during this period that there is an increased possibility for adverse effects anteriorly. At this point, we may elect to reinforce the distal movement of the first molar tooth with daytime use of elastics and nighttime use of high-pull headgear. The headgear appliance may also help with the uprighting movement of the molar roots as they move distally. When it is time to retract the second bicuspids, the root ratio is 1:5. The elastics or headgear may be discontinued at this point, because they are no longer as necessary to reinforce the anchorage requirements. It is the distal movement of the molar teeth that is most critical. If one wants to ensure that no anchorage loss will occur during this period (3 to 4 months for each molar: total 6 to 8 months), especially in a full class II case, then headgear is advised. The patient is still happy because he or she does not have to wear the headgear for the full 2 years of therapy, unless an orthopedic (skeletal) effect is desired.

Figure D8.18 The distal movement of the bicuspid teeth can be reinforced with a Sentalloy (GAC) closed coil spring that extends from the first molar hook to a hook on the bicuspid bracket. The stop in the archwire right in front of the first molar prevents its movement mesially.

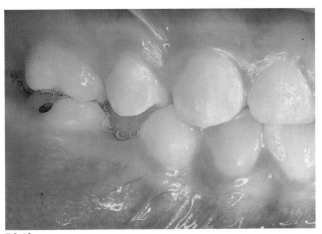

D8.19

Figure D8.19 This is a case of unilateral maxillary right second bicuspid impaction due to premature exfoliation of the second primary molar and mesial drift and rotation of the first permanent molar, which brought this tooth in contact with the first bicuspid. The mesial rotation also brought the first molar into a class II 50% relationship with the mandibular molar. Note the class I cuspid relationship and normal overjet.

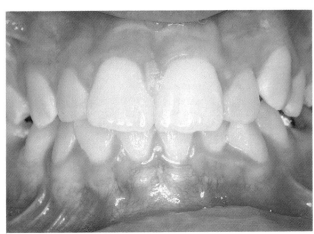

D8.20

Figure D8.20 Anterior view. Note the normal overbite.

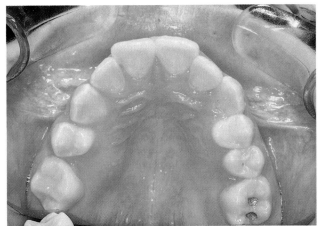

D8.21

Figure D8.21 It was decided to use a flexible NiTi coil spring to move the right first molar tooth distally.

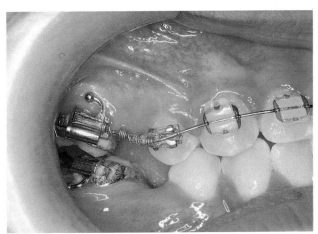

D8.22

Figure D8.22 After only 5 weeks, on return of the patient for her first adjustment appointment, the molar had moved distally more than 4 mm! The cuspid was still in a class I occlusion and the overjet was the same as before, thus emphasizing that the adverse effects of this system (increase in the overjet, flaring of the anterior teeth) are kept to a minimum or that they do not have the time to express themselves before the desired distal molar movement takes place.

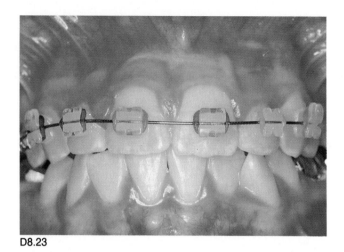

D8.23

Figure D8.23 Anterior view. Note that the overbite has decreased due to initial alignment and leveling.

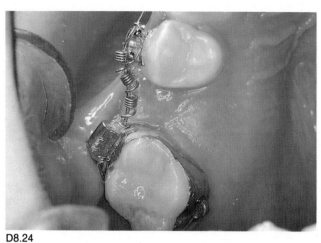

D8.24

Figure D8.24 Closer view of the space that has been created.

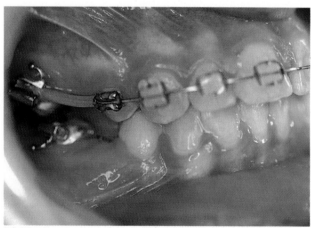

D8.25

Figure D8.25 Three months into treatment and the molar tooth has been moved distally 7 mm! The coil spring has been substituted with plastic tube that maintains the opened space.

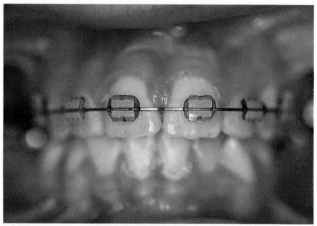

D8.26

Figure D8.26 The anterior view shows that the overjet is normal (2 mm).

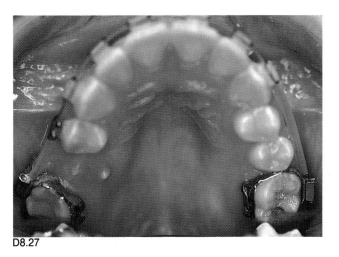

D8.27

Figure D8.27 The occlusal view shows that the second bicuspid is erupting on its own in the space that has been provided for it.

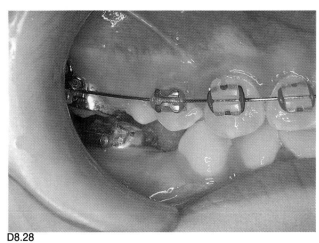

D8.28

Figure D8.28 Five months into treatment, the newly erupted second bicuspid can be seen from the buccal view. Note the full class I cuspid relationship.

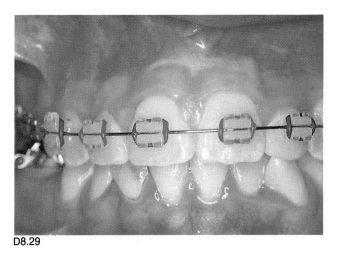

D8.29

Figure D8.29 Anterior view. Note the stable normal overbite.

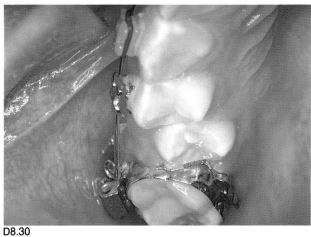

D8.30

Figure D8.30 Closer view of the erupting second bicuspid.

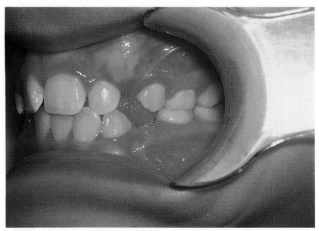

D8.31

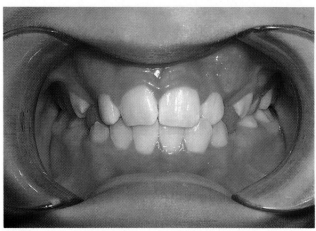

D8.32

Figures D8.31 and D8.32 This patient demonstrates a malocclusion of minor to moderate (5 mm) crowding in the maxillary arch in the cuspid region, just enough to block the cuspid teeth from erupting in their normal positions.

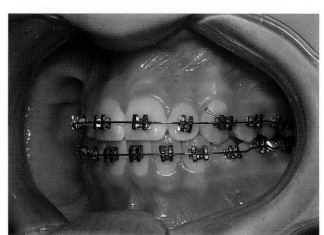

D8.33

Figure D8.33 Use of coil springs between the lateral incisors and first bicuspid teeth provides the extra 2 mm needed on each side to accommodate the cuspid teeth, which otherwise would have stayed in the labial position as they erupted through the soft tissue. The use of flexible NiTi wires brought the cuspid teeth into their final position in the arch. The total treatment time is kept again to less than a year.

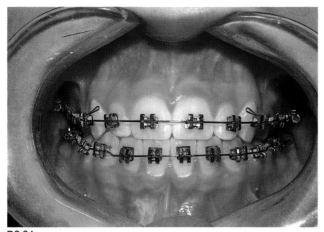

D8.34

Figures D8.34 and D8.35 Anterior view. The overbite has decreased by 1 mm due to the patient's slight vertical growth pattern.

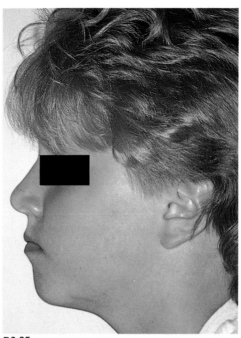

D8.35

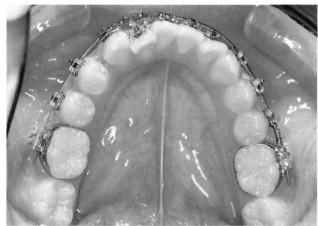

D8.36

Figure D8.36 Use of a NiTi coil spring in the anterior region to move the left cuspid distally and provide space for the lateral incisor.

References

1. Gianelly AA, Bednar J, and Dietz VS: Japanese NiTi coil used to move molars distally. Am J Orthod Dentofacial Orthop 99:564–566, 1991.
2. Miura F, Mogi M, Ohura Y, and Karibe M: The super-elastic Japanese NiTi alloy wire for use in orthodontics. Am J Orthod Dentofacial Orthop 94:89–96, 1988.
3. Gianelly A: Class II nonextraction treatment using Sentalloy coils. Summarized by Hawley BP, Pacific Coast Society of Orthodontists Bulletin 50–51, 1991.

Chapter 9

Elastometric Chain Modules

Elastomeric chain modules (power chains or C-chains) are used in sliding mechanotherapy primarily to close spaces.[1-4] The elastic chain is hooked on the most posterior molar tooth that is banded and is then stretched and placed on every bracket of each tooth all the way around the arch to the most posterior molar tooth (Figs. D9.1 through D9.10). The "pull" of the chain has two major side effects: mesial molar rotation and lingual "dumping" of all the teeth of the arch. These are counteracted with a distal "toe-in" bend in a rectangular stainless steel archwire in the molar region and an increased curve of Spee in the upper and reverse curve in the lower wire.

When attempting to correct the rotation of various teeth, one may easily do so with the help of elastic chains, in addition to the full engagement of the rectangular NiTi superelastic wire in the bracket slots. No wire-tie should be placed on the tooth to be rotated, so that the moment created by the force vector of the elastic chain may "spin" the tooth freely around its axis. The other side of the chain will be placed on a tooth that is wire tied onto the rectangular superelastic wire, unless this also needs to rotate, but in the opposite direction (Figs. D9.11 through D9.35).

Elastomeric chains should be changed every 4 to 5 weeks. If they are replaced every 2 to 3 weeks, initial tipping occurs, but the tooth does not have time to upright[2] (root movement) as the force of the chain dissipates, thus accentuating the tipping of teeth during space closure and not promoting the desired bodily tooth movement.

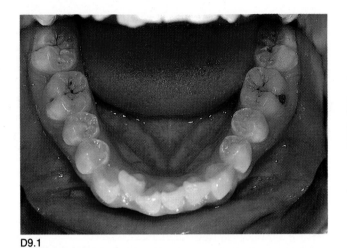

D9.1

Figure D9.1 This patient presented with bimaxillary dentoalveolar protrusion that led to the extraction of the upper first and lower second bicuspid teeth (despite the moderate crowding).

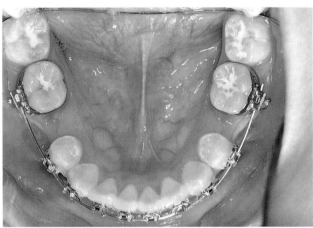

D9.2

Figure D9.2 Two months into treatment, the teeth were aligned with a 0.016×0.022-inch^2 rectangular Neosentalloy (GAC) wire.

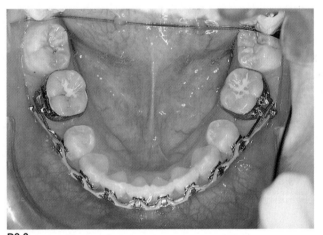

D9.3

Figure D9.3 Elastomeric chains were placed from molar to molar. Shown here is 4 months into treatment. The archwire is a finishing stainless steel 0.016×0.022 inch^2.

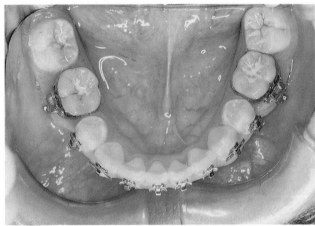

D9.4

Figure D9.4 Monthly change of the chains led to almost completion of space closure 8 months into treatment. Reverse curve of Spee added to the flat archwire. Note the slight lingual rotation of the left first molar from the "pull" of the chain due to the absence of a "toe-in" bend in the wire in front of the molar.

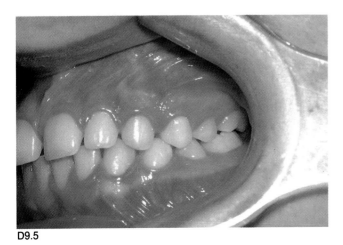

D9.5

Figure D9.5 This is a case of generalized spacing on both arches, with a solid class I molar and cuspid relationship.

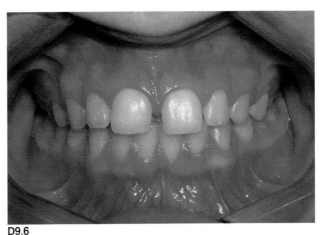

D9.6

Figure D9.6 The OB/OJ relationship is normal (2 mm).

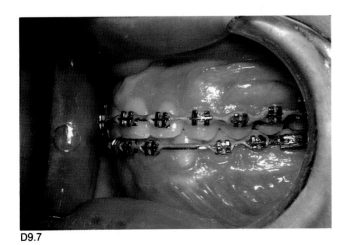

D9.7

Figure D9.7 Ideal bracket placement and the use of two sets of wires, a rectangular 0.016×0.022-inch^2 NiTi for initial alignment and a 0.016×0.022-inch^2 rectangular stainless steel with elastic chains to close the spaces, brought this case to completion in less than a year.

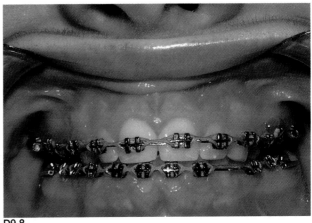

D9.8

Figure D9.8 No bends in the archwire were made. The only adjustments were monthly changes of the chains (done by the assistant) and a slight increase of the curve of Spee of the straight archwires to avoid lingual tipping of teeth during space closure.

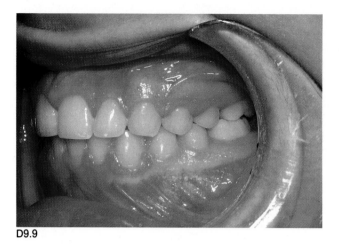

D9.9

Figure D9.9 Patient after 8 months of active treatment.

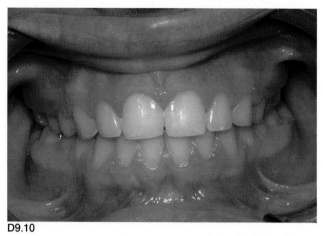

D9.10

Figure D9.10 The OB/OJ relationship has remained normal (2 mm).

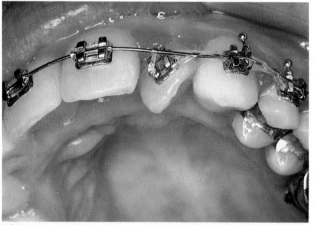

D9.11

Figure D9.11 Placement of elastic chain from the lateral incisor to the ipsilateral first molar for the correction of the rotation on the incisor teeth. Note the "stretch" of the chain around the bracket wings.

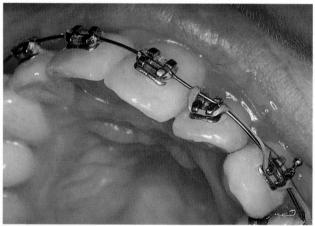

D9.12

Figure D9.12 Two months into treatment (chain was changed once). Note that half of the rotation has been corrected.

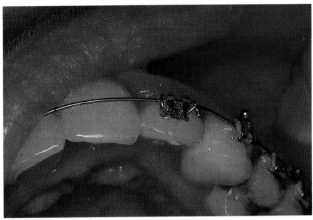

D9.13

Figure D9.13 The incisor rotation was corrected in 4 months. The anchorage of the posterior teeth did not allow them to rotate during this procedure.

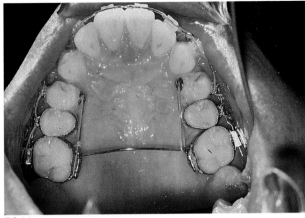

D9.14

Figure D9.14 Lingual buttons on the first bicuspid teeth and the addition of elastic chains to "spin" the teeth around their long axis, with the help of the TPA appliance.

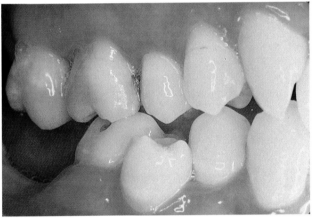

D9.15

Figures D9.15 through D9.19 This adult patient has a class I molar relationship on the right side and a class III 50% on the left with moderate maxillary and severe mandibular crowding, 7 and 10 mm, respectively. Due to the severe crowding and the blocked-out lower second bicuspids, all second bicuspids were extracted in order to be able to end up with a class I cuspid relationship. Although the upper first bicuspids could have been extracted instead of the second, it was estimated that it would be rather simple to obtain a solid class I relationship on both sides with sliding mechanotherapy while keeping the extractions symmetrical. Note that the cuspids are in a class II 50% relationship due to the blocked-out second mandibular bicuspids that have allowed the teeth anterior to them to slip distally.

Illustrations continued on following page.

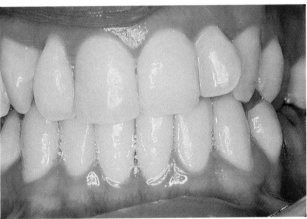

D9.16

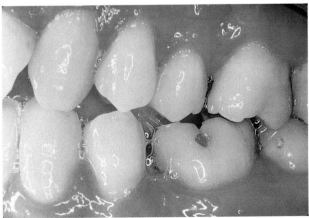

D9.17

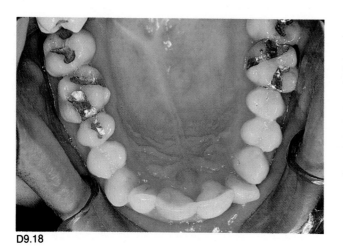

D9.18

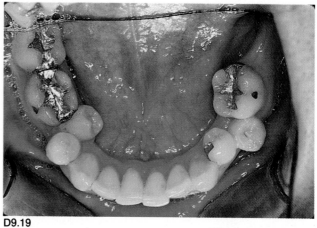

D9.19

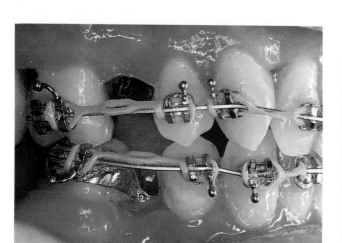

D9.20

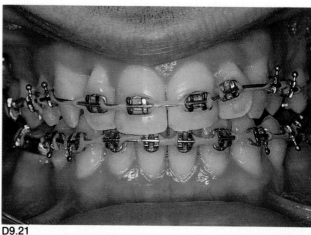

D9.21

Figures D9.20 through D9.22 It was decided to treat this case with only two sets of wires: an initial 0.016×0.022-inch^2 superelastic Neosentalloy-NiTi rectangular wire, which would allow for torque control from the onstart of treatment, and a finishing 0.016×0.022-inch^2 stainless steel rectangular wire. Shown here are the initial superelastic wires engaged in the bracket slots without any deformation. The superelasticity of these wires allows for a gentle rotation and leveling of the teeth during the initial phases of treatment. The elastic chains help in the derotation of the teeth by the simple pull that they exert on the teeth as they force them to rotate around themselves (their long axis). The upper and lower right first bicuspids are being pulled by the three-unit c-chains attached to the molars; the four-unit c-chain from the left upper cuspid to the opposite central helps derotate the cuspid tooth (the central is wire tied with a ligature wire around the main archwire so that it will not rotate itself); the upper right lateral derotates with the help of the five-unit chain that extends all the way to the upper right molar tooth; the lower right cuspid as well as the opposite left first bicuspid both rotate around their long axes from the equal and opposite forces exerted by the elastic chain.

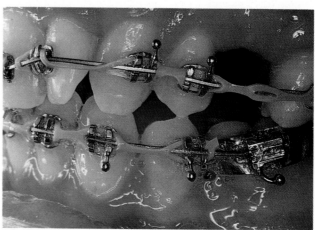

D9.22

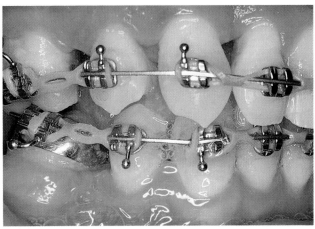

D9.23

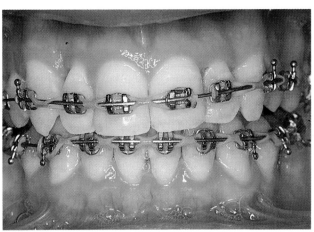

D9.24

Figures D9.23 through D9.25 The result of the effect of the elastic chains: complete rotation of the teeth after 2 months of treatment.

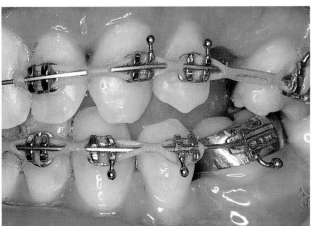

D9.25

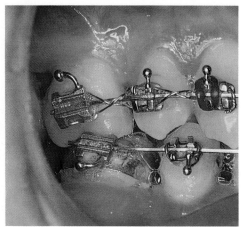

D9.26

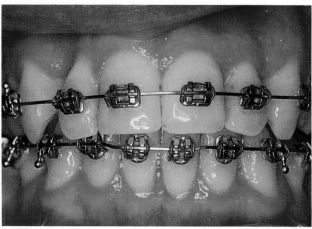

D9.27

Figures D9.26 through D9.28 A class I molar and cuspid relationship has been achieved and the midlines are on; 5 months into treatment.

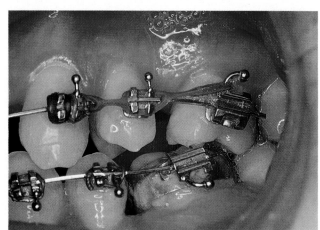

D9.28

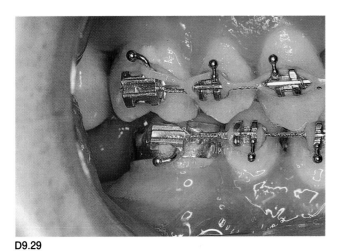

D9.29

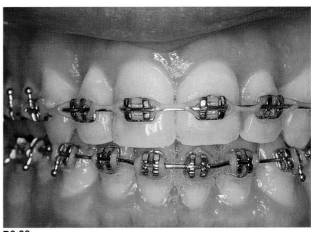

D9.30

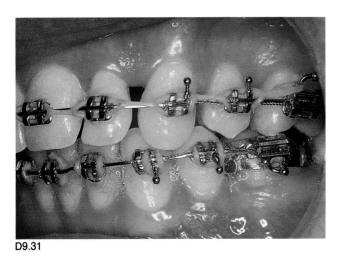

D9.31

Figures D9.29 through D9.31 Ten months into treatment. Elastomeric chains help close any remaining spaces. Note the good class I intercuspation.

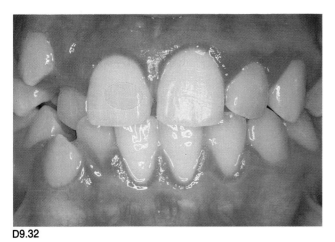

D9.32

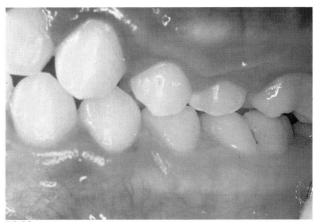

D9.33

Figures D9.32 and D9.33 This patient has an asymmetry of the dental arches, which led to the extraction of the left first bicuspids.

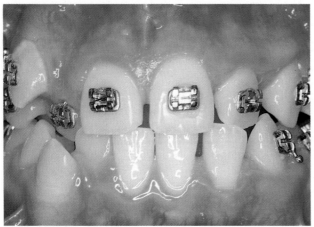

D9.34

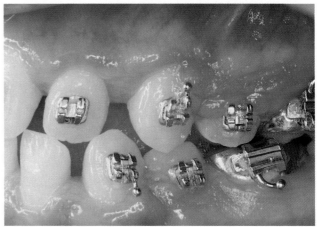

D9.35

Figures D9.34 and D9.35 After the cuspid teeth were retracted, note how the lateral incisors drifted distally (causing spacing in the arch) on their own without any orthodontic mechanotherapy. This is "free" movement, which one should be aware of and take advantage of during treatment.

References

1. Graber LW: *Orthodontics—State of the Art, Essence of the Science.* St. Louis, MO: C.V. Mosby Co., 1986.
2. Graber TM, and Swain BF: *Orthodontics—Current Principles and Techniques.* St. Louis, MO: C.V. Mosby Co., 1985.
3. Alexander RG: *The Alexander Discipline.* Glendora, CA: Ormco Co., 1986.
4. McLaughlin RP, and Bennet TC: The transition from standard edgewise to preadjusted appliance systems. J Clin Orthod 23:142–153, 1989.

Chapter 10

Orthodontic Elastics

Elastics have been a valuable adjunct of any orthodontic treatment for many years.[1-4] Their use, combined with good patient cooperation, provides the clinician with the ability to correct both anteroposterior and vertical discrepancies.[1-4] They are used primarily with rectangular archwires.[1-4] The introduction of the flexible rectangular NiTi wires allows the clinician to obtain immediate torque control from the onset of orthodontic mechanotherapy and thus use elastics from the beginning of treatment.[5]

The following elastics are suggested for clinical use.

Anteroposterior Elastics

Class I Elastics (Fig. D10.1) extend within each arch (intra-arch elastics) and are primarily used to close spaces, in aid of the elastomeric chains.

Class II Elastics (Figs. D10.2 and D10.3) extend from the lower molar teeth to the upper cuspids (interarch elastics). They are primarily used to cause anteroposterior tooth changes; *i.e.,* aid in obtaining a class I cuspid relationship from a class II relationship. If the lower second molars are banded and included in the treatment mechanotherapy, it is best to extend the elastic from the first molar to the cuspid tooth to avoid extrusion of the second molar and the creation of an open bite anteriorly. If the lower second molars are not banded, it is best to extend the elastics from the second bicuspids to the upper cuspids (or even to the lateral incisors for a longer horizontal vector) if they are to be used for over 2 months of treatment. If elastics are to be used for 2 to 6 weeks only, then one may extend them from the lower first molars to the upper cuspid teeth. This treatment regimen minimizes the side effects from the use of elastics (extrusion of the lower posterior teeth and labial tipping of the lower anterior teeth, lowering of the anterior occlusal plane and the creation of a gummy smile). If any temporomandibular joint discomfort occurs, elastics should be discontinued, at least temporarily.

Class III Elastics (Figs. D10.4 and D10.5) are the exact opposite of the class IIs: they extend from the upper molars to the lower cuspids and are used in the treatment of class III cases. They promote extrusion of the upper posterior teeth and flaring of the upper anteriors, along with lingual tipping of the lower anteriors. The same principles discussed above apply for class III elastics as well.

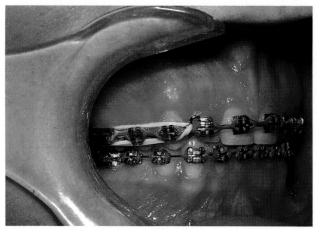

D10.1

Figure D10.1 Class I elastic from the upper first molar to the cuspid tooth.

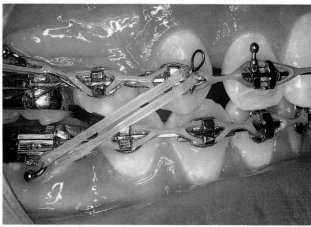

D10.2

Figure D10.2 Class II elastic from the lower first molar to the upper cuspid.

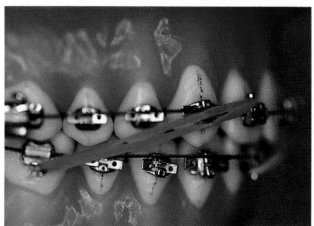

D10.3

Figure D10.3 Long class II elastic (used to increase the horizontal effect of the elastic).

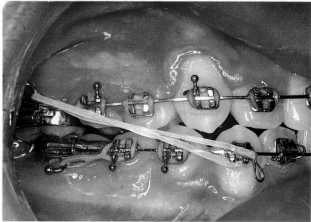

D10.4

Figure D10.4 Class III elastic from the upper first molar to the lower cuspid.

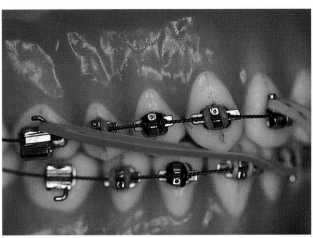

D10.5

Figure D10.5 Long class III elastic (for increased horizontal effect).

Vertical Elastics

Triangle Elastics (Figs. D10.6 through D10.13) aid in the improvement of class I cuspid intercuspation and increasing the overbite relationship anteriorly by closing open bites in the range of 0.5 to 1.5 mm. They extend from the upper cuspid to the lower cuspid and first bicuspid teeth.

Box Elastics (Figs. D10.14 and D10.15) have a box-shape configuration and can be used in a variety of situations to promote tooth extrusion and improve intercuspation. Most commonly, they include the upper cuspid and lateral incisor to the lower first bicuspid and cuspid (class II vector) or to the lower cuspid and lateral incisor (class III vector). All bicuspid teeth of one side can be extruded as well.

Text continued on page 194.

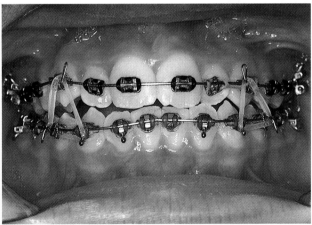

D10.6

Figure D10.6 Triangular vertical elastics. Note the slight open bite.

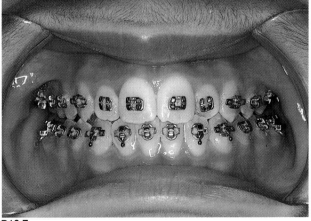

D10.7

Figure D10.7 Within 2 months, the open bite is closed. Rectangular Neosentalloy (GAC) NiTi wires are the archwires used in both arches from the start of treatment.

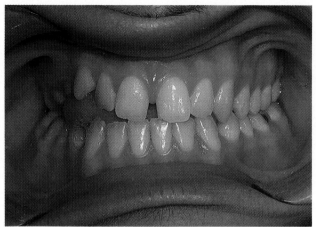

D10.8

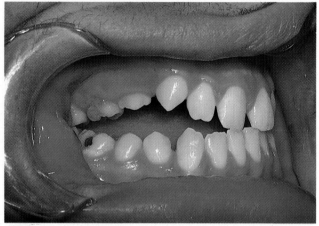

D10.9

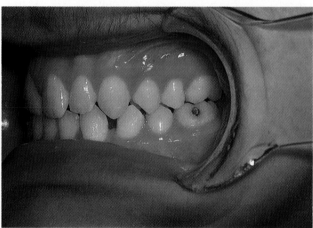

D10.10

Figures D10.8 through D10.10 This case demonstrates a severe right posterior open bite caused by the ankylosed, retained primary first and second molars (no successors were present). Note the almost ideal class I occlusion of the patient's left side. It was decided not to remove the deciduous teeth because of the possible high position of the osseous defect that may have been created. Therefore, extractions of these teeth were postponed until after the open bite has been significantly reduced with vertical elastics.

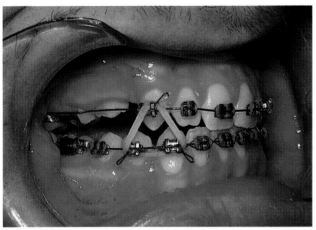

D10.11

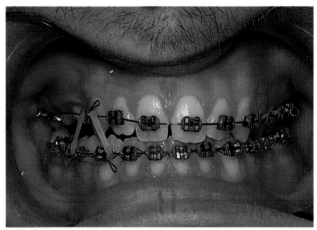

D10.12

Figures D10.11 through D10.13 A 0.016-inch flexible Sentalloy (GAC) round NiTi wire is placed on the maxillary arch and a rigid 0.016×0.022-inch^2 rectangular stainless steel wire on the mandibular arch. This way, the upper cuspid may be extruded without any extrusive side effects of the lower dentition. A heavy triangular elastic is worn 24 h/ day. Note the significant closing obtained in the first 6 months of treatment. The patient is still in therapy.

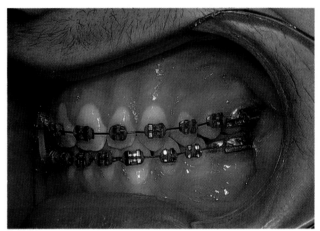

D10.13

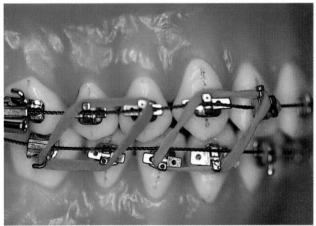

D10.14

Figure D10.14 Box elastics (class II vector).

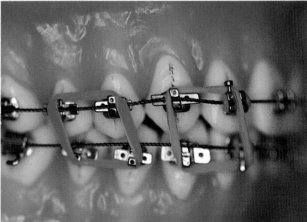

D10.15

Figure D10.15 Box elastics (class III vector).

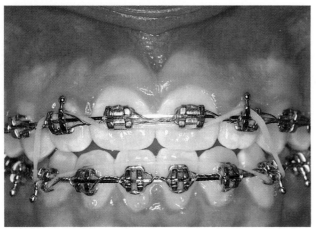

D10.16

D10.17

Figure D10.16 Anterior elastics used toward the end of treatment to close this minimal open bite.

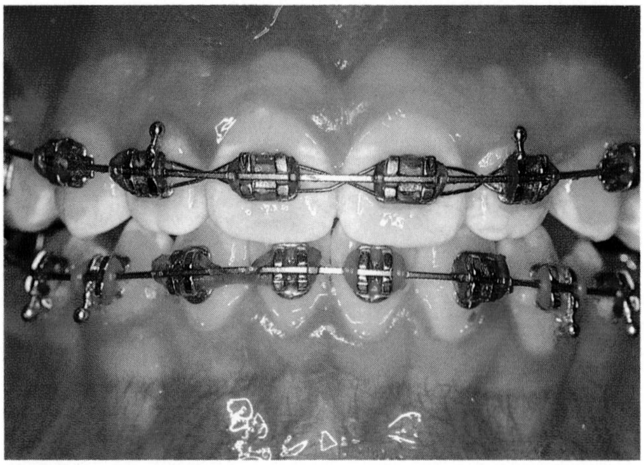

Figure D10.17 After 2 months of elastic wear.

Anterior Elastics (Figs. D10.16 through D10.18) are used to improve the overbite relationship of the incisor teeth. Open bites up to 2 mm may be corrected with these elastics. They may extend from the lower lateral incisors to the upper laterals or central incisor teeth or from the lower cuspids to the upper laterals.

Other Elastics

Asymmetrical Elastics (Fig. D10.19) are usually class II on one side and class III on the other. They are used to correct dental asymmetries. If a significant dental midline deviation is present (2 mm or more), an anterior elastic from the upper lateral to the lower contralateral lateral incisor should also be used.

Finishing Elastics (Figs. D10.20 and D10.21) are used at the end of treatment for final posterior settling. In class II cases, the elastic begins on the maxillary cuspid and continues to the mandibular first bicuspid, and in the same "up-and-down" fashion it finishes at the ballhook of the mandibular first molar band. In an open-bite or class III case, the elastic begins at the lower cuspid, continues to the maxillary cuspid (see below), and finishes at the maxillary molar.

The elastics are attached to ballhooks on the brackets or to K-hooks (heavy ligature wires with an extension). They should preferably be worn full time (24 h/day) for maximum effect, although 12 h/day wear may be indicated to minimize their side effects (Figs. D10.22 through D10.35). They should be changed once or twice a day because the elastics fatigue rapidly (in contrast to the elastomeric chains, which last 3 to 5 weeks). The recommended sizes for the various elastics are (a) *anteroposterior elastics:* $\frac{1}{4}$-inch, 3.5 oz (light) or $\frac{1}{4}$-inch, 6 oz (heavy); (b) *vertical elastics:* $\frac{1}{8}$-inch, 3.5 oz (light) or $\frac{3}{16}$-inch, 6 oz (heavy); and (c) *finishing elastics:* $\frac{3}{4}$-inch, 2 oz.

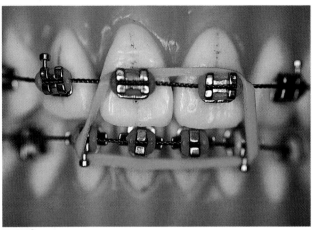

D10.18

Figure D10.18 Anterior elastic from lower laterals to the upper centrals. The effect of the elastic primarily would be on the upper central incisors.

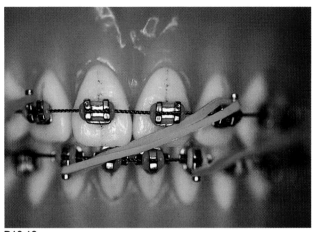

D10.19

Figure D10.19 Asymmetrical elastic to "shift" the midline over to the left.

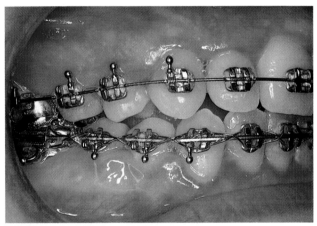

D10.20

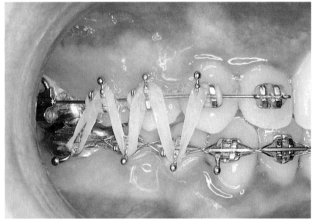

D10.21

Figures D10.20 and D10.21 Finishing elastics. Note the improved intercuspation of the bicuspids after 6 weeks of wear (14 to 16 hr/day).

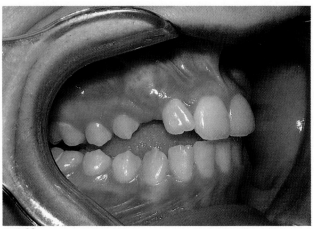

D10.22

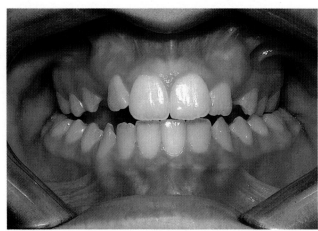

D10.23

Figures D10.22 and D10.23 A 16-year-old girl presented with a class II 50% molar malocclusion, a 4-mm posterior open bite, a borderline anterior open bite, impacted maxillary cuspids, and a bilateral edge-to-edge posterior crossbite. The treatment objective was to close the open bite solely by extruding the maxillary dentition, without undesirable extrusion or tipping of the lower teeth.

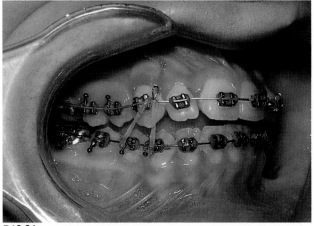

D10.24

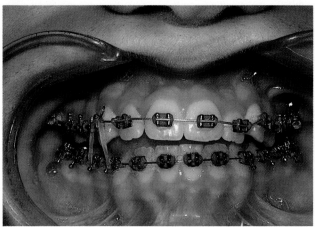

D10.25

Figures D10.24 and D10.25 After initial uncovering of the impacted cuspid, a light (100-g) Neosentalloy (GAC) rectangular NiTi archwire was placed in the upper arch, and a 0.016×0.016-inch^2 stainless steel archwire in the lower. Light triangular vertical elastics were worn full-time, helping to bring the exposed cuspids into the arch. A transpalatal arch, designed to correct the posterior crossbite, initially opened the bite further, as it is shown here 2 months after bracket placement.

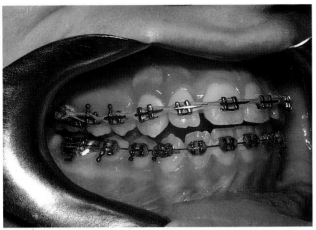

D10.26

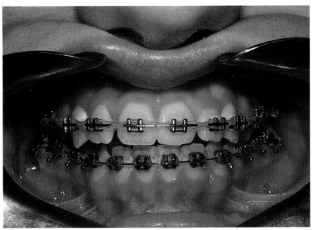

D10.27

Figures D10.26 and D10.27 Three months into treatment, the cuspid teeth are in alignment. Elastomeric chains help consolidate spaces in the upper arch. Elastics (rubber bands) are still being worn to help bring the whole upper dentition more occlusally, because they pull it against the much stiffer lower archwire.

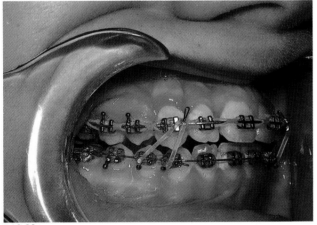

D10.28

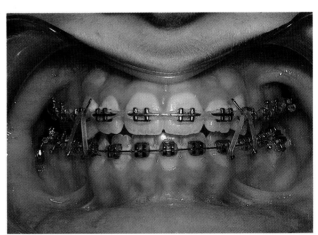

D10.29

Figures D10.28 and D10.29 After 5 months of treatment the posterior open bite had closed significantly. The light elastics continued to be worn full-time.

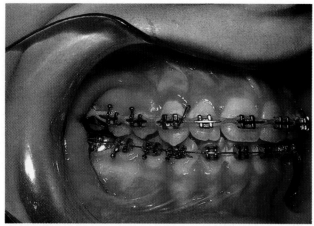

D10.30

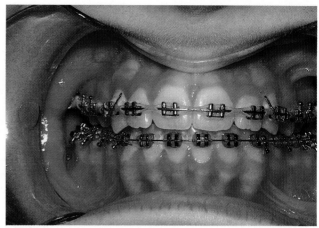

D10.31

Figures D10.30 and D10.31 After 8 months, a harmonious occlusion is almost achieved. Final detailing is to be accomplished with upper and lower 0.016×0.022-inch² stainless steel archwires. This case should be completed in less than a year.

References

1. Proffit WR: *Contemporary Orthodontics.* St. Louis, MO: C.V. Mosby Co., 1986.
2. Alexander RG: *The Alexander Discipline: Contemporary Concepts and Philosophies.* Glendora, CA: Ormco Co., 1986.
3. Alexander RG: Countdown to retention. J Clin Orthod 21:526–527, 1987.
4. Steffen JM, and Haltom FT: The five cent tooth positioner. J Clin Orthod 21:525–529, 1987.
5. Viazis AD: Clinical application of the rectangular NiTi wires. J Clin Orthod 25:370–374, 1991.

Chapter 11

Class I Cuspid Relationship

The first objective of orthodontic mechanotherapy in the anteroposterior dimension is the attainment of a class I cuspid relationship.[1,2] This will not only result in a stable, functional occlusion, but it will also ensure a good overbite (OB) and overjet (OJ) relationship when no tooth size discrepancy is present. The upper central and lateral incisor roots should be slightly convergent, and the remaining upper teeth should show a distal inclination, except for the second molars, which should be mesially tilted. The lower incisors should be upright, and the other lower teeth should be increasingly distally inclined as one moves posteriorly.

In most instances, in order to obtain a class I cuspid relationship, the cuspid tooth needs to move into the extraction space of the first bicuspid without loss of anchorage (Figs. D11.1 through D11.10). All the clinician has to consider is the number of roots to be placed in opposition with each other in each unit. For example, if the posterior unit is composed of the first molar (three roots) and the second bicuspid (one root) and the anterior unit is the cuspid (one large root) and the incisor teeth (two roots), we have a total of four posterior roots against three anterior roots. This will cause both units to move into the extraction space, thus resulting in anchorage loss. When, conversely, individual cuspid retraction is used (one anterior root) and the posterior unit is composed of the second and first molars and the second bicuspid (a total of seven posterior roots), one may easily comprehend that the cuspid tooth will move posteriorly without almost any anchorage loss (*i.e.,* mesial movement of the upper posterior teeth).

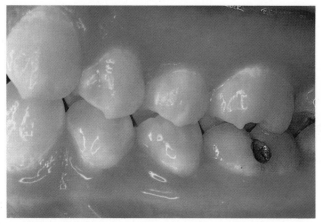

D11.1

Figures D11.1 and D11.2 This patient presents with a class II 50% (end-to-end) molar and cuspid relationship with a midline deviation of 3 mm to the right (the right side is class I). Due to the increased proclination of the dentition, fullness of the profile, the protrusive lips, and the general bimaxillary dentoalveolar outlook of the patient, extractions of the upper first and the lower second bicuspids were performed (the lower first bicuspids could have been extracted instead).

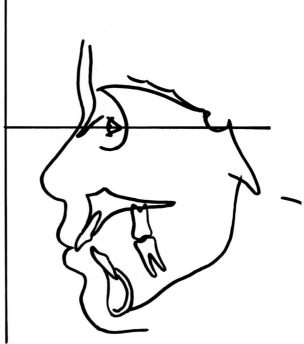

D11.2

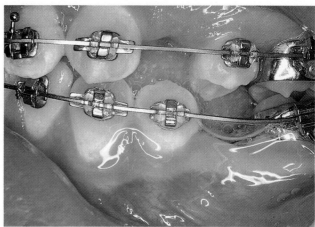

D11.3

Figures D11.3 through D11.8 Rectangular Neosentalloy NiTi (0.016 × 0.022 inch²) initial archwires were placed on both arches. One month into treatment, the teeth are aligned. The next objective of the mechanotherapy is to obtain a class I cuspid relationship. This is very easily done with a superelastic NiTi coil spring between the lateral and cuspid and an elastic chain from the molar to the cuspid tooth. Note that the lateral is wire tied to avoid unnecessary rotation of that tooth. The spring (shown here after 2 months) is left in place until completion of the movement, whereas the elastic chain is changed once a month.

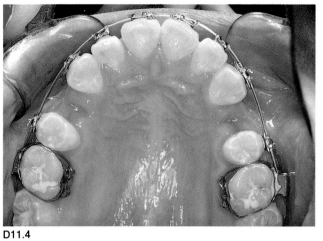

D11.4

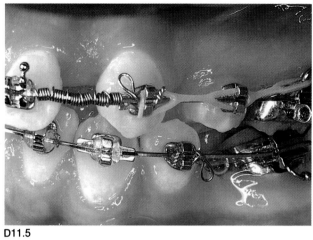

D11.5

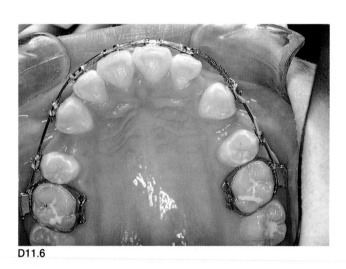

D11.6

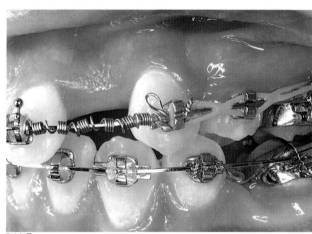

D11.7

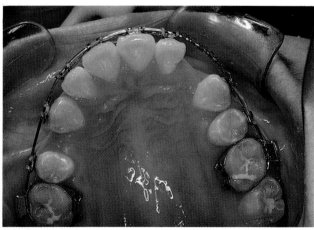

D11.8

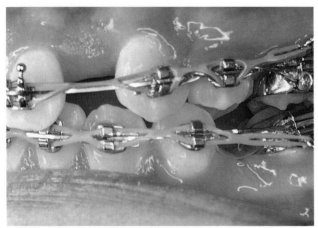

D11.9

Figure D11.9 Five months into treatment, the left cuspid has been moved bodily into a class I relationship and is part of the posterior anchor unit (it is wire tied with a ligature to the posterior teeth). Note that there was no increase in the overjet relationship from the reaction force of the coil spring to the anterior dentition.

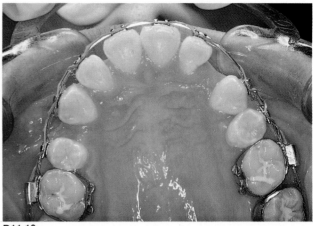

D11.10

Figure D11.10 General space closure may be initiated with elastic chains from molar to molar, upper and lower. Class II elastics are also used at night.

References

1. Proffit WR: *Contemporary Orthodontics.* St. Louis, MO: C.V. Mosby Co., 1984.
2. Graber T, and Swain BF: *Orthodontics: Current Principles and Techniques.* St. Louis, MO: C.V. Mosby Co., 1985.

Part **E**

Adjunctive Appliances

Chapter 1

Rapid Maxillary Expansion (RME) Appliances

One of the first objectives in orthodontic treatment is the correction of any skeletal or dental discrepancies in the transverse dimension. If there is a single-tooth crossbite, dental in nature, full archwire engagement will, in most cases, correct the problem. If the crossbite is skeletal, either bilateral or unilateral in nature, rapid maxillary expansion (RME)[1-14] should be attempted at the start of treatment.

Maxillary expansion appliances may be used to correct unilateral or bilateral posterior crossbites involving several teeth when the discrepancy between the maxillary and mandibular first molar and bicuspid widths is 4 mm or more.[1] The applied pressure acts as an orthopedic force that opens the midpalatal suture.[1] The appliance compresses the periodontal ligament, bends the alveolar processes, tips the anchor teeth, and gradually opens the midpalatal suture.[1] The separation is pyramidal in shape, with the base of the pyramid at the oval side of the bone.[1] The amount of sutural opening is reported to be equal to or less than one half the amount of dental arch expansion.[2-4] The increase in the intermolar width can be as much as 10 mm, with a mean increase of 6 mm.[2-4] During the retention period there is uprighting of the buccal segments; therefore, one can appreciate the need for overcorrection of the dental arches[5,6] (Figs. E1.1 through E1.9).

Because the midpalatal suture may ossify as early as age 15 years and as late as age 27 years, the optimal period for sutural expansion is between 8 and 15 years of age.[7] The appliance should never be regularly activated for a period longer than 1 week against an unyielding suture in the hope of achieving maxillary separation.

It is believed that, during active suture opening, the incisors separate approximately half the distance the screw has been opened.[8] The incisors also upright or tip lingually. This is thought to be caused by the stretched circumoral musculature.[5] On completion of the expansion, the transseptal fibers pull first the crowns and then the roots to their original axial inclinations.[1]

Parallel to the changes in the transverse dimension, the maxilla consistently moves inferiorly and anteriorly to a varying degree, approximately 1 mm.[9,14] The inferior movement of the maxilla,[14] as well as the correction of the crossbites, account for the consequential opening of the mandibular plane angle.[9] The anterior open-bite tendency is sometimes successfully masked by the uprighting incisors.

Advocates of rapid expansion (1 to 4 weeks) believe that it results in minimum tooth movement (tipping) and maximum skeletal displacement (each turn of the screw opens the appliance 0.25 mm). Advocates of slow expansion (2 to 6 months) believe that it produces less tissue resistance in the circummaxillary structures and better bone formation in the intermaxillary suture, and that both factors help to minimize postexpansion relapse.[1]

It has been shown that RME results in concurrent expansion of the lower arch. Haas observed an increase of as much as 4 mm and 6 mm of lower intercuspid and intermolar width, respectively.[5,8] He advocated that the mandibular arch tends to

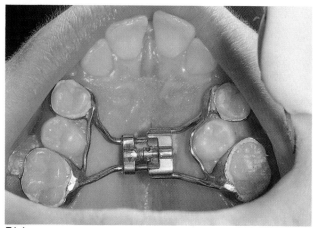

E1.1

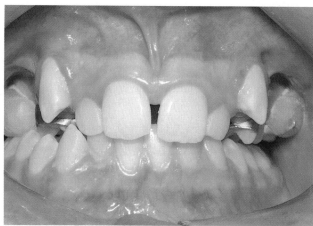

E1.2

Figures E1.1 and E1.2 A 13-year-old boy with bilateral posterior crossbite and a constricted maxilla. A typical Hyrax RME appliance is banded on the first bicuspids and first permanent molars. The screw is activated twice a day (every 12 hours), two turns each time (each turn causes 0.25 mm of expansion). A total of 0.5 mm per day is the desired rate of expansion. Within a week, a midline diastema is created (as shown here). If not, the expansion should be abandoned.

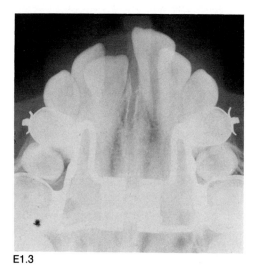

E1.3

Figure E1.3 Opening of the midpalatal suture (radiograph from another patient).

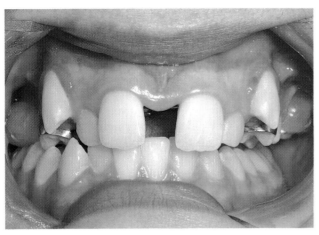

E1.4

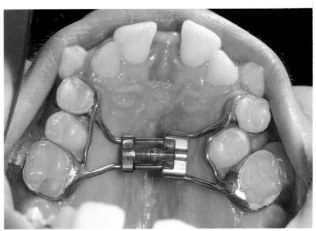

E1.5

Figures E1.4 and E1.5 After $2\frac{1}{2}$ weeks of expansion. Note the significant midline diastema and the increase in arch width. The same result may be achieved within 1 month if the screw is turned only once per day.

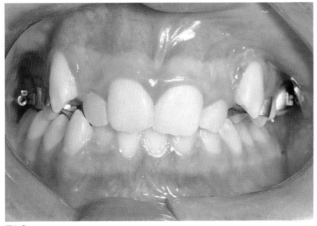

E1.6

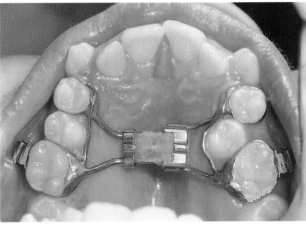

E1.7

Figures E1.6 and E1.7 Within 2 to 3 weeks of expansion, the transeptal fibers have pulled the central incisor teeth together and closed the unesthetic diastema. Acrylic has been added to the screw to keep it in its open position.

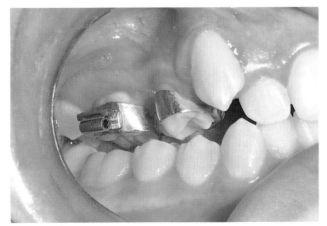

E1.8

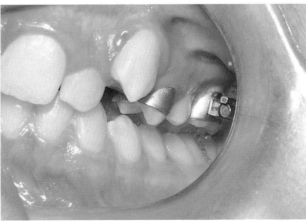

E1.9

Figures E1.8 and E1.9 Overcorrection of the buccal segments should be such that the lingual cusps of the maxillary teeth reach the buccal of the mandibular ones.

follow the maxillary teeth by tipping laterally and that the mandibular intercuspid width in the non-grower may be increased if the maxillary complex is widened. Sandstrom et al.[10] found a statistically significant increase of the mandibular intercuspid (1.1 mm) and intermolar width (2.8 mm) after RME.

RME also has been an accepted procedure to relieve deficiencies in arch perimeter. With the increasing emphasis on nonextraction therapy, the procedure has gained popularity because of the relief it provides in cases of crowding (Figs. E1.10 through E1.25). RME with the Hyrax appliance produces increases in maxillary arch perimeter at the rate of approximately 0.7 times the change in the first bicuspid width.[11] Slight palatal movement of the maxillary incisors and mild buccal tipping of the anchor teeth, as well as slight compensatory buccal uprighting of the mandibular posterior teeth, are also noted.[11]

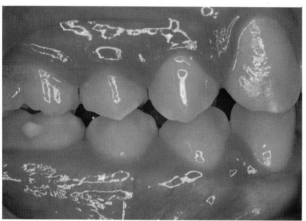

E1.10

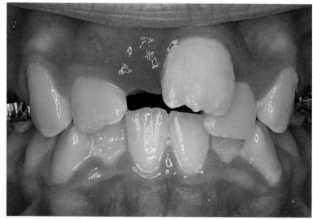

E1.11

Figures E1.10 through E1.14 Although this patient has a normal buccolingual occlusion (no crossbite present), it was decided to attempt to create space for the impacted central incisor with an RME appliance. Note the short root of the impacted tooth in Figure E1.14.

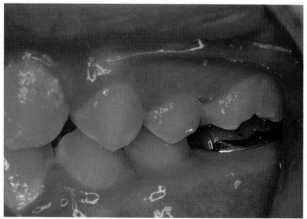

E1.12

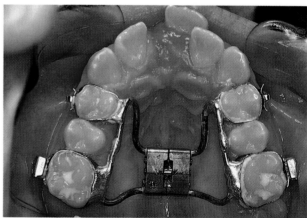

E1.13

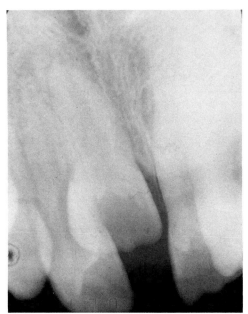

E1.14

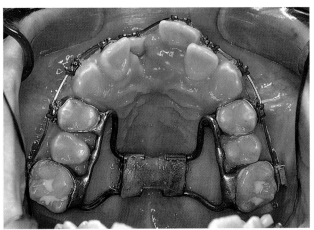

E1.15

Figures E1.15 through E1.17 After 2 weeks, the expansion was terminated; acrylic was placed over the screw to stabilize it in its position, and the impacted incisor was surgically uncovered. Note the open midpalatal suture on the radiograph. The teeth were bonded and an initial 0.016×0.022 inch^2 Neosentalloy (GAC) light (100 g) rectangular NiTi wire was placed in all the teeth but the right lateral incisor (to avoid unnecessary tipping of that tooth).

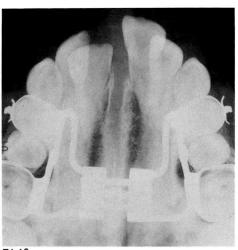

E1.16

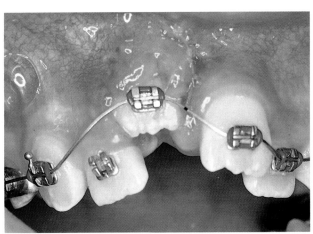

E1.17

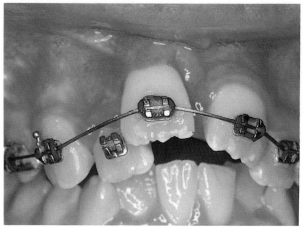

E1.18

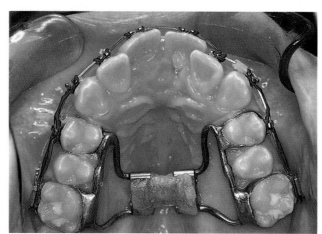

E1.19

Figures E1.18 and E1.19 One month later, the right central incisor had come closer to the occlusal plane (from the continuous light force of the flexible wire), at which point the lateral was attached to the wire.

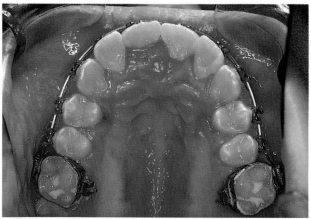

E1.20

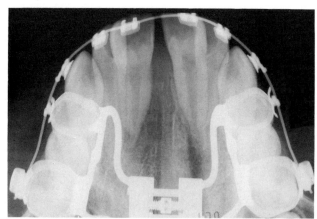

E1.21

Figures E1.20 through E1.22 Three months from the beginning of treatment, the right central incisor has assumed its position in the arch. The midpalatal suture has begun to ossify. Note the normal bone structure around the small, deformed root of the right central in Figure E1.22.

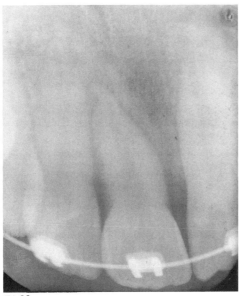

E1.22

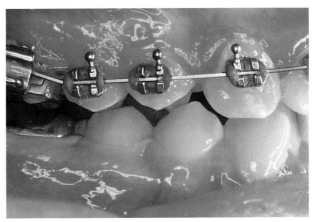

E1.23

Figures E1.23 through E1.25 The posterior buccal crossbites that had been created from the expansion (for the sake of space gaining for the impacted tooth) were corrected by simply allowing the teeth to return to their pretreatment positions (the expansion was not retained posteriorly). The RME appliance was removed after the expansion, and the same day/fixed appliances were bonded on the patient's teeth. Note the normal overbite relationship. Further treatment will finish the nonextraction case.

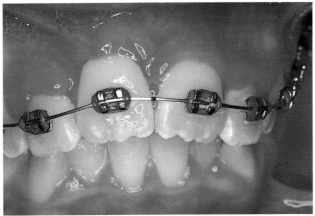

E1.24

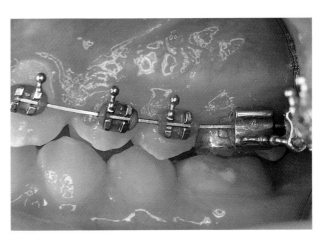

E1.25

In a study of the skeletal changes in vertical and anterior displacement of the maxilla with bonded RME appliances,[9] it was found that inferior movement of the jaw is lessened, and that there is a slight upward posterior movement at the posterior nasal spine (PNS) with a downward and posterior displacement at anterior nasal spine (ANS) that carries the upper central incisors in a clockwise rotation. RME, as it expands the maxilla and tips the dentition outward, causes the lingual cusps of the upper posterior teeth to move downward, thus opening the bite. It is suggested that bonded appliances instead of banded ones are indicated in open-bite tendency cases (long lower face, high mandibular plane angle), where extrusion of the maxilla or maxillary dentition would worsen the open-bite situation and create a more difficult vertical pattern to treat. The 2 to 3 mm of bonded acrylic introduces a passive stretch of elevator and retractor musculature that provides an apically directed (intrusive) force to the maxilla and the mandible, which limits changes in the vertical direction[9] (Fig. E1.26).

RME causes extensive buccal root resorption.[12] Repair of defects occurs by deposition of cementum. The clinician has no way of estimating the full extent of the resorption.[12] The expansion should be retained for about 3 months to allow for bone regeneration in the midpalatal suture and to avoid collapse of the maxilla to its original state.

Correction of the transverse maxillary deficiency, where a constricted upper arch occludes with a normal mandibular arch demonstrated with a bilateral posterior crossbite, is attempted surgically when the patient is generally age 16 years or older and the transverse discrepancy exceeds 4 mm.[1] An RME appliance is activated at the time of surgery to keep the upper arch in its expanded position postsurgically, or the patient is instructed to activate it four turns a day for 1 to 2 weeks postsurgery.[16] The procedure is called surgically assisted rapid palatal (or maxillary) expansion and involves surgical relief of the zygomatic buttresses[13] (Figs. E1.27 through E1.29). It can be done on an outpatient basis in the beginning of treatment. It may also be incorporated into the overall treatment plan of a more complicated skeletal problem (class II or III), when total maxillary or mandibular osteotomies are needed. It should be noted that the mandible's tendency to rotate backward in conventional RME also applies to the surgically assisted procedure, especially in patients with open-bite tendencies.[17]

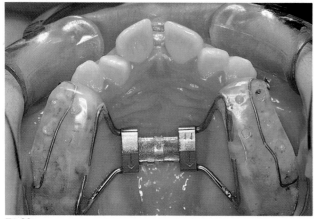

E1.26

Figure E1.26 A bonded RME appliance with acrylic coverage of the posterior teeth and a screw conformed 3 mm off the palate. Note the cold-cure acrylic placed in the screw to hold the appliance in its expanded position.

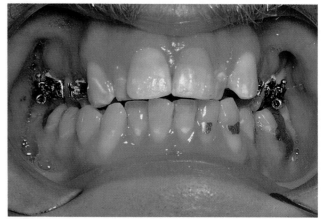

E1.27

Figure E1.27 Adult patient with bilateral posterior crossbite.

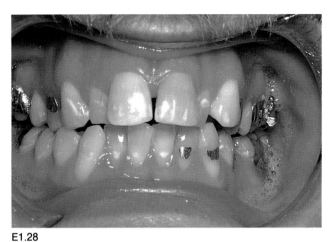

E1.28

Figure E1.28 After surgically assisted RME.

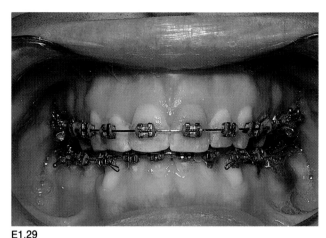

E1.29

Figure E1.29 Patient toward the end of treatment.

References

1. Bishara SE, and Staley RN: Maxillary expansion: Clinical implications. Am J Orthod Dentofacial Orthop 91:3–14, 1987.
2. Krebs A: Expansion of the midpalatal suture studied by means of metallic implants. Transactions, European Orthodontic Society 34:163–171, 1958.
3. Krebs AA: Expansion of midpalatal suture studied by means of metallic implants. Acta Odontol Scand 17:491–501, 1959.
4. Krebs AA: Rapid expansion of mid palatal suture by fixed appliance. An implant study over a 7 year period. Transactions, European Orthodontic Society 40:141–142, 1964.
5. Haas AJ: The treatment of maxillary deficiency by opening the midpalatal suture. Angle Orthod 35:200–217, 1965.
6. Wertz RA: Skeletal and dental changes accompanying rapid midpalatal suture opening. Am J Orthod 58:41–66, 1970.
7. Persson M, and Thilander B: Palatal suture closure in man from 15–35 years of age. Am J Orthod 72:42, 1977.
8. Haas AJ: Rapid expansion of the maxillary dental arch and nasal cavity by opening the midpalatal suture. Angle Orthod 31:73–90, 1961.
9. Sarver DM, and Johnston MW: Skeletal changes in vertical and anterior displacement of the maxilla with bonded rapid palatal expansion appliances. Am J Orthod Dentofacial Orthop 95:462–466, 1989.
10. Sandstrom RA, Klaper L, and Papaconstantinou S: Expansion of the lower arch concurrent with rapid maxillary expansion. Am J Orthod Dentofacial Orthop 94:296–302, 1988.
11. Adkins MD, Nanda RS, and Currier GF: Arch perimeter changes on rapid palatal expansion. Am J Orthod Dentofacial Orthop 97:194–199, 1990.
12. Barber AF, and Sims MR: Rapid maxillary expansion and external root resorption: An SEM study. Am J Orthod 79:630–652, 1981.
13. Wintner MS: Surgically assisted palatal expansion: An important consideration in adult treatment. Am J Orthod Dentofacial Orthop 99:85–90, 1991.
14. daSilva OG, Boas MCV, and Capelozza L: RME in the primary and mixed dentitions: A cephalometric evaluation. Am J Orthod Dentofacial Orthop 100:171–181, 1991.
15. Timms DJ: *Rapid Maxillary Expansion.* Chicago: Quintessence Publishing Co., 1981.
16. Turpin DL: Case report. Angle Orthod 59:155–159, 1990.
17. Woods MG, Swift JQ, and Markowitz NR: Clinical implications of advances in orthognathic surgery. J Clin Orthod 23:420–429, 1989.

Lip Bumper

The lip bumper is a very popular appliance for expansion of the mandibular arch and thus for gaining space as a result of the transverse changes, as well as from the distal uprighting movement of the lower molar teeth and forward movement of the incisor teeth[1,2] (Figs. E2.1 through E2.6). Based on various recent studies, the mandibular first molars tip back about 1.5 mm on each side and are 8 degrees more upright.[2] The incisors tip forward approximately 1.4 mm.[2] Depending on whether the lip bumper is passive or expanded on its insertion in the molar buccal tubes, the transverse changes range from 2 to 2.8 mm, 2.5 to 4 mm, and 2 to 5.5 mm in the cuspid, first bicuspid, and first molar regions, respectively.[1-4] The total arch length increase ranges from +7.45 mm to +18 mm.[1-4]

The lip bumper can maximize space gain in the lower arch, and—in conjunction with class III elastics—it can effectively correct tooth malpositions in special situations and help to determine the shape of the lower arch.[3,4] It is important to seat the bumper into the second molars if they can be banded (in deep-bite cases).[4] Mandibular right and left second molars are rotated until their lingual surfaces are parallel, and this positioning has an important effect on the eventual arch form.[4] When this rotation is completed, a lip bumper is fitted against the first molars.[4] Later, the bicuspids are rotated mesiobuccally with fixed appliances and then moved toward the first molars.[4]

The lip bumper should be worn full-time for a period of 6 to 18 months, depending on the amount of tooth movement and correction required. It is an effective appliance in mixed dentition therapy.

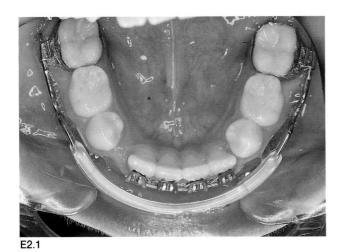

E2.1

Figure E2.1 The lip bumper appliance in place in the lower first molar auxiliary tubes. Note the distance from the anterior teeth: the lip bumper should be 5 to 7 mm anterior to the teeth in order to avoid injury to the gingiva as the appliance progressively moves posteriorly with molar movement.

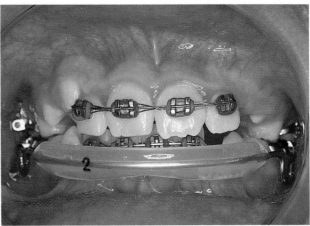

E2.2

Figure E2.2 The lip bumper wire embedded in the acrylic should be at the level of the CEJ of the lower incisors. Note the loops on the side, which, along with the acrylic anteriorly, keep the soft tissue (lips and cheeks) away from the alveolus, thus allowing for natural transverse expansion. The loops also help increase the length of the appliance.

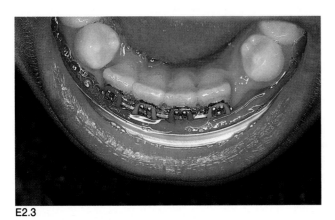

E2.3

Figures E2.3 through E2.6 When the lip bumper is properly placed, the lower lip should very easily cover the appliance and rest (without any effort from the patient) against it.

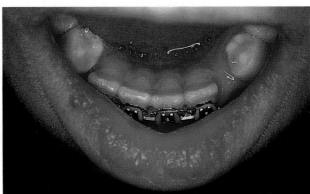

E2.4

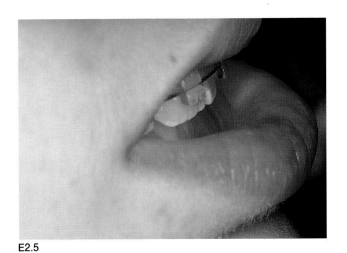

E2.5

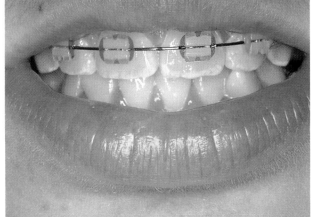

E2.6

References

1. Osborn WS, Nanda RS, and Currier GF: Mandibular arch perimeter changes with lip bumper treatment. Am J Orthod Dentofacial Orthop 99:527–532, 1991.
2. Nevant CT, Buschang PH, Alexander RG, and Steffen JM: Lip bumper therapy for gaining arch length. Am J Orthod Dentofacial Orthop 100:330–336, 1991.
3. Cetlin NM, and Ten Hoeve A: Nonextraction therapy. J Clin Orthod 17:396–413, 1983.
4. Ten Hoeve A: Palatal bar and lip bumpers in nonextraction treatment. J Clin Orthod 19:272–291, 1985.

Chapter 3

Headgear

Extra-oral anchorage or headgear mechanics are primarily used in cases of maxillary protrusion where the objectives are to restrict forward growth of the maxilla while the mandible continues its growth (skeletal effect) and to move the maxillary molar teeth distally (dental effect).[1-10]

The headgear has two bows: an outer bow, which connects to the head (high pull) or neck (cervical) strap, and an inner bow, which is inserted into the tube of the upper first molar.[2,3] There are various types of headgear; the one used the most with the least side effects is the high-pull headgear (composed of a head strap that is connected to the facebow)[3] (Fig. E3.1). This produces a distal and upward force on the first molar teeth that causes a slight intrusion of these teeth. A cervical headgear (around the neck) tends to significantly extrude the molar teeth, which even in some deep-bite patients may be contraindicated. A more occipital type of a force vector (instead of a high-pull) may be used in such cases.[3]

In order to obtain a skeletal effect with headgear mechanics, the extraoral appliance should be worn around 12 to 14 hr/day (during sleeping hours) with a force of about 10 to 16 oz (400 to 450 g) per side.[1] Hyalinization due to the excessive forces exerted on the first molars limits dental movement and promotes the skeletal effect (because the force would be transmitted to the skeletal substrate). After 2 years of treatment, a total of 5 to 7 mm of molar position change may be expected: 3 to 4 mm from retardation of maxillary growth relative to the mandible and 2 to 3 mm from actual distal tooth movement.[1] The total force to the maxilla should not exceed 2 to 3 lb.[1-3] To produce bodily movement of the molar teeth, the line of force (defined by the direction of pull by the strap to the outer bow) should pass through the center of resistance of the first molars[3] (Figs. E3.2 through E3.4). If the length of the bow or its position creates a line of force above or below the center of resistance, tipping will occur because of the movement that is produced.

When a headgear appliance is worn, the patient should not engage in any activities that might promote accidental release of the facebow and damage to the face (especially the eyes). This is the reason for the recent development of "safety" headgear products.[4]

Headgear therapy can most readily be achieved in the early mixed dentition.[11] The bones are less mineralized and therefore more easily deformed; sutures and ligaments are more cellular, resulting in more rapid biological responses; and growing tissues are generally more responsive to external forces.[11] The best orthopedic results are obtained when growth is most active and the juvenile period has greater growth on the average at its beginning.[11] The headgear can be used as a retainer-appliance for the first year after treatment for 4 to 5 hr/day or every other day if the anteroposterior correction was a full class II or 50% class II, respectively. This retention plan will not only keep the molar teeth in their overcorrected position, but also will help in the final class II skeletal correction postretention. Nonextraction edgewise therapy combined with extraoral force (headgear) on a class II, division 1 malocclusion inhibits the forward growth of the maxilla and allows the downward and forward growth of the mandible, thus resulting in the correction of the class II malocclusion into a class I.[12] It should be noted that the inner bow of the headgear appliance may sometimes cause the first molars to tip buccally (due to the heavy wire, even the slightest activation will cause tooth movement). In order to avoid this, a transpalatal bar (TPA) made of 0.036-inch round wire should be inserted in the lingual sheaths of the upper first molars. TPAs are available prefabricated and in various sizes. Another way to avoid buccal tipping is to constrict the inner bows of the headgear.

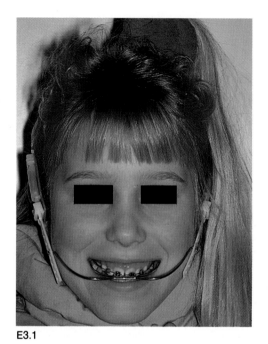

E3.1

Figure E3.1 The high-pull headgear appliance.

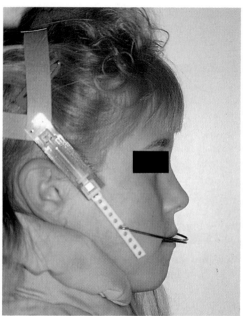

E3.2

Figure E3.2 The line of force, as defined by the direction of pull by the white strap to the outer bow, should pass through the center of resistance of the first molars located at the trifurcation of the roots of these teeth. This can be checked with a cephalometric radiograph.

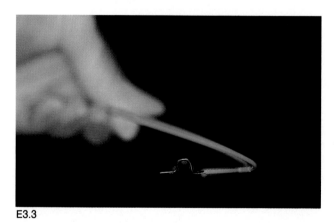

E3.3

Figure E3.3 The outer bow should be bent upward in a high-pull headgear appliance system.

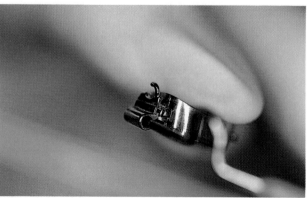

E3.4

Figure E3.4 The inner bow is inserted in the molar band headgear tube.

References

1. Wieslander L: The effect of force on craniofacial development. Am J Orthod 65:531–538, 1974.
2. Armstrong MM: Controlling the magnitude, direction and duration of extraoral force. Am J Orthod 59:217–243, 1971.
3. Jacobson A: A key to the understanding of extraoral forces. Am J Orthod 75:361–386, 1979.
4. Mossey PA, Hodgkins IFW, and Williams P: Clinical technique, a safety adaptation to Interlandi headgear. Br J Orthod 18:131–133, 1991.
5. Wieslander L: Dentofacial orthopedics: Headgear-Herbst treatment in the mixed dentition. J Clin Orthod 18:551–564, 1984.
6. Teuscher U: An appraisal of growth and reaction to extra oral anchorage. Am J Orthod 89:113–121, 1986.
7. Teuscher U: A growth-related concept for skeletal class II treatment. Am J Orthod 74:258–275, 1978.
8. Teuscher U, and Stockli P: Combined activator-headgear orthopedics. In *Orthodontics: Current Principles and Techniques.* St. Louis: C.V. Mosby Co.; 1985, pp 405–480.
9. Van Beek H: Combination headgear activator. J Clin Orthod 18:185–189, 1984.
10. Chabre C: Vertical control with a headgear-activator combination. J Clin Orthod 24:618–624, 1990.
11. King GJ, Keeling SD, Hocevar RA, and Wheeler TT: Timing of treatment for Class II malocclusions in children—a literature review. Angle Orthod 60:87–97, 1990.
12. Canglialosi TJ, Meistrell ME, Leung MA, and Ko JY: A cephalometric appraisal of edgewise class II nonextraction treatment with extraoral force. Am J Orthod Dentofacial Orthop 93:315–324, 1988.

Chapter 4

Removable Appliances

A removable orthodontic appliance is composed of (1) a retentive part, which consists of the various clasps (circumferential, Adam's, or ball clasp) that hold the appliances in place; (2) the acrylic component, which gives it its particular size and shape; and (3) the active or passive wire component (bow, spring, screws) that expresses the action of the appliance on the teeth.[1-3]

The biggest advantage of removable appliances is that they can be removed by the patient whenever the social environment indicates it.[1-3] Conversely, this presents their major disadvantages: patient compliance and interrupted tooth movements.[1-3] Most removable appliances need to be worn either full-time or for a number of consecutive hours during the day in order to obtain the desired treatment outcome. Unless the patient agrees to cooperate fully, the treatment objectives will not be met. In addition, removable appliances mainly have a tipping effect on the teeth.[1-3] Comprehensive major bodily tooth movement is almost always obtained with fixed appliances.

The most popular removable appliances are the various modifications of the Hawley appliances. The Hawley-type appliance has two primary purposes: as a retainer, to maintain a status quo; or as an active spring appliance, to achieve tooth movement (Figs. E4.1 through E4.6).

As a retainer, it must retain the teeth in their proper positions, permit the forces of physiologic activity to act on the teeth when desired, and be hygienic, strong, and esthetically and physiologically acceptable.

As a tooth-moving appliance, the Hawley appliance can be considered a limited correction device. Realistic treatment objectives for Hawley-type appliances are usually limited to tipping movements of the teeth.

Individual incisor movement by tipping can be easily done with a flexible spring (0.014-inch or 0.016-inch stainless steel wire with loops) behind the tooth (spring retainer) (Fig. E4.3). Arch expansion in the lower arch can be obtained with a screw, embedded in the acrylic of a lower retainer, which is activated by either the doctor or the patient. Most screws provide 1 mm of tooth movement per one complete revolution. A single quarter-turn of the screw would produce 0.25 mm of expansion. Because this type of space gaining through tipping is very unstable and relapse is high, the rate of active tooth movement should not exceed 1 mm/month and not more than a few millimeters of total expansion.

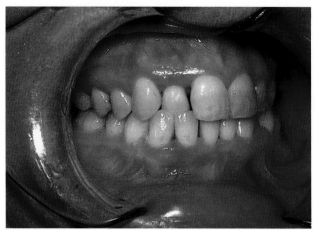

E4.1

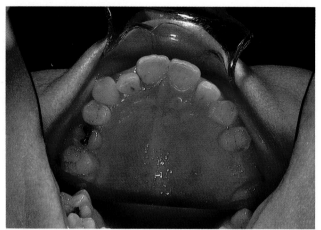

E4.2

Figures E4.1 through E4.3 A single tooth crossbite in the anterior maxillary region, such as the right upper lateral incisor presented in this case, may easily be corrected with a Hawley-type retainer with a helical spring made of 0.014-inch round stainless steel wire and activated as much as the tooth needs to come out of the crossbite. This case is ideal for this treatment because not only is there space mesial to the lateral, but also because this tooth is too upright compared to its contralateral counterpart, thus allowing the tipping movement provided by the spring retainer to bring it to its correct inclination. The appliance shown here is from another patient for correction of the centrals. The labial wire is an 0.030-inch round retainer wire. The lingual springs are made of 0.016-inch round wire.

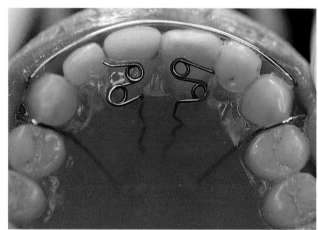

E4.3

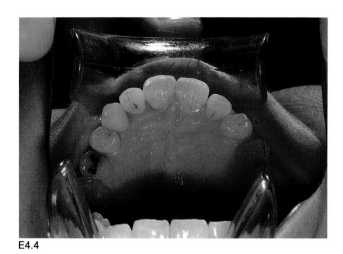

E4.4

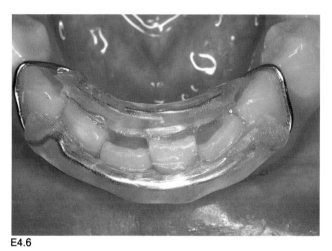

E4.5

Figures E4.4 and E4.5 After 3 months of full-time appliance wear. Note the excellent inclination of the lateral incisor.

E4.6

Figure E4.6 A lower spring retainer placed on lower anteriors with minor crowding (1 to 2 mm). It should be removed at night to avoid swallowing. The wire is a 0.030-inch round retainer wire.

References

1. Proffit WR: *Contemporary Orthodontics.* St. Louis, MO: C.V. Mosby Co., 1986.
2. Graber TM, and Swain BF: *Orthodontics: Current Principles and Techniques.* St. Louis, MO: C.V. Mosby Co., 1985.
3. Moyers RE: *Handbook of Orthodontics,* 3rd edition, Chicago: Year Book Medical Publishers, 1984.

Chapter 5

Functional Appliances

Growth modification is theoretically expressed in the following three ways:[1] (1) by an increase or decrease in the size of the jaws; (2) by redirection, even if the absolute size remained the same; and (3) by acceleration of growth. Although histologically evident and statistically significant, an absolute change in size is clinically insignificant. Redirecting growth in another direction has been shown to be of some value. A patient with a severely prognathic mandible might benefit from redirection of his or her growth in a more downward than forward manner.[1] Acceleration of growth shortens treatment time and provides a better jaw relationship sooner. Correcting a skeletal problem through growth modification should begin 1 to 3 years before the adolescent growth spurt, so that the maximum effect may be obtained in the shortest possible time frame. This is done by usage of functional[1-20] and extraoral appliances.[1]

The term "functional appliance" refers to a variety of removable appliances designed to alter the arrangement of the various muscle groups that influence the function and position of the mandible in order to increase its length. A number of clinicians believe that this is best achieved by 2 to 3 mm incremental advancements of the mandible every 4 to 5 months, because this decreases the risk of muscular fatigue as each new forward position of the mandible results in renewed growth stimulation of the condyle.[21]

In general, the use of functional appliances remains very controversial. Minimal bone growth increase (2 mm), along with the creation of dual bites in patients, put them in an unfavorable position in the armamentarium of the modern practitioner.[21]

Most functional appliances induce mandibular function in a predetermined position, usually 3 to 8 mm anteriorly to the centric relation position (class II correction).[12-19] This stretches the soft tissue and muscles, which in turn transmit the resulting forces to the teeth (dentoalveolar changes) and to the skeletal substrate.[22] Functional appliances may retard maxillary growth in the same modality as headgear.[22] In addition, it has been shown histologically that new bone is formed in the posterior aspect of the glenoid fossa, which usually resorbs after the stimulus (anterior repositioning of mandible) is taken away.

The correlation between condylar growth and lateral pterygoid muscle activity was a constant finding in animal studies.[7-10] It was proven that increased activity of this muscle was correlated with increased condylar growth. Rather, it might be the tension in the posterior part of the condylar capsule—caused by the activity of the lateral pterygoid muscle—that may be responsible for increased condylar growth.[22] The resultant tension of structures in the posterior part of the capsule decreased after a maximum level of activity 6 to 8 weeks after the start of treatment. A constant reactivation may, therefore, be important in obtaining a maximum condylar growth response.[22]

Tipping of teeth and dentoalveolar changes are the effects of functional appliances.[22] Class II correction comes from nearly 50% skeletal and 50% dental changes.[22] Functional appliances that promote a class II dentoalveolar correction are the Activa-

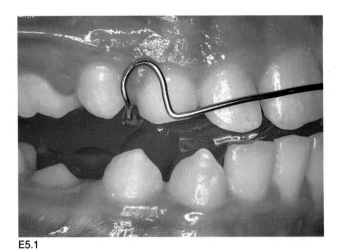

E5.1

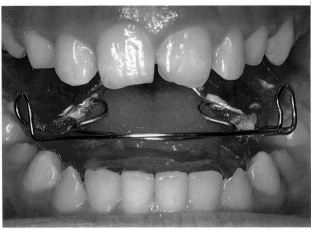

E5.2

Figures E5.1 and E5.2 The Bionator functional appliance. Note the anterior (end-to-end) position of the mandible relative to the maxilla. The patient bites into this anteriorly directed position and thus theoretically stimulates bone growth. Also note the bulky acrylic in the patient's mouth.

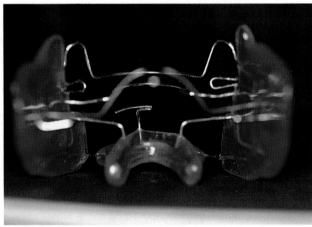

E5.3

Figure E5.3 The Fränkel functional appliance has buccal and lip pads to keep the soft-tissue pressures off the teeth and thus promote arch development. It, like the bionator, keeps the mandible in a more anterior position.

tor, the Bionator (Figs. E5.1 and E5.2), the Fränkel (Fig. E5.3), the Herbst, and the Jasper Jumper (Figs. E5.4 through E5.7). The last two are fixed—not removable— appliances. Appliances that help to correct a class III problem use lip and buccal shield pads to relieve the maxillary dentoalveolar complex from any extreme pressure, so that it may grow to its full potential (Fränkel III). Such appliances require extreme patient cooperation to have any effect. A number of studies have shown that the average increase in mandibular growth was 2 mm.[1,12-16,22] At the end of treatment with functional appliances, one might achieve a mean growth modification of 2 mm, which is clinically insignificant (6 mm of bone growth to correct a full class II malocclusion into a class I).[23]

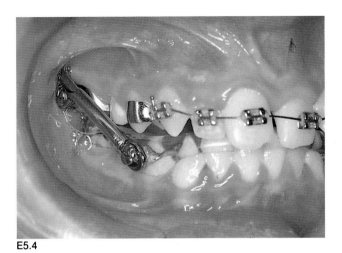

E5.4

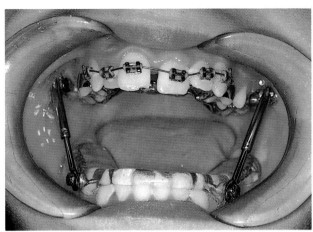

E5.5

Figures E5.4 and E5.5 The Herbst appliance is a fixed functional appliance (cemented onto the teeth with bands or acrylic) that solves the problem of patient cooperation. Its effect in actual bone growth is, like all other functional appliances, questionable for the majority of patients.

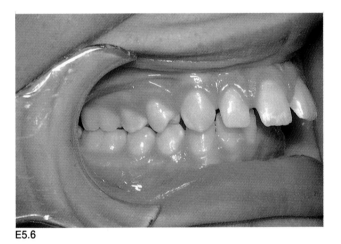

E5.6

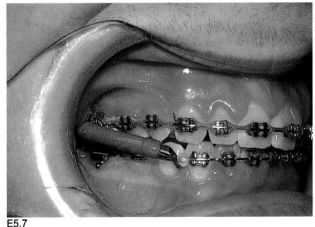

E5.7

Figures E5.6 and E5.7 The Jasper Jumper (American) appliance is a modification of the Herbst appliance. It is actually attached onto the main archwire and, like the previous appliances, keeps the mandible in a forward position.

The best controlled clinical studies of functional appliance therapy have been unable to show clinically useful increases in mandibular length.[24] Recently, it has been shown that bone formation at a histologic level does take place in the glenoid fossa after functional appliance therapy. The increased fibrous tissue of the disk posterior to the condyle appears to stabilize the anterior condylar displacement. This fibrous overgrowth (in conjunction with possible muscle splinting) may explain why the mandible cannot be manipulated back after functional appliance therapy, thus giving the false impression of a class II correction. Within a matter of months, such fibrous tissue resorbs and the mandible partially returns to its original position.[24]

The dramatic results shown in some European studies required more than 2 years of full-time appliance wear.[1-5] Other studies[24-29] have demonstrated the effects of a headgear/functional appliance combination with similar results: improvement of the occlusal discrepancies, but with great cooperation and the necessity to use fixed appliances to finish the cases ideally. If this type of therapy is to be attempted, then the growth potential in the early mixed dentition would be as favorable or even better than in the pubertal age groups.[2]

The full correction of class II, division 2 malocclusions into a class I through the use of the bionator functional appliance has been demonstrated in the literature; but, again, after very lengthy treatments of as much as 7 years (8 to 15 years of age) with 15 to 18 hours of wear a day.[31] Arch expansion gained with the Fränkel appliance through the action of the vestibular shields (that displace the attachment of the lips and cheeks at the sulci in an outward direction, thus allowing the development of the apical base) seems to be more stable than expansion seen with fixed appliance treatment. Again, the major disadvantage of the Fränkel therapy is the length of full-time wear (2.5 to 4 years) of a bulky appliance to obtain this desired result.

In a recent study on the changes in mandibular length before, during, and after successful orthopedic correction of class II malocclusions using a functional appliance, it was found that there is no significant difference after 4 years between the control and treated individuals.[20] In addition, it was concluded that the greater the result, the greater the relapse potential.[20] The main causes of relapse after Herbst treatment were a persisting lip–tongue dysfunction habit and an unstable cuspal interdigitation after treatment.[35] In general, functional appliances have only a temporary impact on the existing skeletofacial growth pattern.[20] In other words, the inherent morphogenetic pattern dominates over the treatment procedure.[20]

Functional appliances have been shown to be of clinical use in certain cases of hemifacial microsomia.[36-38] The generation of normal muscle balance in the absence of a condyle results in sufficient bone apposition to restore symmetry. It is speculated that the less severe the deformity, the greater the likelihood of a favorable response. Although still controversial, persons who have small mandibles may benefit more from functional appliance therapy than patients with normal-sized mandibles.[39]

A functional appliance that is simple and not bulkier than a pair of upper and lower Hawley retainers is the modified Chateau (Great Lakes) appliance.[40] It simply has a wire configuration that comes down from the maxillary Hawley appliance toward the lingual of the lower incisors and slides down the acrylic of the lower Hawley on the lingual side, thus forcing the mandible to be in a protruded position. The patient believes that he or she has retainers and does not object to wearing the appliance 24 hr/day (see Figs. F1.30 through F1.35).

References

1. Proffit WR: *Contemporary Orthodontics.* St. Louis, MO: C.V. Mosby Co., 1986.
2. Fränkel R: The treatment of class II, division 1 malocclusion with functional correctors. Am J Orthod 55:265–275, 1969.
3. Fränkel R: Guidance of eruption without extraction. Transactions, European Orthodontic Society 303–315, 1971.
4. Fränkel R: Decrowding during eruption under the screening influence of vestibular shields. Am J Orthod 65:372–406, 1974.
5. Fränkel R: A functional approach to treatment of skeletal open bite. Am J Orthod 84:54–68, 1983.
6. Stockli PW, and Willert HG: Tissue reactions in the temporomandibular joint resulting from anterior displacement of the mandible in the monkey. Am J Orthod 60:142–155, 1971.
7. McNamara JA, Jr.: *Neuromuscular and Skeletal Adaptations to Altered Orofacial Function.* Ann Arbor, MI: Monograph 1, Craniofacial Growth Series, Center for Human Growth and Development, University of Michigan, 1972.
8. McNamara JA, Jr., Connelly T, and McBride MC: *Histological Studies of Temporomandibular Joint Adaptations. Determinants of Mandibular Form and Growth.* Ann Arbor, MI: Monograph 4, Craniofacial Growth Series, Center for Human Growth and Development, University of Michigan, 1975.

9. McNamara JA, Jr., and Carlson DS: Quantitative analysis of temporomandibular joint adaptations to protrusive function. Am J Orthod 76:593–611, 1979.

10. McNamara JA, Jr.: Functional determinants of craniofacial size and shape. Eur J Orthod 2:131–159, 1980.

11. Wieslander L, and Lagerstron L: The effect of activator treatment on class II malocclusions. Am J Orthod 75:20–26, 1979.

12. Pancherz H: Treatment of class II malocclusions by jumping the bite with the Herbst appliance: A cephalometric investigation. Am J Orthod 76:423–441, 1979.

13. Pancherz H, and Anehus-Pancherz J: Muscle activity in class II, division 1 malocclusions treated by jumping the bite with the Herbst appliance: An electromyographic study. Am J Orthod 78:321–329, 1980.

14. Pancherz H, and Anehus-Pancherz J: The effect of continuous bite jumping with the Herbst appliance on the masticatory system: A functional analysis of treated class II malocclusions. Eur J Orthod 4:37–44, 1982.

15. Langford NM, Jr.: The Herbst appliance. J Clin Orthod 15:558–561, 1981.

16. Langford MN, Jr.: Updating fabrication of the Herbst appliance. J Clin Orthod 16:173–174, 1982.

17. Howe RP: The bonded Herbst appliance. J Clin Orthod 16:663–667, 1982.

18. Ekstrom C: Facial growth rate and its relation to somatic maturation in healthy children. Swed Dent J (Suppl 11) 1982.

19. Pancherz H, and Fackel V: The skeletofacial growth pattern pre- and post-dentofacial orthopaedics. A long-term study of class II malocclusions treated with the Herbst appliance. Eur J Orthod 12:209–218, 1990.

20. DeVincenzo JP: Changes in mandibular length before, during and after successful orthopedic correction of Class II malocclusions, using a functional appliance. Am J Orthod Dentofacial Orthop 99:241–257, 1991.

21. Bishara SE, and Ziaga RR: Functional appliances—A review. Am J Orthod Dentofacial Orthop 95:250–258, 1989.

22. Wieslander L: Dentofacial orthopedics: Headgear-Herbst treatment in the mixed dentition. J Clin Orthod 18:551–564, 1984.

23. Melsen B: *Current Controversies in Orthodontics.* Chicago: Quintessence Publishing Co., 1991.

24. Woodside DG, Metaxas A, and Altuna G: The influence of functional appliance therapy on glenoid fossa remodeling. Am J Orthod Dentofacial Orthop 92:181–189, 1987.

25. Teuscher U: An appraisal of growth and reaction to extraoral anchorage. Am J Orthod 89:113–121, 1986.

26. Teuscher U: A growth-related concept for skeletal class II treatment. Am J Orthod 74:258–275, 1978.

27. Teuscher U, and Stockli P: Combined activator, headgear orthopedics. In *Orthodontics: Current Principles and Techniques.* St. Louis, MO: C.V. Mosby Co., 1985, pp 405–480.

28. Van Beek H: Combination headgear activator. J Clin Orthod 18:185–189, 1984.

29. Chabre C: Vertical control with a headgear-activator combination. J Clin Orthod 24:618–624, 1990.

30. Valant JR, and Sinclair PM: Treatment effects of the Herbst appliance. Am J Orthod Dentofacial Orthop 95:138–147, 1989.

31. Rutter RR, and Witt E: Correction of class II, division 2 malocclusions through the use of the bionator appliance. Am J Orthod Dentofacial Orthop 97:106–112, 1990.

32. Fränkel R: Decrowding during eruption under the screening influence of vestibular shields. Am J Orthod Dentofacial Orthop 65:372–406, 1974.

33. Hine DL, and Owen AH III: The stability of the arch expansion effects of Fränkel appliance therapy. Am J Orthod Dentofacial Orthop 98:437–445, 1990.

34. Blackwood HO III: Clinical management of the Jasper Jumper. J Clin Orthod 25:755–760, 1991.

35. Pancherz H: A cephalometric long-term investigation on the nature of class II relapse after Herbst appliance treatment. Am J Orthod Dentofacial Orthop 100:220–233, 1991.

36. Kaplan RG: Induced condylar growth in a patient with hemifacial microsomia. Angle Orthod 59:85–90, 1990.

37. Melsen B, Bjerrejaard J, and Bundgaard M: The effect of treatment with functional appliance on a pathologic growth pattern of the condyle. Am J Orthod 90:503, 1986.

38. Epker BN, and Fish LC: *Dentofacial Deformities: Integrated Orthodontic and Surgical Correction,* vol. II. St. Louis, MO: C.V. Mosby Co, 1986.

39. Mamandras AH, and Allen LP: Mandibular response to orthodontic treatment with the bionator appliance. Am J Orthod Dentofacial Orthop 97:113–120, 1990.

40. Chateau M: *Orthopedie Dentofaciale. Bases Fondamentales.* Paris: Julien Prélat, 1975.

Chin-Cup Therapy

Strong orthopedic forces in the range of 400 to 800 g might be used to reduce a mandibular prognathism with the use of the "chin-cup" appliance[1-10] (Fig. E6.1). Although a number of significant craniofacial alterations have been noted in patients who underwent orthopedic chin-cup therapy (*i.e.,* retardation of mandibular growth),[5,6] it seems that a complete inhibition of mandibular growth is difficult to achieve.[8] Growth always continues when a chin cup was worn for 12 to 14 hours per day, which seems to be the most practical length of time to expect most patients to wear this appliance.[1-4,8] Alteration of the direction was limited to the period that the force was applied.[8] Inherited growth direction seems to be maintained and to recover when the mechanical intervention is removed.[8]

Chin-cup therapy does not necessarily guarantee positive correction of skeletal profile after complete growth, because the skeletal profile is greatly improved during the initial stages of chin-cup therapy but is often not maintained thereafter.[8] In order to have any permanent results, the patient would have to wear the appliance for many years, well past the completion of growth. Although there have been promising reports in the literature on the combination of chin-cup therapy followed by headgear for vertical control (open-bite cases), the long-term effects of chin-cup therapy for class III treatment is still questionable.[9] In addition, although in a recent study it was concluded that chin-cup therapy does not seem to present a functional risk,[10] one cannot ignore the fact that its posteriorly directed force puts a strain on the temporomandibular joint (especially if the chin cup is worn for a number of years). The chin-cup appliance needs to be worn well past the cessation of mandibular growth (about 10 years of wear, from 5 to 15 years of age or even more!), something that may not be very practical or easily accepted by the patient. Alternative treatment methods certainly need to be investigated.

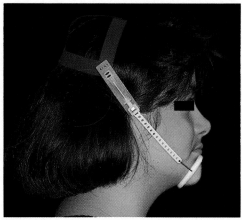

E6.1

Figure E6.1 Chin-cup appliance in place.

References

1. Irie M, and Nakamura S: Orthopedic approach to severe skeletal class III malocclusion. Am J Orthod 67:377–392, 1975.
2. Mitani H: Occlusal and craniofacial growth changes during puberty. Am J Orthod 72:76–84, 1977.
3. Sakamoto T: Effective timing for the application of orthopedic force in the skeletal class III malocclusion. Am J Orthod 80:411–416, 1981.
4. Mitani H: Prepubertal growth of mandibular prognathism. Am J Orthod 80:546–553, 1981.
5. Graber LW: Chin cup therapy for mandibular prognathism. Am J Orthod 72:23–41, 1977.
6. Wendell PD, Nanda R, Sakamoto T, and Nakamura S: The effects of chin cup therapy on the mandible: A longitudinal study. Am J Orthod 87:265–274, 1985.
7. Mitani H, and Sakamoto T: Chin cup force to a growing mandible. Angle Orthod 54:93–122, 1984.
8. Sugawara J, Asano T, Endo N, and Mitani H: Long-term effects of chin cup therapy on skeletal profile in mandibular prognathism. Am J Orthod Dentofacial Orthop 98:127–133, 1990.
9. Pearson LE: Vertical control in fully-banded orthodontic treatment. Angle Orthod 205R–224, 1986.
10. Gavakos K, and Witt E: The functional status of orthodontically treated prognathic patients. Eur J Orthod 13:124–128, 1991.

Thumb Sucking and Habit Control

Prolonged digit- or pacifier-sucking and tongue-thrusting habits have long been believed to be causative factors in a variety of malocclusions. The most common form of digit sucking is thumb sucking.[1-5] Graber[1] points out that three modifying factors—duration, frequency, and intensity—are extremely important and must be recognized and evaluated before the question of damage to the teeth and the tissues is answered.[2] Dental effects include (1) labial inclination or displacement of maxillary incisors with increased overjet, (2) overeruption of posterior teeth, (3) decreased overbite or anterior open bite, (4) linguoversion of mandibular incisors, (5) posterior crossbite, and (6) class II molar relationship. Skeletal effects include a lowered mandibular posture and autorotation. Spontaneous correction of some components of dental malocclusion is likely if the habit stops by the early mixed dentition.

Tongue thrusting may be defined as an abnormal tongue, perioral, and facial muscle posture and activity during deglutition or at rest. A direct cause-and-effect relationship between tongue posture, tongue thrust, swallowing, and malocclusion certainly must be questioned.[4] With the increase in overjet that accompanies so many finger-sucking habits, normal swallowing patterns become increasingly difficult. Perioral muscle aberrations, compensatory tongue thrust during swallowing, and abnormal mentalis activity may accelerate the malocclusion.[2]

Treatment for chronic digit sucking and tongue thrusting during the mixed dentition should begin with the simplest form of therapy. For digit-sucking habits, behavior modification may be attempted first, using rewards, encouragement, and reminders. The success of these treatment modalities is judged by both cessation of the habit and significant improvement of the malocclusion. In their article on the effectiveness of various methods of treatment of thumb sucking, Haryett et al.[3] suggest that palatal crib treatments are more effective than psychologic treatment or palatal arch treatment. They also found that the majority of those treated with the crib stopped the habit in 7 days, and mannerisms did not develop more frequently than in those subjects whose habits had remained active. It should be noted that good rapport with the patient might reduce the incidence of mannerisms and arrest other associated habits. These findings are in accordance with Graber's view that thumb sucking is a simple learned habit (learning theory) without an underlying emotional disturbance.

If the simple attempts fail, then one may try the Thumbsucking Control Appliance (TCA) (GAC) (Figs. E7.1 through E7.7). It can be very easily constructed by bending two to three consecutive loops on an 0.036-inch wire that is designed to fit into the lingual sheaths of the upper first molar bands, just like a regular transpalatal arch (TPA).[5] This requires minimal chairside time (3 to 5 minutes) and can be adjusted to cover the whole span of the patient's open bite, making insertion of the thumb in the mouth very difficult. It is also available in various sizes (preformed).

Bands are fitted on the first maxillary molars and the TCA is inserted late on a Friday afternoon. The child is advised that if he or she quits the habit, the TCA will be removed Monday morning before he or she goes to school, but the bands will be

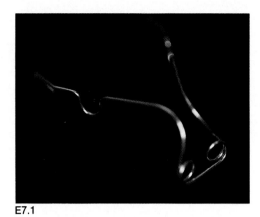

E7.1

Figure E7.1 The TCA (GAC) appliance.

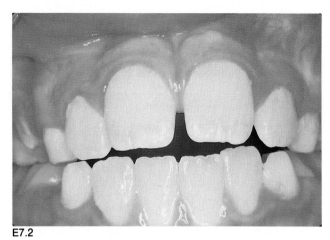

E7.2

Figure E7.2 Open bite from chronic thumb sucking and subsequent tongue thrust.

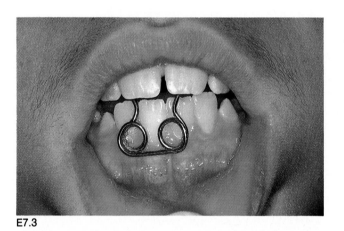

E7.3

Figure E7.3 The TCA (GAC) in place. The loops block the entrance of the thumb (or any other object) in the mouth. The patient may still eat comfortably from the side.

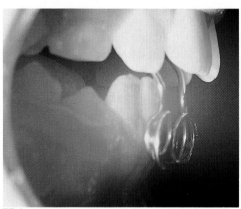

E7.4

Figure E7.4 The appliance comes passively over the lower incisors (without touching them) and terminates at the vestibule (without contacting the soft tissue). The palatal segment of the wire behind the upper incisors prevents any tongue thrust.

left in place for at least 1 to 2 months. If the habit is initiated again, it is very easy to re-insert the same appliance in the mouth. The child usually complies with this treatment and looks forward to Monday morning. The open bite from the habit should show improvement after cessation of the thumb sucking, within 2 to 4 months. Oral hygiene instructions, along with the recommendation that the parent watch the patient on occasion during sleeping hours to make sure that the patient is not sucking his or her thumb, are part of the therapy plan.

It should be noted that this appliance will work if there is significant overbite and a marked overjet. There must be enough so that it will not interfere with mandibular function. The clinician should be cautioned not to allow the lower incisors to impinge on the wire; otherwise, a functional retrusion would be enhanced.

The TCA can also serve as a tongue block, as the tongue contacts the palatal wire of the appliance upon swallowing (tongue thrust prevention). It can also be expanded to alleviate any crossbites in the first molar region, just like a transpalatal arch (TPA). When used as a tongue thrust control appliance, the TCA should be left in place for 2 to 4 months (so that the tongue can "learn" to obtain a new position upon swallowing).

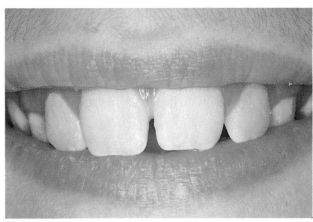

E7.5

Figure E7.5 The patient dislikes the appliance, but he can still hide it upon smiling.

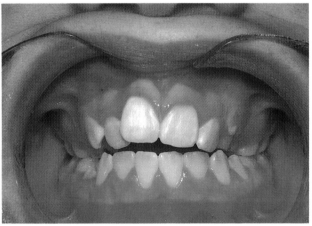

E7.6

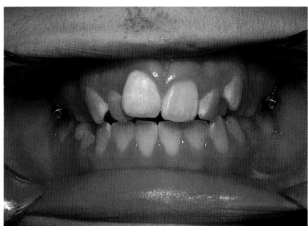

E7.7

Figures E7.6 and E7.7 A 3-mm open bite was significantly reduced within 3 months after insertion of the habit appliance and cessation of the habit. (Reproduced from Viazis AD: The Triple-loop corrector (TLC): A new thumbsucking habit control appliance. Am J Orthod Dentofacial Orthop July:91–92, 1991. With permission of Mosby-Year Book, Inc.)

References

1. Graber TM: Thumb and finger sucking. Am J Orthod 45:259–264, 1959.
2. Popovich F, and Thompson GW: Thumb and finger sucking: Its relation to malocclusion. Am J Orthod 63:148–155, 1973.
3. Haryett RD, et al.: Chronic thumbsucking: The psychological effects and relative effectiveness of various methods of treatment. Am J Orthod 53:569–585, 1967.
4. American Association of Orthodontists: Oral habits: Non-nutritive sucking and tongue thrusting. Orthodontic Dialogue 4:2–3, 1991.
5. Viazis AD: The triple-loop corrector. Am J Orthod Dentofacial Orthop 100:91–92, 1991.

Chapter 8

Protraction Facemask

Maxillary deficiency occurs in a large percentage of class III skeletal malocclusions (20% to 50%).[1,2] It is indicated by a straight vertical shadow from the infraorbital margin, through the alar base of the nose, to the corner of the mouth. The reverse-pull facemask in combination with a fixed palatal expansion appliance is proposed as the treatment method of choice for early interception of class III malocclusions[1-10] (Figs. E8.1 through E8.6). Treatment should begin as soon as the maxillary central and lateral incisors and maxillary first molars have completely erupted.[9] Rapid palatal expansion can produce a slight forward movement of point A and a slight downward and forward movement of the maxilla.[3,4] The effect of such expansion is to disrupt the maxillary sutural system, thus possibly enhancing the orthopedic effect of the facial mask by making sutural adjustments occur more readily.[8]

Several investigators have demonstrated the dramatic skeletal changes that can be obtained in animals with continuous protraction forces to the maxilla.[3-5] The entire maxilla is displaced anteriorly, with significant effects as far posteriorly as the zygomaticotemporal suture.[3-5]

The facial mask is secured to the face by stretching elastics from the hooks on the maxillary splint to the crossbow of the facial mask. Heavy forces are generated, usually through the use of ⅝-inch, 14-oz elastics bilaterally. The current version of the facial mask is made of two pads that contact the soft tissue in the forehead and chin regions.[6-9]

In instances in which no transverse change is necessary, the expansion appliance is activated once a day for a week to produce a disruption in the sutural system that facilitates the action of the facemask. A week later, the facemask therapy is initiated. The position of the crossbar is similarly adjusted in the vertical dimension to allow the elastics to pass through the interlabial gap without producing discomfort to the patient. The elastics travel in an inferomedial direction anteriorly from the hooks on the splint to the crossbar (Fig. E8.5).[10] If the tendency of an anterior open bite is suspected in a patient, an anterior site of protraction is required (bicuspid or even in front of the cuspid) (Fig. E8.4). Care must be taken that the elastics do not cause irritation to the corners of the mouth. The patient should wear the facemask on a full-time basis, except during meals. Young patients (5 to 9 years old) can usually follow this regimen, particularly if the patient is told that the full-time wear will last only 3 to 5 months.

The patient should be seen every 3 or 4 weeks to check on the condition of the splint and to evaluate the hard- and soft-tissue changes. The facial mask is usually worn until a positive overjet of 2 to 4 mm is achieved interincisally.

The possible treatment effects include[6-8] a forward and downward movement of the maxilla, a forward and downward movement of the maxillary dentition, and a downward and backward redirection of mandibular growth.

Although several investigators have claimed definite orthopedic advancement of the maxilla with reverse-pull mechanics, the proof of such movement is somewhat questionable because the same results have also been observed in patients who had only palatal expansion. The increase in maxillary length could also be attributed to growth.[10]

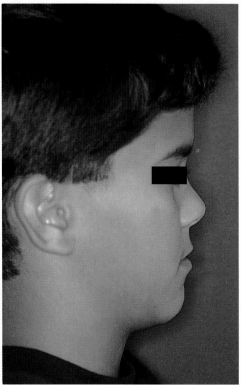

E8.1

Figure E8.1 Patient with a slightly deficient maxilla, which can be detected clinically by blocking out the mandible and noticing a straight line that comes vertically from the eyebrows to the cheek contour—normally the cheek should project 3 to 4 mm in front of this imaginary line.

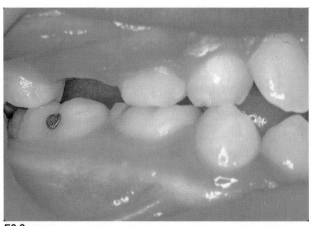

E8.2

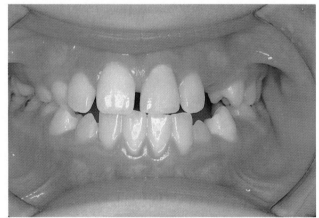

E8.3

Figures E8.2 and E8.3 A class III occlusion. Note the end-to-end incisor relationship. Also note the flared upper incisors (this is a contraindication to further dental tipping to correct the malocclusion).

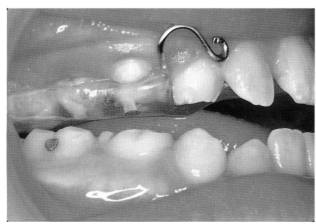

E8.4

Figure E8.4 Bonded rapid maxillary expansion (RME) with a hook in front of the cuspid to receive the elastics.

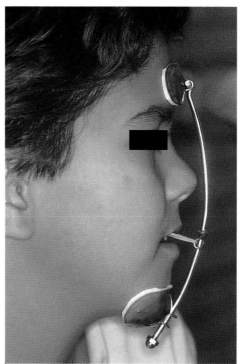

E8.5

Figure E8.5 The protraction facemask in place. Note the inferior direction of the elastics.

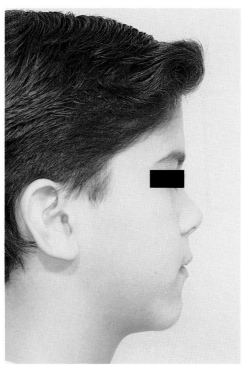

E8.6

Figure E8.6 The patient's profile shows improvement 3 months into treatment.

References

1. Guyer EC, Ellis EE, McNamara JA, and Behrents RG: Components of class II malocclusion in juveniles and adolescents. Angle Orthod 56:7–30, 1986.
2. Ellis E, and McNamara JA: Components of adult class III malocclusion. J Oral Maxillofac Surg 42:295–305, 1984.
3. Jackson GW, Kokich VG, and Shapiro PA: Experimental response to anteriorly directed extraoral force in young *Macaca nemestrina.* Am J Orthod 75:319–333, 1979.
4. Kambara T: Dentofacial changes produced by extra-oral forward force in the *Macaca irus.* Am J Orthod 71:249–277, 1977.
5. Nanda R: Protraction of maxilla in rhesus monkeys by controlled extraoral forces. Am J Orthod 74:121–131, 1978.
6. Turley PK: Orthopedic correction of class III malocclusion with palatal expansion and custom protraction headgear. J Clin Orthod 22:314–325, 1988.
7. Nanda R: Biomechanical and clinical considerations of a modified protraction headgear. Am J Orthod 78:125–138, 1980.
8. McNamara JA: An orthopedic approach to the treatment of class III malocclusion in young patients. J Clin Orthod 21:598–608, 1987.
9. Campbell PM: The dilemma of class III treatment. Angle Orthod 53:175–191, 1983.
10. Mermigos J, Full CA, and Andreasen G: Protraction of the maxillofacial complex. Am J Orthod Dentofacial Orthop 98:47–55, 1990.

Chapter 9

Active Vertical Corrector

The characteristics of skeletal open bite may be recognizable at early ages, especially in patients with long lower faces.[1-4] Such patients would benefit from early treatment and force distribution designed to hold, restrict, or redirect vertical growth,[4] especially because these subjects appear to reach their adolescence at an early age. The timing of initiation of treatment in long faces in this sense is similar to that for a class III malocclusion. Conversely, deep-bite patients experience late pubertal growth spurts and can be treated later. They often require prolonged retention to ride the wave of continued post-adolescence growth.[4]

Treatment of skeletal open bites at young ages can be done with magnetic appliances.[5-14] The most popular one is the Active Vertical Corrector (AVC) appliance.[8] The AVC[8] is a simple, fixed (24 hr/day) orthodontic appliance with magnets that intrudes the posterior teeth in both the maxilla and mandible by reciprocal forces[8] (Figs. E9.1 through E9.4). By the use of effective posterior intrusion of teeth, the mandible is allowed to rotate in upward and forward directions. The uniqueness of this appliance is that it allows the clinician to correct anterior open-bite problems by actually reducing anterior facial height. The AVC is an adaptation of present-day bite-block therapy. The AVC works as an energized bite block. The energy system is obtained by the repelling force of samarium cobalt magnets. A specially designed headcap and chin strap may be worn during sleep and at all other times deemed socially fitting by the patient to help keep the mouth closed. Follow-up on cases 3 years out of AVC treatment has shown little tendency for teeth to re-erupt. A high-pull headgear can be used in the retention phase for 6 to 12 months.

It has been found that posterior teeth intrude an average of 1.5 mm, thus resulting in an average of 3 mm of anterior open-bite closure over an 8-month treatment period (600 g of repelling force/side).[5,8,13,14] Additional significant contributions to the correction of the open bite were due to maxillary incisor eruption and lingual tipping combined with mandibular incisor lingual movement.[8,14] A small amount of mandibular bite-closing rotation and a decrease in anterior facial height have been noted, but there were only minimal skeletal changes in the sagittal direction attributable to AVC therapy.[8,14] Any side effects of AVC therapy (*i.e.,* creation of buccal crossbites from the repelling force system) could possibly be diminished by using a less powerful magnet system or decreasing the treatment time.[13] Treatment of severe open bites that are skeletal in nature has been reported in the literature.[13-16]

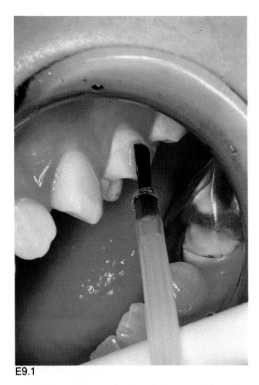

E9.1

Figure E9.1 The AVC appliance is bonded by etching the buccal and lingual surfaces of the posterior teeth (just like a bonded rapid maxillary expansion (RME) appliance).

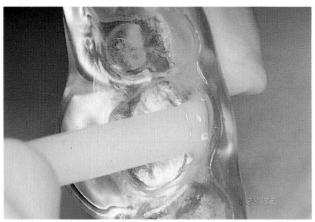

E9.2

Figure E9.2 Adhesive is placed in the buccal and lingual sides of the appliance and is later light-cured in the mouth.

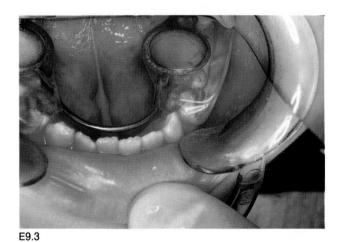

E9.3

Figure E9.3 The lower bonded AVC in place.

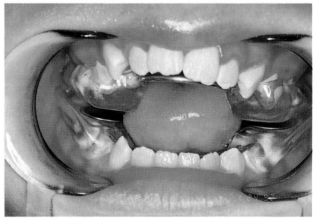

E9.4

Figure E9.4 The complete AVC in place. The repelling forces from the magnets will intrude the posterior teeth 1 to 2 mm over 3 to 5 months of wear.

References

1. Nanda SK, and Rowe TK: Circumpubertal growth spurt related to vertical dysplasia. Angle Orthod 59:113–122, 1989.
2. Chafari J, Clark RE, Shofer FS, and Bernan PH: Dental and occlusal characteristics of children with neuromuscular disease. Am J Orthod Dentofacial Orthop 93:126–132, 1988.
3. Nanda SK: Patterns of vertical growth of the faces. Am J Orthod Dentofacial Orthop 93:103–116, 1988.
4. Bishara SE, Jamison JE, Peterson LC, and DeKock WH: Longitudinal changes in standing height and mandibular parameters between the ages of 8 and 17 years. Am J Orthod 80:115–135, 1981.
5. Kalra V, Burstone CJ, and Nanda R: Effects of a fixed magnetic appliance on the dentofacial complex. Am J Orthod Dentofacial Orthop 95:467–478, 1989.
6. Pearson LE: Vertical control through use of mandibular posterior intrusive forces. Angle Orthod 43:194–200, 1973.
7. Pearson LE: Vertical control in treatment of patients having backward-rotational growth tendencies. Angle Orthod 48:132–140, 1978.
8. Dellinger EL: A clinical assessment of the Active Vertical Corrector—A nonsurgical alternative for skeletal open bite treatment. Am J Orthod Dentofacial Orthop 89:428–436, 1986.
9. Kalra V, Burstone CJ, and Nanda R: Effects of a fixed magnetic appliance on the dentofacial complex. Am J Orthod Dentofacial Orthop 95:467–478, 1989.
10. Vardimon AD, Graber TM, Voss LR, and Verrusio E: Magnetic versus mechanical expansion with different force thresholds and points of force application. Am J Orthod Dentofacial Orthop 92:455–465, 1987.
11. Vardimon AD, Graber TM, and Voss LR: Stability of magnetic versus mechanical palatal expansion. Eur J Orthod 11:107–115, 1989.
12. Woods MG, and Nanda RS: Intrusion of posterior teeth with magnets. An experiment in growing baboons. Angle Orthod 58:136–150, 1988.
13. Kilaridis S, Egermark I, and Thilander B: Anterior open bite treatment with magnets. Eur J Orthod 12:447–457, 1990.
14. Barbre RE, and Sinclair PM: A cephalometric evaluation of anterior open bite correction with the magnetic active vertical corrector. Angle Orthod 61:93–102, 1991.
15. Martina R, Laino A, and Michelotti A: Class I malocclusion with severe open bite skeletal pattern treatment. Am J Orthod Dentofacial Orthop 97:363–373, 1990.
16. Takeyama H, Houzawa O, Hozaki T, and Kiyomura H: A case of open bite with Turner's syndrome. Am J Orthod Dentofacial Orthop 97:505–509, 1990.

Orthodontic Treatment Modalities

Chapter 1

Early Treatment

Early orthodontic treatment at 3 to 8 years of age is directed toward preventing dysplastic growth of both the skeletal and dentoalveolar components.[1,2] It alleviates functional posterior crossbites that can develop from cuspal interferences and the mandibular shift that accompanies the crossbites. It prevents habits that can develop as a result of tooth interferences and incorrect occlusion. Because crossbites are seldom self-correcting owing to the relationship of the permanent to the primary predecessors, early treatment can re-establish proper muscle balance and thus prevent adjustment of the jaw muscles on the position that results from the habitual posturing of the mandible (Figs. F1.1 through F1.20).

Early treatment (phase I) can also prevent potential injury of protruding incisors in severe overjet class II cases (Figs. F1.21 through F1.29). The clinician can also take advantage of the juvenile growth spurt to attempt functional appliance or headgear therapy at age 8 to 10 years (Figs. F1.30 through F1.35). Early treatment may be done for esthetic considerations as well (Figs. F1.36 through F1.38).

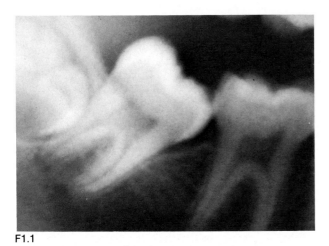

F1.1

Figure F1.1 Dislodging a second molar stuck underneath the distal surface of the first molar is quite easy to accomplish.

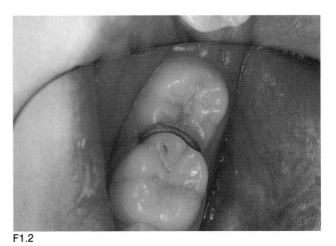

F1.2

Figure F1.2 Placement of an orthodontic elastic separator between these two teeth.

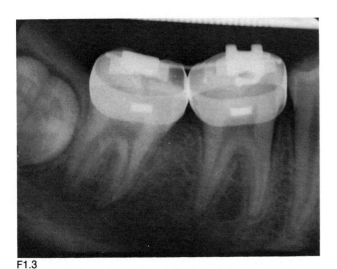

F1.3

Figure F1.3 If the second molar maintains its excessive mesial inclination, molar bands may be fitted on the two teeth, and a flexible 0.016-inch NiTi wire will slowly upright the second molar in 2 months.

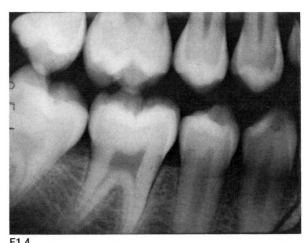

F1.4

Figure F1.4 Posttreatment periapical radiograph showing the uprighted second molar.

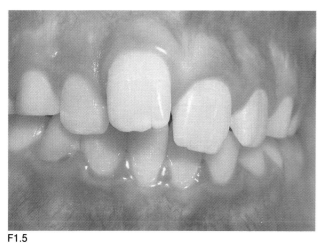

F1.5

Figure F1.5 This patient is in the mixed dentition and demonstrates a labially displaced right central incisor due to a pencil-biting habit, which has been discontinued.

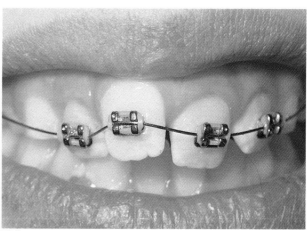

F1.6

Figure F1.6 A simple 2 × 4 appliance (2 bands on the upper first permanent molar teeth and 4 brackets on the upper permanent incisors) with a 0.016-inch round flexible NiTi wire in place.

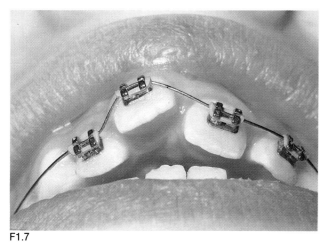

F1.7

Figure F1.7 Occlusal view. The wire is fully engaged without any deformation. Its elastic pull will gradually bring the tooth into alignment with the rest of the incisors.

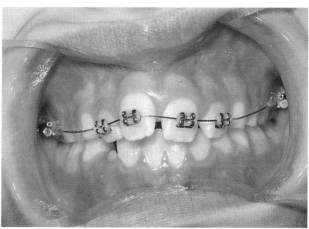

F1.8

Figure F1.8 After 1 month of treatment.

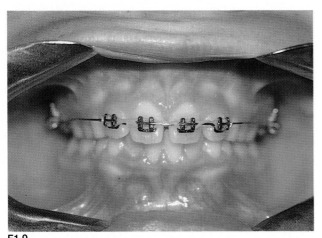

F1.9

Figure F1.9 After 3 months of treatment. A four-unit elastic chain (C-chain) has been placed to close the existing spaces. The laterals (the most outer teeth of the C-chain) have been wire tied with ligature ties to prevent any undesirable rotation of those teeth.

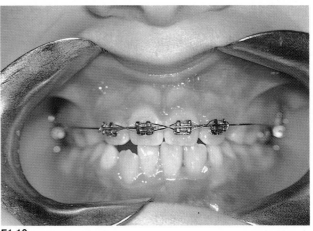

F1.10

Figure F1.10 After space closure is completed, the teeth are tied together in a figure-8 fashion and held in place (from another patient).

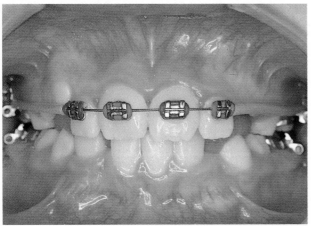

F1.11

Figure F1.11 Plastic tubes may be placed to prevent irritation of the cheeks from the long wire span.

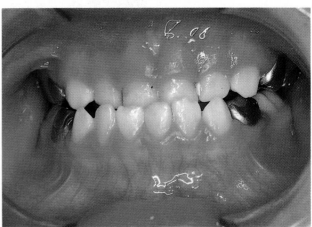

F1.12

Figure F1.12 A 3-year-old boy presented a complete anterior crossbite from lateral to lateral with a 1-mm negative overjet. Upon manipulation of the mandible, the incisors obtained an end-to-end relationship, indicative of a dental problem. (Reproduced from Vadiakas G, and Viazis AD: Anterior crossbite correction in the early primary dentition. Am J Orthod Dentofacial Orthop 102:160–162, 1992. With permission of Mosby-Year Book, Inc.)

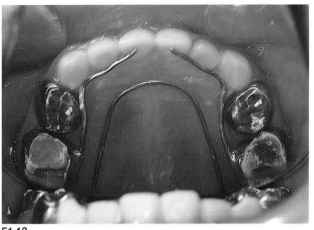

F1.13

Figure F1.13 A fixed (due to the age of the patient) W-arch with extended arms to the maxillary incisors was inserted. The arms were activated 1.5 mm in an anterior direction. (Reproduced from Vadiakas G, and Viazis AD: Anterior crossbite correction in the early primary dentition. Am J Orthod Dentofacial Orthop 102:160–162, 1992. With permission of Mosby-Year Book, Inc.)

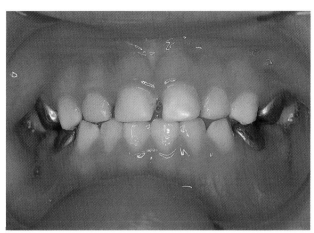

F1.14

Figure F1.14 After 4 months, the patient was out of crossbite through tipping of the anterior maxillary teeth. (Reproduced from Vadiakas G, and Viazis AD: Anterior crossbite correction in the early primary dentition. Am J Orthod Dentofacial Orthop 102:160–162, 1992. With permission of Mosby-Year Book, Inc.)

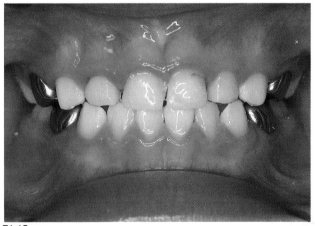

F1.15

Figure F1.15 Six months after the appliance was removed, the patient's bite was quite normal with an improved overbite relationship. (Reproduced from Vadiakas G, and Viazis AD: Anterior crossbite correction in the early primary dentition. Am J Orthod Dentofacial Orthop 102:160–162, 1992. With permission of Mosby-Year Book, Inc.)

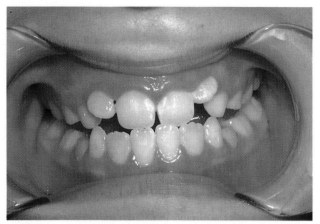

F1.16

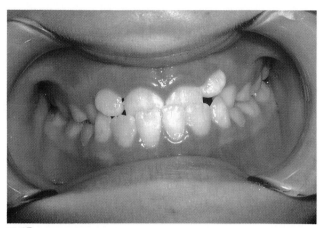

F1.17

Figures F1.16 through F1.18 This patient in the mixed dentition has an end-to-end incisor relationship that slides into an anterior crossbite (underbite), giving him a pseudo class III mandibular prognathism appearance.

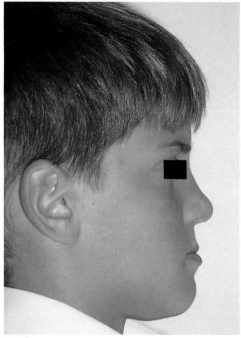

F1.18

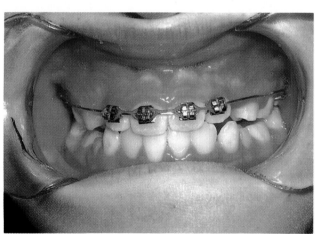

F1.19

Figure F1.19 A 2 × 4 appliance (2 bands on the two first permanent molars and 4 brackets on the incisors) and an 0.014-inch stainless steel archwire were inserted. A stop (similar to the one used to hold the molars back after their distal movement with coil springs) was placed in the archwire next to the molars, which kept the wire 2 mm anterior to the brackets. It took 2 months for the activated wire to bring the four teeth out of crossbite. Note the uneven incisal edges of the central incisors due to incorrect bracket placement on the left central incisor.

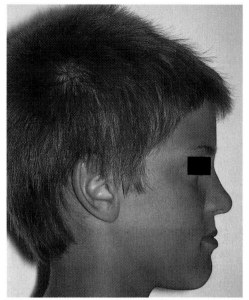

F1.20

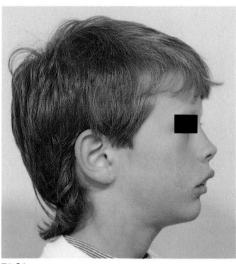

F1.21

Figure F1.20 Patient after treatment. Note the improvement of the patient's profile. Had this crossbite not been corrected, the functional effect of the forced position of the patient's mandible anteriorly could have resulted in a significant skeletal problem a few years later.

Figure F1.21 The severe class II, division 1 malocclusion of this case made a phase I treatment imperative for this patient.

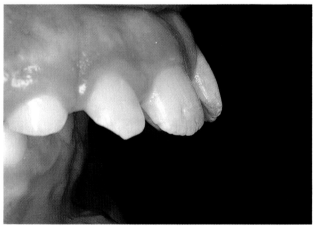

F1.22

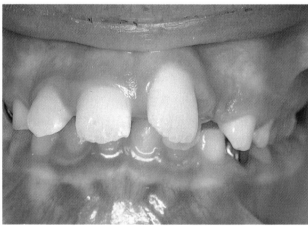

F1.23

Figures F1.22 and F1.23 The patient presents with a 16-mm overjet, a full step class II molar relationship, a lingually displaced permanent lateral incisor, and uneven gingival contours of the upper anterior teeth.

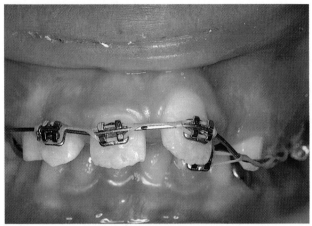

F1.24

Figure F1.24 A 2 × 4 appliance with a 0.016 × 0.022 inch² rectangular Neosentalloy NiTi wire and elastic chains were all that was needed to alleviate the generalized spacing and severe overjet. The right three-unit elastic chain is used to derotate the left central and close the midline diastema. Note that the wire in the right lateral is wire tied to the bracket to prevent rotation of this tooth. The contralateral central is not tied in order to have just that effect of rotation.

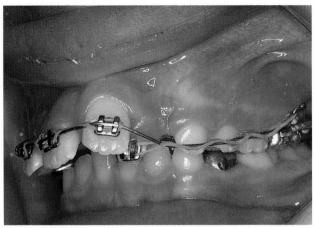

F1.25

Figure F1.25 The left elastic chain is placed along the main archwire and serves to bring the left lateral labially.

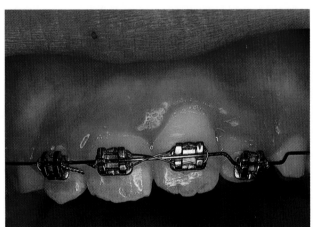

F1.26

Figure F1.26 Two months later, the anterior spaces are closed. Note the second-order bend placed to bring the left lateral into proper alignment with the incisal edges of the rest of the permanent anteriors. The bracket on this tooth is placed too far incisally, due to the gingival overgrowth in that area.

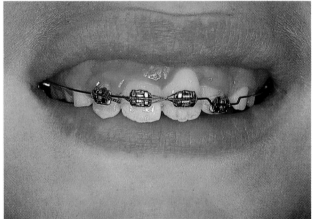

F1.27

Figure F1.27 At this point, the patient was referred to the periodontist. The uneven gingival contours before periodontal plastic surgery give this patient a very unpleasant smile.

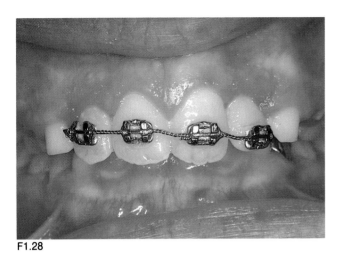

F1.28

Figure F1.28 After periodontal plastic surgery. Note the difference in the gingival contours.

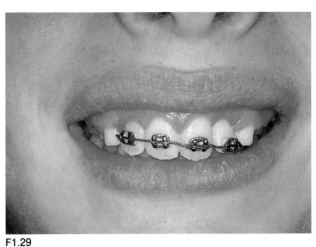

F1.29

Figure F1.29 The smile has improved significantly.

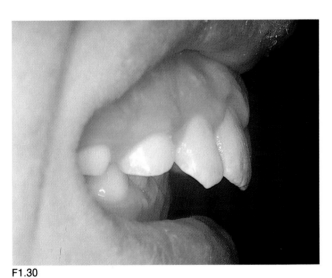

F1.30

Figure F1.30 After the 2 × 4 phase I treatment, the overjet is reduced but is still significant because of the mandibular retrognathism.

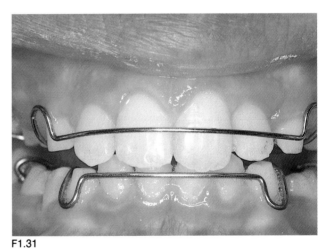

F1.31

Figure F1.31 The patient is given a functional appliance that is composed of maxillary and mandibular Hawley retainers (modified Chateau).

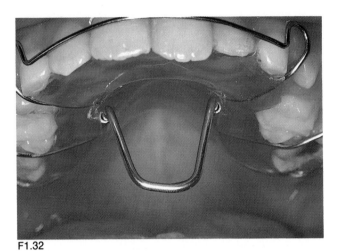

F1.32

Figure F1.32 The maxillary Hawley has a 0.036-inch round wire that comes out of two tubes embedded in the acrylic and is directed toward the floor of the mouth. The wire can come out of the tubes, if desired.

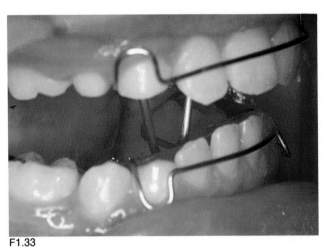

F1.33

Figure F1.33 As the patient closes his mouth, the wire slides along the lingual side of the lower Hawley, thus directing the mandible anteriorly.

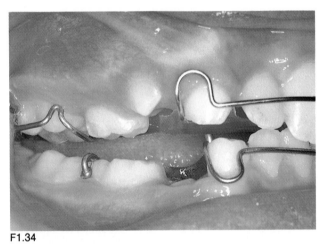

F1.34

Figure F1.34 The appliance in place. Note the normal overbite and overjet relationship. The acrylic should be adjusted occasionally to facilitate tooth eruption.

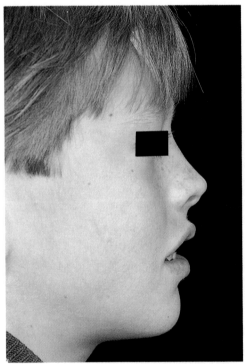

F1.35

Figure F1.35 Note the dramatic improvement of the patient's profile with the appliance in place.

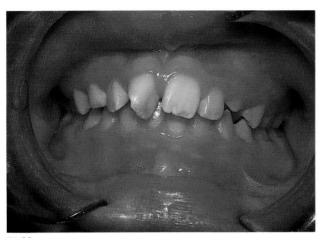

F1.36

Figure F1.36 This patient could not afford a full orthodontic treatment. Her chief complaint was the severely rotated right central maxillary incisor (almost 90 degrees).

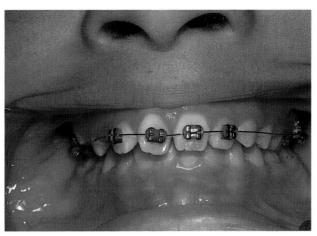

F1.37

Figure F1.37 A simple 2 × 4 appliance with a single archwire (0.016-inch round NiTi) was used for a minimal treatment fee.

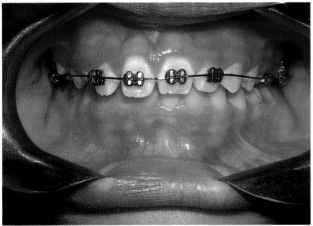

F1.38

Figure F1.38 In just 3 months, the chief complaint was addressed. The patient was extremely happy, and the patient's mother was grateful for the treatment.

References

1. Graber LW: Orthodontics—State of the Art, Essence of the Science. St. Louis, MO: C.V. Mosby, 1986.
2. Proffit WR, and White RP: *Surgical Orthodontic Treatment.* St. Louis, MO: Mosby-Year Book, 1991.

Chapter 2

Tooth Guidance
(Serial Extraction)

The premature extraction of deciduous teeth to correct the alignment of the permanent incisors is done under the assumption that it is possible to predict at a very early age that the alveolar ridge will not develop sufficiently to accommodate all the permanent teeth.[1] Recontouring the proximal surfaces of deciduous teeth instead of extractions is based on the same assumption.[2] Once serial extraction is initiated, more often than not bicuspids will have to be extracted owing to a deficiency in arch length,[1] which probably is the direct result of the extraction of the primary teeth.

Alignment of the permanent lower incisors depends more on arch width (intercuspid width) than on arch length.[1] It appears that the deciduous cuspids have a significant influence on the development of the alveolar arches by maintaining integrity of contact from the permanent molars forward.[1] Extraction of the deciduous cuspids causes a break in the contact with apparent adverse influence on the development of the alveolar arch. The embryonic position of the lower lateral incisors is to the lingual, and thus lower lateral incisors erupting lingually should be known as anatomically correct.[1] As the lateral incisors move labially, the deciduous cuspids will be made to move sideways, which creates more space for the accommodating of all anterior teeth.

The profile of a patient with a long lower face, high mandibular plane angle, an open-bite tendency, and severe crowding is an ideal case for a tooth-guidance procedure (Figs. F2.1 through F2.7). It must be emphasized that the exact same situation in a patient with a deep bite (short lower face height) would be a contraindication for serial extractions. In such a case, mechanics to gain arch length through expansion or distal movement of the posterior teeth should be the treatment of choice, because extraction even of only the primary cuspids would deepen the bite.

In a tooth-guidance procedure, teeth adjacent to the extraction sites do not move equally into the extraction space. Teeth anterior to the extraction sites move distally about twice as much as posterior teeth move mesially.[2] In addition, there is no advantage in early removal of bicuspids.[2]

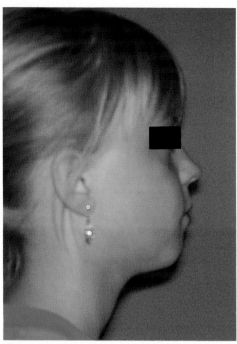

F2.1

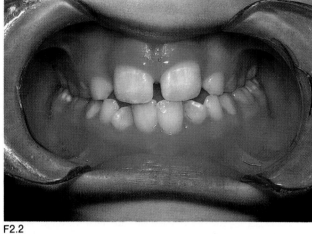

F2.2

Figures F2.1 through F2.4 Patient with a long lower face, minimal to 0 mm overbite, and severe crowding. This is an ideal case for a tooth-guidance procedure.

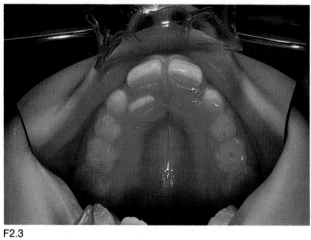

F2.3

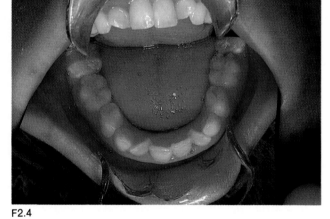

F2.4

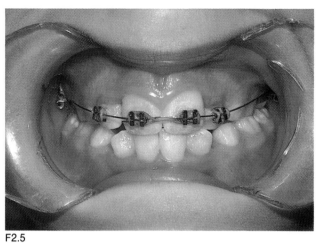

F2.5

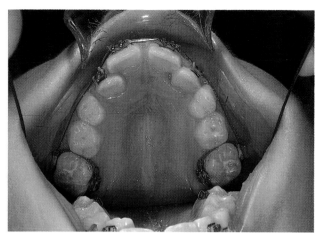

F2.6

Figures F2.5 through F2.7 After extraction of the primary cuspids, fixed appliances were placed (0.016-inch NiTi in a 2 × 4) to align the upper incisors. Note that the lower incisors align on their own as space is provided for them. Also note the positive overbite relationship that was obtained. The extraction of the primary first molars and first bicuspids will follow later in treatment.

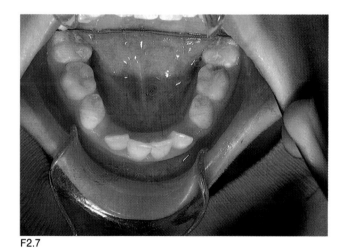

F2.7

References

1. Lee PK: Behavior of erupting crowded lower incisors. J Clin Orthod 14:24–33, 1980.
2. Creekmore TD: Teeth want to be straight. J Clin Orthod 16:745–764, 1982.

Chapter 3

Tooth Recontouring

Interproximal reduction was once limited to the mandibular incisors but has recently been extended to the posterior teeth with a technique called air-rotor stripping (ARS).[1,2] I prefer to call this technique tooth recontouring (TR). This method resolves mild (1 to 3 mm) to moderate (4 to 7 mm) crowding by reducing enamel where the greatest amount of enamel is present—distal to the cuspids.[1,2] A fine diamond bur is used to remove 0.25 mm to 0.5 mm from each side of the posterior teeth, after adequate space has been opened up with a Sentalloy (GAC) coil spring. As much as 0.5 to 1 mm is removed from each tooth, thus allowing for about 3 mm of space in each quadrant. This space is used to alleviate anterior crowding (Figs. F3.1 through F3.17).

There are two ways to protect the recontoured surfaces.[3-8] One is by polishing with an instrument such as a superfine diamond bur or a paper disc, followed by application of fluoride. The other is to apply a sealant after etching.[5] The second technique is much faster but raises questions such as how long the sealant lasts and what condition the enamel will be in once the sealant has dissipated. Results of a recent study indicate that the roughness produced by recontouring does not predispose to caries.[4] Remineralization appears after 9 months.[4] These findings substantiate those of other studies that found no increased susceptibility to caries or periodontal disease after stripping.[6,7] Therefore, a sealant would only delay the remineralization that occurred between 6 and 9 months.[4] However, topical application of fluoride after recontouring should be encouraged.[4]

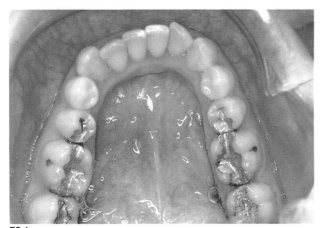

F3.1

Figure F3.1 The moderate crowding of this lower arch (5 mm) makes it ideal for tooth recontouring.

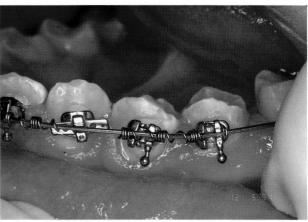

F3.2

Figure F3.2 In the TR technique, an NiTi coil spring is placed first between the first molar and the second bicuspid. After 2 weeks, a 2-mm space has been created. The mesial of the molar and the distal of the second bicuspid are recontoured with a fine diamond bur; 0.25 mm of enamel is removed from each side. The next step is to place the coil spring between the first and second bicuspid. Note the coil spring in its passive state. It extends from the mesial of the second to the mesial of the first bicuspid.

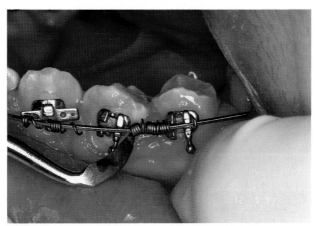

F3.3

Figure F3.3 A scaler pushes the coil spring between the two bicuspids.

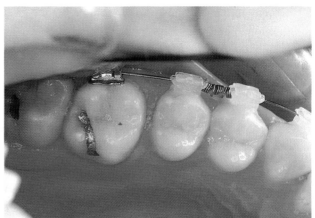

F3.4

Figure F3.4 Occlusal view from another case, showing the compressed coil spring between the two bicuspids.

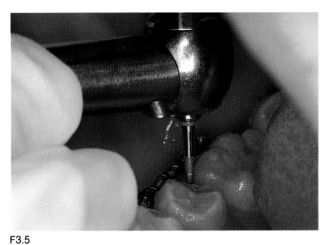

F3.5

Figure F3.5 The fine diamond bur as it recontours the teeth (care should be taken to avoid undercuts and steps at the gingival margin).

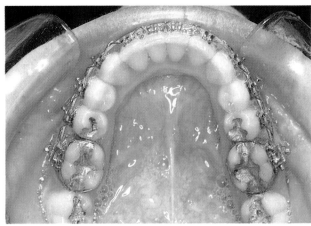

F3.6

Figure F3.6 The case presented in Figure F3.1 after completion of TR.

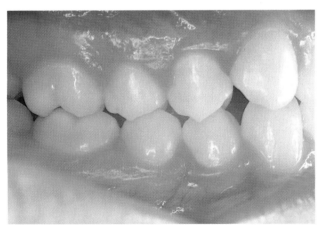

F3.7

Figure F3.7 Patient with a class II 50% cuspid and class I molar relationship due to oversized bicuspids.

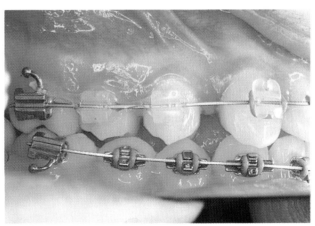

F3.8

Figure F3.8 After TR, a space is created distal to the cuspid. Elastic chains will bring it into a class I occlusion.

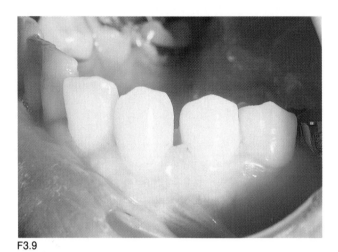

F3.9

Figure F3.9 Recontouring of individual teeth can be done in the space provided by 1 week of wear of a separator.

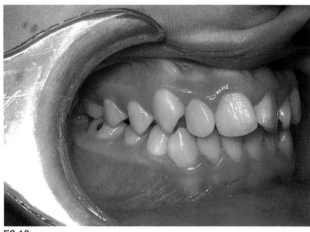

F3.10

Figures F3.10 through F3.13 This patient demonstrates a class I occlusion, a normal growth pattern, and moderate crowding in both arches (5 to 6 mm). The tooth recontouring technique was the treatment of choice for this case.

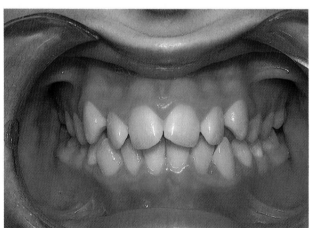

F3.11

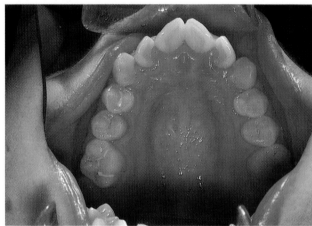

F3.12

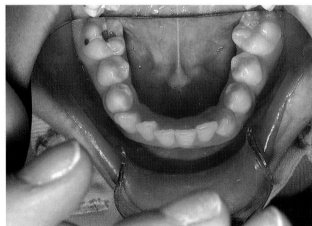

F3.13

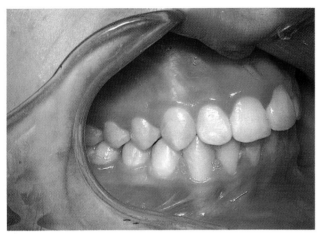

F3.14

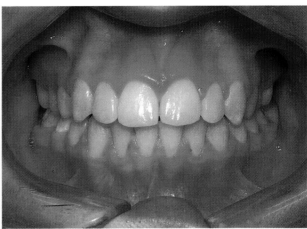

F3.15

Figures F3.14 through F3.17 At the end of the orthodontic treatment, a little over a year later. Note the solid class I cuspid relationship. The anterior teeth were retracted posteriorly, in the spaces provided from the recontouring of the posterior teeth.

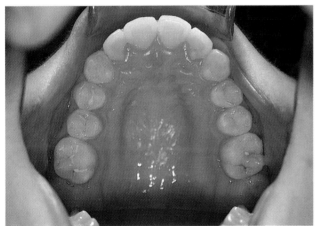

F3.16

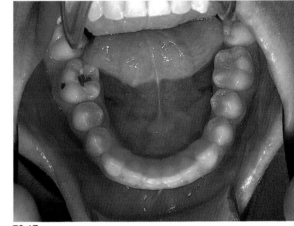

F3.17

References

1. Sheridan JJ: Air-rotor stripping. J Clin Orthod 19:43–59, 1985.
2. Sheridan JJ: Air-rotor stripping update. J Clin Orthod 21:781–788, 1987.
3. Philippe T: A method of enamel reduction for correction of adult arch-length discrepancy. J Clin Orthod 25:484–489, 1991.
4. El-Mangoury NH, Moussa MM, Mostafa YA, and Girgis AS: In-vivo remineralization after ARS. J Clin Orthod 25:75–78, 1991.
5. Sheridan JJ, and Ledoux PM: Air-rotor stripping and proximal sealants—An SEM evaluation. J Clin Orthod 23:790–794, 1984.
6. Crain G, and Sheridan JJ: Susceptibility to caries and periodontal disease after posterior air-rotor stripping. J Clin Orthod 24:84–85, 1990.
7. Radlanski RJ, Jager A, Schwestka R, and Bertzbach F: Plaque accumulation caused by interdental stripping. Am J Orthod 94:416–420, 1988.
8. Carter RN: Reproximation and recontouring made simple. J Clin Orthod 23:636–637, 1989.

Chapter 4

Treatment Planning in the Permanent Dentition

The first and foremost objective in orthodontics is the attainment of a class I cuspid relationship after treatment, when the upper cuspid occludes in the embrasure between the lower first bicuspid and cuspid. With this goal in mind, the following general treatment patterns may be applied in orthodontics.[1-12]

Class I

The majority of patients with class I cases who seek orthodontic therapy have minor, moderate, or severe crowding, accompanied by various intra-arch discrepancies that are easily corrected orthodontically (Figs. F4.1 through F4.33). Minor and moderately crowded cases are usually resolved with the tooth recontouring (TR) technique. When we have a class I extraction case (severe crowding, impacted teeth, bimaxillary protrusion, dental open bite or open-bite tendency cases), the objective is the presence of the class I cuspid and molar relationship (Figs. F4.34 through F4.59). If there is severe crowding in both arches, extraction of all first bicuspids[11] will alleviate the problem and the class I cuspid and molar relationship can be maintained.[3-5] If there is severe crowding on the upper or lower arch only, then the first bicuspids in both arches may need to be extracted in order to preserve a class I cuspid relationship.

Class II

Class II cases are either division 1 (flared upper incisor, excess overjet) or division 2 (retroclined upper central incisors, labially displaced laterals, and no overjet). By uprighting the retroclined upper central incisors in a division 2 case, we turn it into a division 1 case. Therefore, the treatment approach for both is similar. The treatment strategy with such cases depends on the patient's age.[13-15] In mixed dentition, nonextraction mechanotherapy that would move the upper posterior teeth distally is the treatment of choice. In the adolescent permanent dentition, some clinicians may try to do the same as in the mixed dentition, whereas others would extract the upper first bicuspids and finish a class II molar and class I cuspid relationship. In the adult patient, the ideal treatment in most cases would be nonextraction, uprighting of the central incisors, followed by a mandibular advancement orthognathic surgical procedure that would improve facial esthetics. (Class II patients usually have a retrognathic mandible.) If the patient refuses surgery, the treatment of choice would be extraction of the upper first bicuspids.

If the crowding is in both arches, extraction of all first bicuspids is necessary (Figs. F4.60 through F4.81). Because we are extracting in both arches in order to end up with a class I cuspid relationship, we must also end up with a class I molar relationship. This is what makes these cases very difficult in modern practice; if we have a full class II molar relationship to start with, in order to obtain a final class I relationship of these teeth, we must achieve a total of 7 mm (the width of a cusp or the difference between a class I and a class II) of molar movement. This is usually done by mesial movement of the mandibular first molar in the range of 3 to 4 mm along with distal movement of the maxillary molar in the range of 2 to 3 mm, either with a

Text continued on page 293.

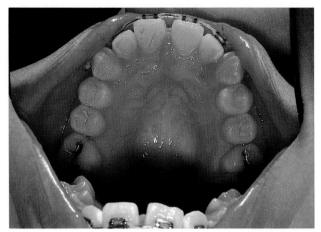

F4.1

Figure F4.1 Limited orthodontic treatment of the adult dentition may be attempted when the patient has realistic expectations and the chief complaint is simple enough. This midline diastema requires minor tooth tipping for correction. In this case, as can be seen from the palatal view, correction of the diastema would provide adequate space in the rest of the anterior area for the alleviation of the minor rotations of the left lateral and cuspid teeth.

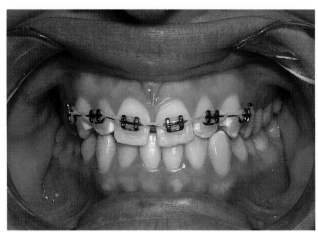

F4.2

Figure F4.2 A 2×6 appliance (two bands on the first molars and six brackets on the anterior teeth) with a Neo-sentalloy (GAC) light (100 g) 0.016×0.022 inch² rectangular NiTi wire along with an elastic chain from cuspid to cuspid was all it took to correct the discrepancy. The cuspid teeth are not wire tied to allow for their rotation from the pull of the elastic chain.

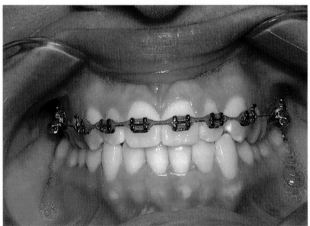

F4.3

Figure F4.3 The diastema is closed in 3 months.

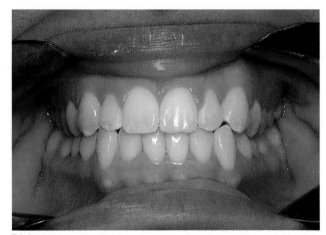

F4.4

Figure F4.4 Patient after appliance removal.

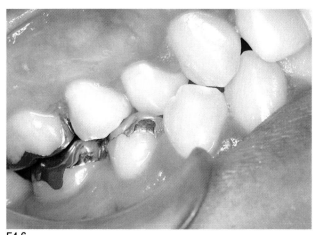

F4.5

Figure F4.5 A permanent retainer wire is bonded on the lingual of the central incisor teeth.

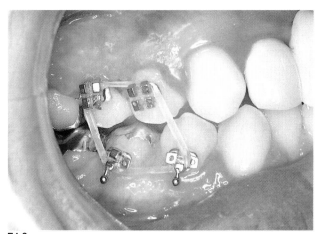

F4.6

Figure F4.6 Single-tooth crossbite of the upper first bicuspid in an otherwise ideal class I occlusion. A limited treatment may be rendered.

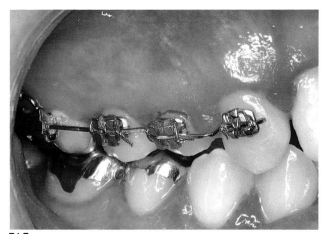

F4.7

Figure F4.7 Four brackets placed from the upper first molar to the ipsilateral cuspid tooth and a 0.016-inch round NiTi wire followed by a 0.016 × 0.022 inch² stainless steel segmental wire was all it took to bring the bicuspid out of the crossbite. Note that, because of the gingival overgrowth over that tooth, the bracket is not high enough on the bicuspid. A step downbent (second order) in the archwire compensated for the improper bracket placement.

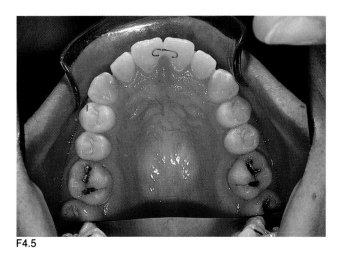

F4.8

Figure F4.8 Use of 24-hour box elastics for 1 week brought the teeth into a solid intercuspation.

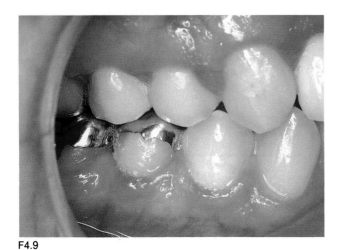

F4.9

Figure F4.9 Total treatment time: 2 months.

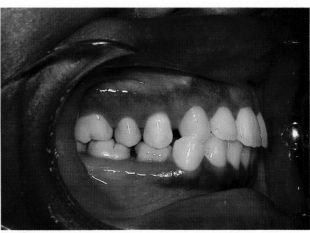

F4.10

Figure F4.10 Right buccal view before treatment. Note the "super" class I molar relationship (20% class III) and the retained mandibular second primary molar. The upper cuspid is in lingual crossbite with the first bicuspid and in a class I relationship with the lower cuspid.

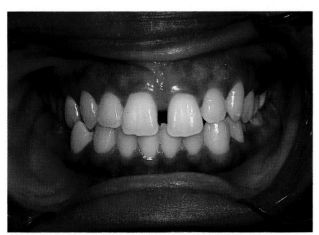

F4.11

Figure F4.11 Anterior view before treatment. Note the midline diastema, which was the patient's chief complaint.

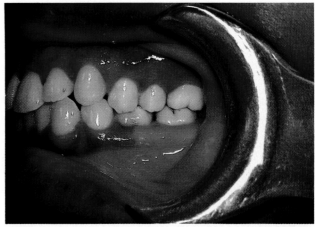

F4.12

Figure F4.12 Left buccal view before treatment. Note the class I molar relationship and the retained mandibular second primary molar.

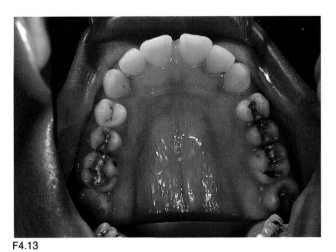

F4.13

Figure F4.13 Upper occlusal view showing a total of 4 mm of spacing.

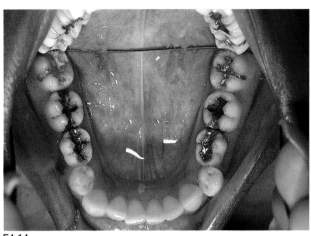

F4.14

Figure F4.14 Lower occlusal view showing a total of 3 mm of crowding.

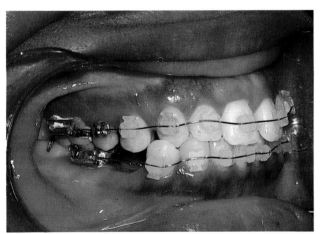

F4.15

Figures F4.15 through F4.17 Immediately after bracket placement. Due to the minor movements planned for this case and the absence of a deep bite, ceramic appliances were placed even on the lower teeth, well away from the line of occlusion, in order to avoid abrasion of the maxillary teeth; 0.012-inch initial round stainless steel archwires were placed on both arches for initial alignment and leveling.

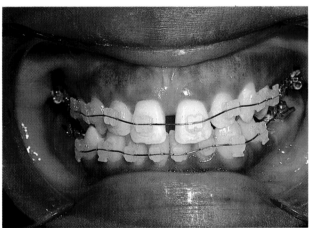

F4.16

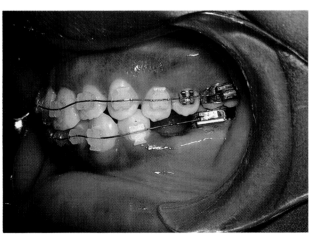

F4.17

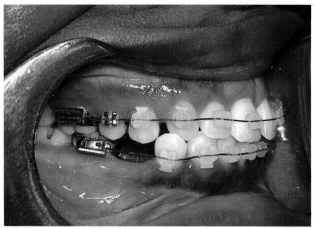

F4.18

Figures F4.18 through F4.20 Round 0.014-inch archwires were placed to continue with the alignment and leveling. The clinician may proceed to the next size of wires when they can be placed in the brackets without deformation of the wires.

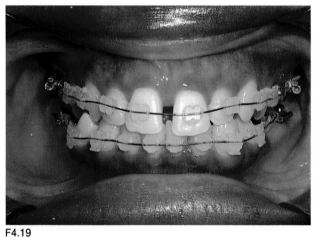

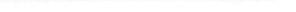

F4.19

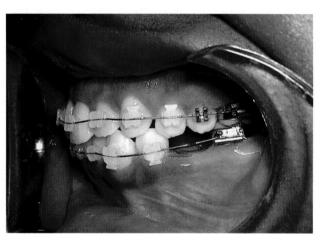

F4.20

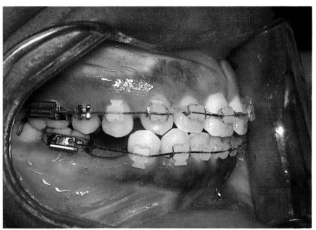

F4.21

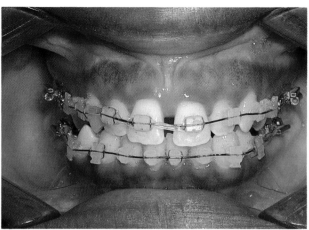

F4.22

Figures F4.21 through F4.23 Round 0.016-inch archwires complete the alignment and leveling. All of the stainless steel archwires used up to now could have been substituted with an 0.016-inch round NiTi wire or even the new rectangular superelastic Neosentalloy (GAC) NiTi wires, which give torque and root control from the start of treatment. Note the elastomeric chains (power or C-chains) from the upper right cuspid to the left central incisor and from the lower left first bicuspid to the left first mandibular molar. The purpose is to bring the upper left incisor closer to the midline and to alleviate the crowding in the lower left area by bringing the bicuspid back 2 mm into the space that has been made available after the extraction of the Es. The ligature wire that ties around the right cuspid, left incisor, and the lower left bicuspid prevents those teeth from rotating from the pull of the elastic chains. Ideally, we would place elastic chains when we are in rectangular wires, but because the tooth movements that are attempted in this case are minor (1 to 2 mm), we can save some treatment time by using only sectional C-chains on round wires. Even if the teeth tip a little, root uprighting will occur when we place the finishing rectangular wires.

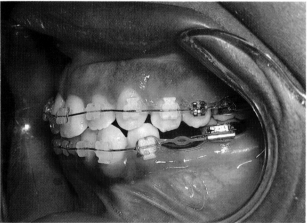

F4.23

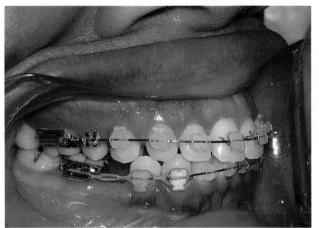

F4.24

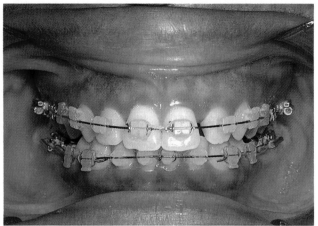

F4.25

Figures F4.24 through F4.26 Rectangular 0.016×0.022 inch^2 finishing archwires placed in the arches with sectional C-chains. Note the closure of the central diastema and the correction of the upper midline (the lower midline was on from the beginning). Also note the correction of the right crossbite between the upper right cuspid and the lower first bicuspid. This was obtained gradually through the archwire changes. Elastic chains (from molar to molar) will close any remaining spaces over the next 4 to 6 months to finish the case.

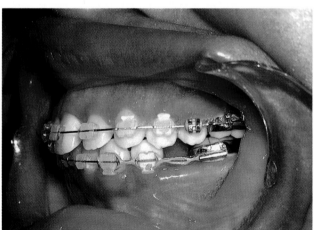

F4.26

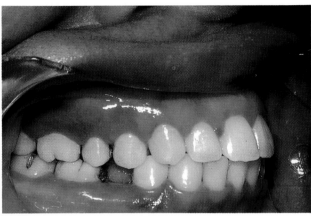

F4.27

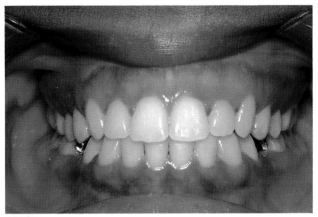

F4.28

Figures F4.27 through F4.31 The patient's occlusion immediately after debonding. Note the slight gingival inflammation, despite the patient's excellent oral hygiene cooperation. The space provided by the extraction of the lower second primary molars was used to alleviate the lower crowding as well as to retract the lower teeth to create 2 mm of overjet and thus all the retraction of the upper teeth to close the spaces in the maxillary arch. (Due to the minimal overjet initially, closure of the midline diastema would not have been possible.) Total treatment time was a little over a year.

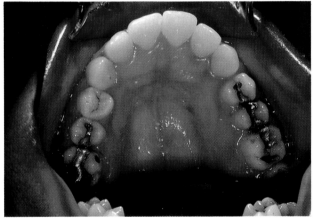

F4.30

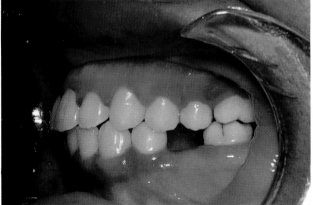

F4.29

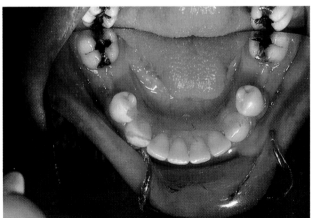

F4.31

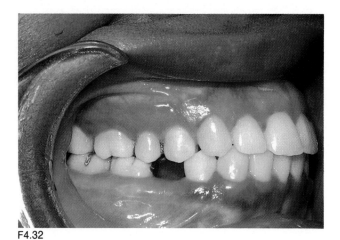

F4.32

Figure F4.32 The patient's occlusion 1 week after debonding.

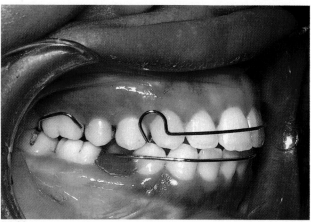

F4.33

Figure F4.33 The maxillary and mandibular Hawley retainers provide posttreatment stability. Note the acrylic to preserve the lower E space until the patient has prosthetic work done.

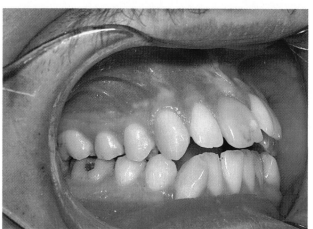

F4.34

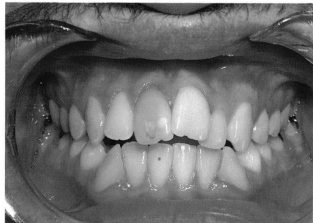

F4.35

Figures F4.34 and F4.35 This is a dental open bite with significant flaring of the anterior teeth. It is obvious that the anterior teeth need to be retracted to their ideal position over the basal bone. The crowding is minor (3 mm) and moderate (6 mm) on the upper and lower dental arches, respectively.

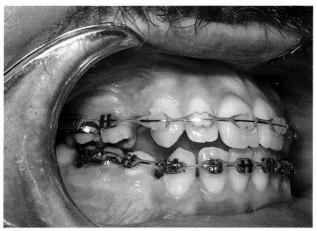

F4.36

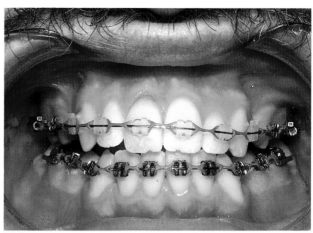

F4.37

Figures F4.36 and F4.37 Extraction of the first bicuspids facilitated the retraction of the anterior teeth with upper and lower 0.016 × 0.022 inch² Neosentalloy (GAC) wires and elastomeric chains. Note the normal OB and OJ relationship of 2 mm that has been established early in treatment (within 3 months).

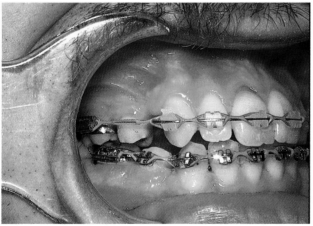

F4.38

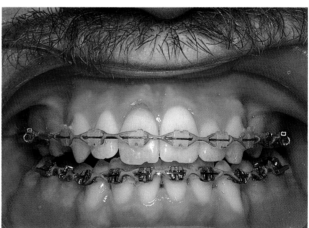

F4.39

Figures F4.38 and F4.39 The bite is continuing to close as further leveling (especially of the upper arch on the right side) is taking place.

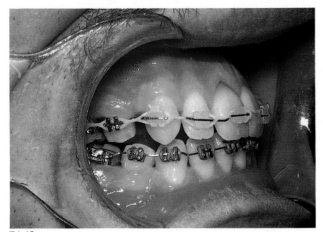

F4.40

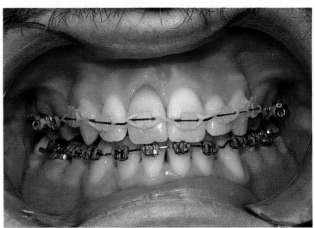

F4.41

Figures F4.40 and F4.41 Finishing stainless steel rectangular wires (0.016×0.022 inch²) are used to place compensating bends as space closure continues with elastomeric chains.

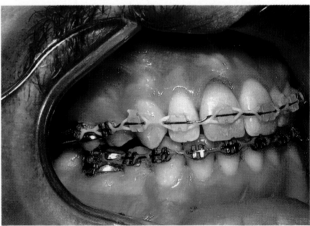

F4.42

Figure F4.42 Toward the end of treatment with space closure almost completed.

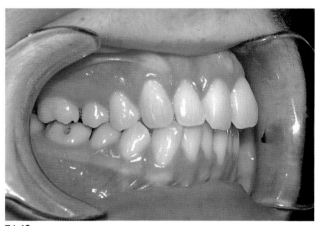

F4.43

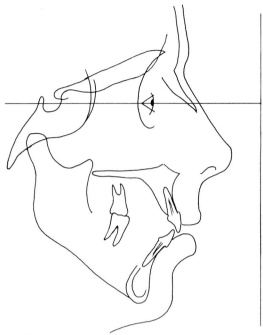

F4.44

Figures F4.43 through F4.46 Patient's occlusion before treatment. Note the class I molar relationship, the open bite tendency, and the mesially tipped bicuspids and cuspids, which make them appear in a class I relationship versus a class II 50% (end-to-end) if they were upright. The crowding is minor (about 3 mm for each arch).

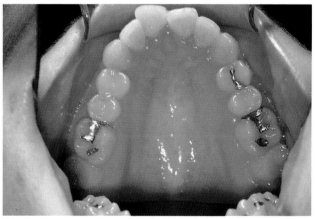

F4.45

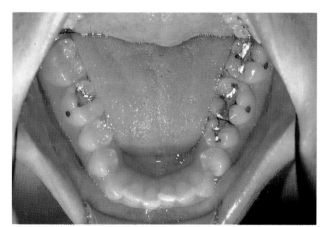

F4.46

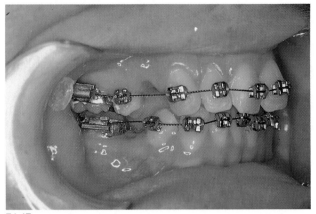

F4.47

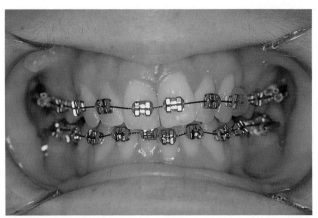

F4.48

Figures F4.47 and F4.48 Although this case could have been treated with TR, the therapy plan here was extraction of the upper first and the lower second bicuspids. This extraction pattern was necessitated by the patient's long lower facial pattern with an open-bite tendency (see Fig. 4.44). Immediately after bracket placement, initial 0.0175-inch braided stainless steel archwires are used (an 0.12-inch stainless steel wire could have been used as well).

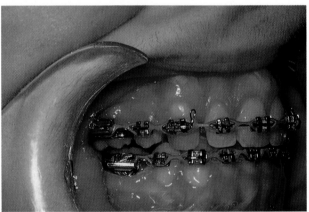

F4.49

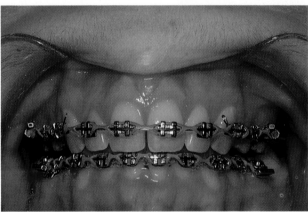

F4.50

Figures F4.49 and F4.50 After having gone through the usual stainless steel round archwire sequence presented previously (0.014-inch, 0.016-inch), 0.016×0.022 inch² finishing rectangular stainless steel archwires were used. The mechanics used for space closure are elastomeric chains from molar to molar and class II elastics (from the lower molar to the upper cuspid), worn full-time or at least at night. Class II elastics were used 24 hours a day for over 3 months (from the lower molar to the upper cuspid), and have a tendency to extrude the lower molars while flaring the lower and tipping back the upper anterior teeth. Elastics should be used only with rectangular archwires to minimize the afore-mentioned side effects and to maximize their use, which is for bodily mesial movement of the lower posterior segments and distal movement of the upper anterior segment.

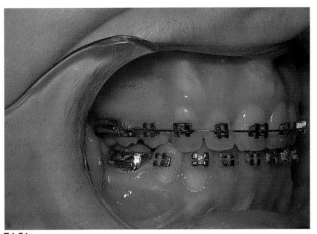

F4.51

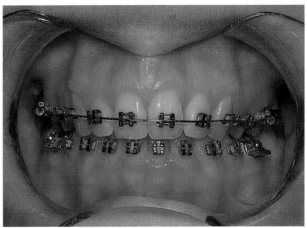

F4.52

Figures F4.51 and F4.52 After the posterior spaces have closed and a class I cuspid and molar relationship has been achieved, C-chains from molar to molar will consolidate tooth contacts and close any remaining spaces; 0.016×0.022 inch² stainless steel archwires with accentuated and reverse curve of Spee on the upper and the lower arches, respectively, are used. These will counteract the lingual tipping of the anterior segments due to the constant pull of the elastic chains over the months of treatment. If this side effect starts to occur, the clinician will notice the creation of an open bite in the bicuspid area and excessive retroclination of the anterior segments.

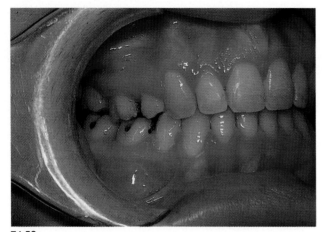

F4.53

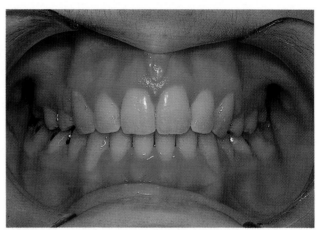

F4.54

Figures F4.53 through F4.56 Patient after appliance removal. Note the 2-mm overbite relationship that has been achieved.

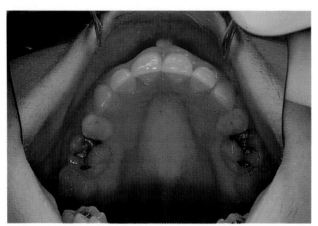

F4.55

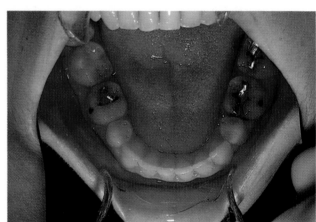

F4.56

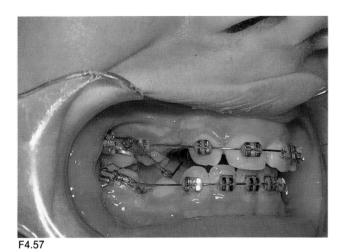

F4.57

Figure F4.57 This patient demonstrated a palatally impacted cuspid that was brought in the arch with a slight modification of the "ballista spring system" (Jacoby H: The "ballista spring" system for impacted teeth. Am J Orthod 75:143–151, 1979). The double-loop spring for initial activation of palatally impacted cuspids is made of 0.016 × 0.022 inch² wire. Its posterior end is inserted into the auxiliary buccal tube of the molar band, while its middle segment forms a 45-degree angle with the main archwire.

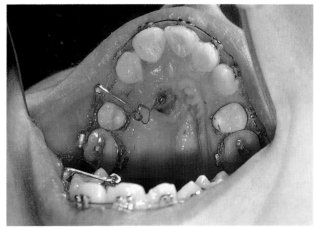

F4.58

Figure F4.58 The anterior segment of the spring forms a 90-degree angle with the rest of the appliance and intersects the occlusal plane toward the palate, where it hooks onto the loop of the ligature tie wire of the bracket that was bonded to the cuspid upon its surgical uncovering.

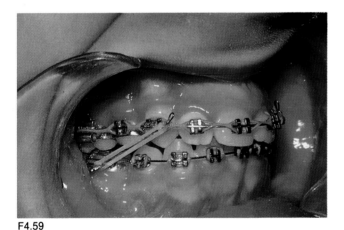

F4.59

Figure F4.59 The activation of the spring helps guide the impacted tooth to its final position in the arch, where elastics may complete its movement.

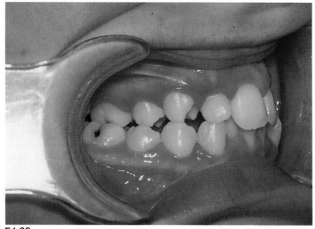

F4.60

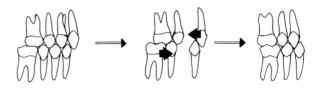

F4.61

Figures F4.60 through F4.63 A case with class II 50% relationship with severe maxillary (16 mm) and mandibular (8 mm) crowding. The crowding can very easily be calculated by eye-balling the arches: the cuspid width is about 8 mm, whereas each incisor overlap is about 2 mm of crowding. With such severe lack of space, extractions are necessary in both arches. This means that, in order to end up with a class I cuspid relationship, we must secure a class I molar relationship as well. In other words, we must make sure that the mandibular first molars come 3 to 4 mm anteriorly, while keeping the maxillary ones where they are, so that a class I relationship may be achieved. The combination of upper first bicuspid and lower second bicuspid extractions brings us closer to our goals: the maxillary cuspids can easily be brought into the space of the first bicuspids, and the mandibular molars can slip anteriorly with sliding mechanics. As shown in the diagram, if we had a full class II (100%) molar relationship, then the total tooth movement would have been even more difficult, because the lower molar would have to move anteriorly even more and the upper cuspid 7 mm distally.

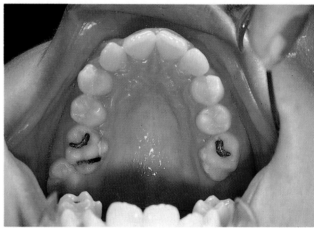

F4.62

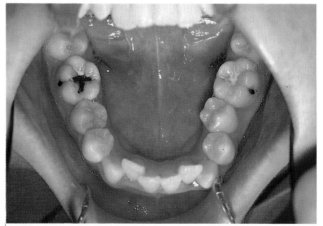

F4.63

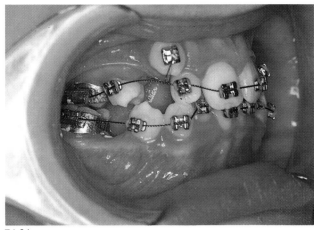

F4.64

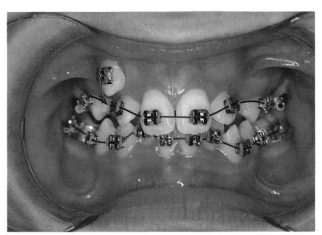

F4.65

Figures F4.64 and F4.65 After banding and bonding, initial 0.175-inch, round, braided archwires are used with a slight vertical activation to the uncovered maxillary cuspid wired with a ligature wire tie. (Rectangular 0.016×0.022 inch^2 superelastic initial wires would be used today.)

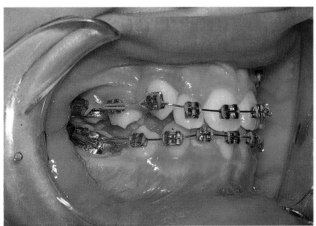

F4.66

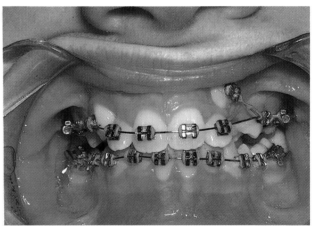

F4.67

Figures F4.66 and F4.67 The second set of wires are 0.014-inch round stainless steel. An elastic chain pulls the maxillary cuspid distally into the extraction space.

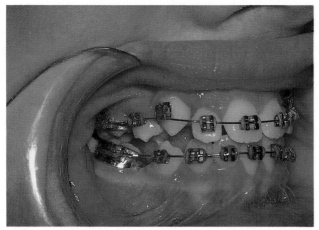

F4.68

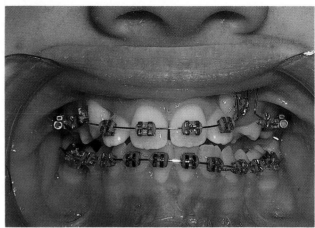

F4.69

Figures F4.68 and F4.69 The third set of wires are 0.016-inch round stainless steel. Note the correction of the crossbite in the molar region that was accomplished with the activation of the TPA. Also note the mesial movement of the mandibular molar that has brought this tooth into a class I relationship with the upper molar, as well as the leveling that has taken place. All the changes that have been achieved up to now in this case with the aforementioned sequence archwires would now be achieved with only one initial archwire: a rectangular NiTi 0.016×0.022 inch^2 superelastic Neosentalloy (GAC).

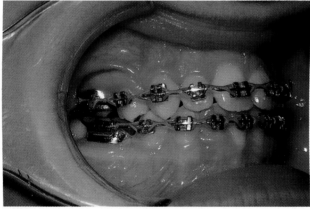

F4.70

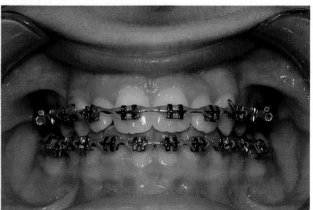

F4.71

Figures F4.70 and F4.71 Finishing archwires—0.016×0.022 inch^2 stainless steel with elastic chains—to close any remaining spaces.

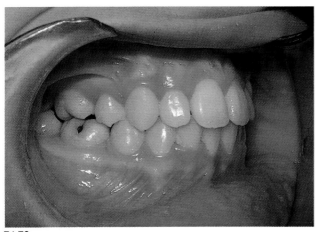

F4.72

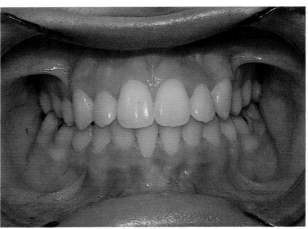

F4.73

Figures F4.72 and F4.73 The occlusion at the time of appliance removal. Note the solid intercuspation of the cuspid teeth in a class I relationship.

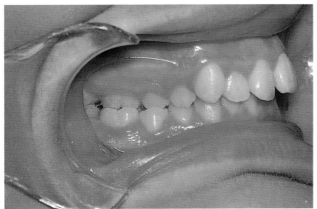

F4.74

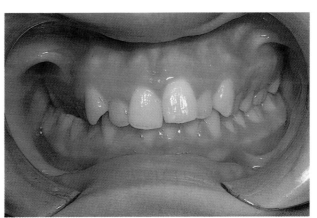

F4.75

Figures F4.74 and F4.75 This class II 50% (end-to-end) adult case is similar to the previous one, but it is treated a little differently in the finishing stages.

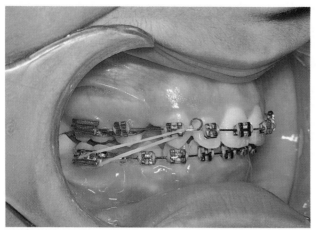

F4.76

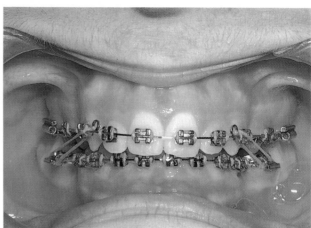

F4.77

Figures F4.76 and F4.77 After alignment and leveling had been completed, a finishing 0.016×0.022 inch^2 rectangular stainless steel archwire with a loop in front of each cuspid was used with class II elastics. This type of mechanotherapy achieves a twofold goal: it protracts the lower molar mesially while it pulls on the whole upper anterior segment (through the loops) distally.

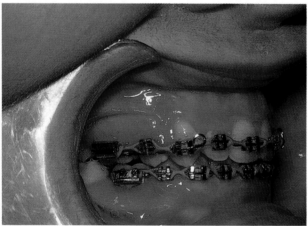

F4.78

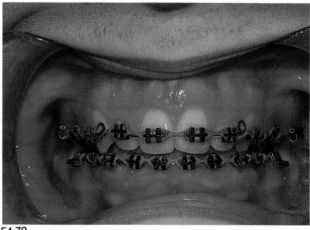

F4.79

Figures F4.78 and F4.79 A class I molar and cuspid relation is achieved with the use of the reciprocal forces exerted by the elastic. Elastomeric chains are used to consolidate any remaining spaces.

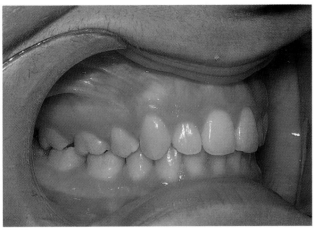

F4.80

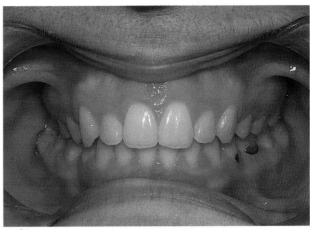

F4.81

Figures F4.80 and F4.81 Occlusion after appliance removal. It should be pointed out that this case was treated before the introduction of the Neosentalloy (GAC) coil springs (for nonextraction treatments). The patient was reluctant to wear a headgear appliance, and thus the extraction of teeth was the most appropriate option for securing a class I cuspid relationship.

coil-spring apparatus[7] or headgear appliance[4,5] (Figs. F4.82 through F4.88). In an adult, this would be done with a 7-mm mandibular advancement orthognathic procedure. If the initial relationship was a class II 50%, then the total correction is much easier (3 to 4 mm of total molar movements).

If there is crowding in the maxillary arch only, extraction of the upper first bicuspids is the extraction pattern of choice. This would result in a class I cuspid occlusion and a class II molar relationship (*i.e.,* the molars are left in class II) (Figs. F4.89 through F4.96). If there is crowding in the mandibular arch only, the extraction of the lower front bicuspids would leave us with two options: (1) to align the lower teeth and perform a mandibular advancement procedure[8] that will result in the class I cuspid relationship or (2) to extract in the upper arch as well and try to finish in a class I occlusion (similar to the class II situation with upper and lower severe crowding). The extractions in the upper arch would be necessary because the upper cuspids would have to be retracted in order to end up with a class I cuspid relationship. This would be a very difficult treatment.

Text continued on page 298.

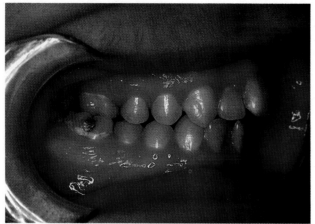

F4.82

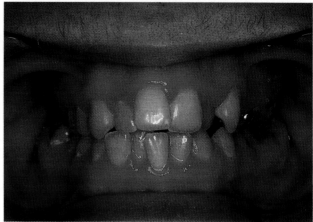

F4.83

Figures F4.82 through F4.84 This is a characteristic dental asymmetry case caused by the previous extraction of the upper left first bicuspid years ago. As a result, the upper dental midline shifted to the left by 4 mm, and the right cuspids ended up in a full step class II relationship, whereas the left ones are in a class I relationship. Had the bicuspid extraction not taken place, there would have been no midline deviation and the cuspids would both be in a class II 50% (end-to-end) relationship. Because the left side is now in a class I cuspid and a solid class II molar relationship without any crowding, the treatment plan should have as a primary objective preservation of these relations on the left side while at the same time attempting to shift the midline toward the right and obtaining a class I cuspid relationship on the right side (from a full class II).

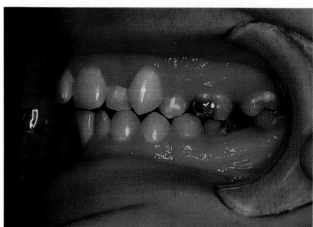

F4.84

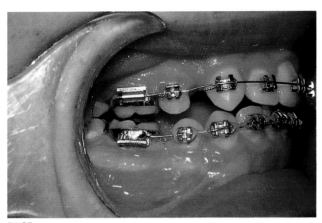

F4.85

Figure F4.85 It is obvious that by extracting the upper right first bicuspid, the aforementioned goals would be achieved. The patient also had a 6.5-mm lower crowding. The choices were to extract a lower incisor and end up with a slightly increased overjet (see Chapter 5) or to extract the lower right second bicuspid and end up with a class I molar relationship on the right side and compromise the lower midline toward the right side (as we alleviate the crowding) but end up with an ideal OB and OJ of 2-mm. The latter approach was chosen. In retrospect, extraction of a lower incisor might have been a better plan. The patient was also given a high-pull (occipital) headgear to wear at night only to try to influence the vertical dimension by keeping the upper molars from extruding (and thus opening more the bite anteriorly) during orthodontic mechanotherapy. (***Remember:*** Teeth always extrude when fixed appliances with continuous or segmental archwires are placed on them, even if the clinician keeps any leveling of the occlusion to a minimum.)

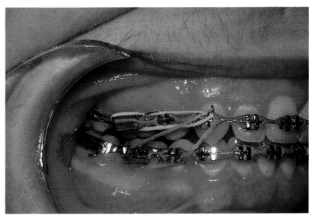

F4.86

Figures F4.86 through F4.88 The patient underwent the normal sequence of round archwire changes (0.012-, 0.014-, 0.016-inch stainless steel). When the finishing 0.016×0.022 inch^2 stainless steel archwires were placed on both arches, elastomeric chains and asymmetrical elastics were used for 4 months to close spaces and secure a class I cuspid relationship on the left side. The class III elastic used on the left side (from the upper molar to the lower cuspid) brings the upper and lower teeth slightly anteriorly and posteriorly, respectively. On the right side, the mechanotherapy used is a little different. The class II elastic (from the lower molar to the upper cuspids, thus having the opposite effect of the class IIIs) has a vertical component to it (by including the lower bicuspid) in an effort to obtain as great an intercuspation as possible during the anteroposterior retraction. The class I elastic (from the upper first molar to the upper cuspid) aids the elastomeric chain during space closure within the same arch (in this case, the space distal to the cuspid). This case will finish far from ideally with a class II 30% right cuspid relationship. Headgear cooperation was fair.

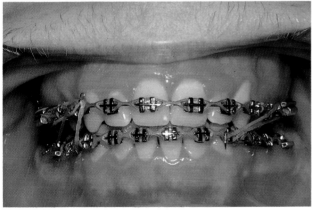

F4.87

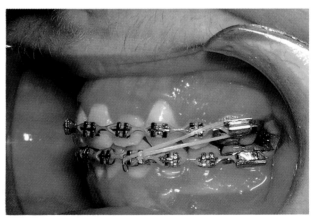

F4.88

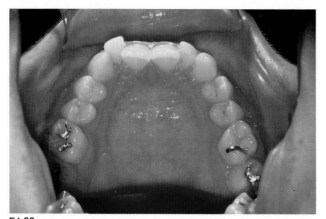

F4.89

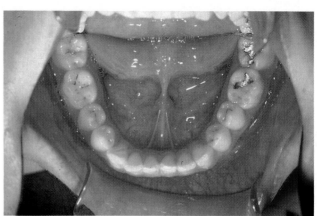

F4.90

Figures F4.89 through F4.92 Typical class II, division 2 mal-occlusion in an adult. Note the lingually retroclined upper central and labially displaced lateral incisors. Although the ideal treatment would have been correction of the inclination of the central incisors and a 7-mm mandibular advancement, extraction of the first bicuspids was done instead because the patient refused the surgical option.

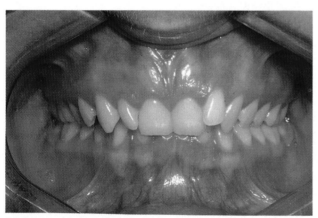

F4.91

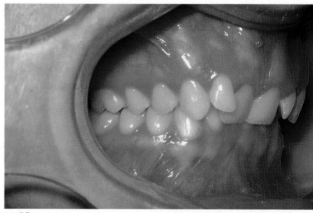

F4.92

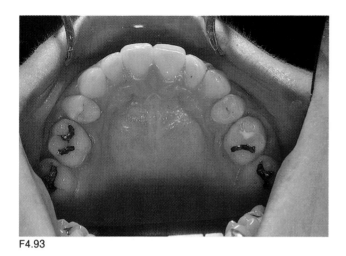

F4.93

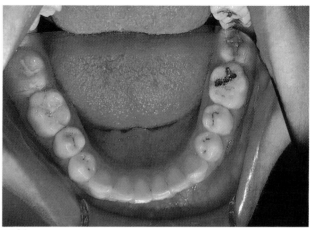

F4.94

Figures F4.93 through F4.96 Posttreatment occlusion. Note the class II molar with class I cuspid relationship.

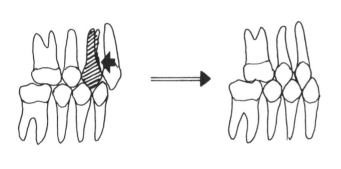

F4.95

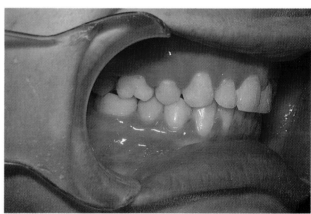

F4.96

Class III

In a recent investigation of 302 adult class III individuals, it was reported that almost one third of the sample had a combination of maxillary retrusion and mandibular protrusion.[16] Maxillary skeletal retrusion with a normally positioned mandible is found in 19.5% to 25% of class II patients.[1,2] Mandibular protrusion, commonly cited as the major skeletal aberration in individuals with class III malocclusion, was found in only 18.7% of the total sample.

In another study, a combination of maxillary retrusion and mandibular protrusion was found in 22.2% of the sample.[17] Forty-one percent of this entire sample (59 of 144) also had long lower face height. Clearly, even in children and adolescents, a class III malocclusion does not indicate some typical facial skeletal pattern. Rather, it can be the result of any of several combinations of aberrations in the craniofacial complex. A tendency exists for a morphologic difference between the mandibles of class III and class I individuals. This difference occurs early. The increase in vertical lower anterior facial growth occurs later and is not typically present in early childhood.[16,17] In young patients (5 to 11 years of age) with maxillary deficiency, the treatment of choice is protraction facemask therapy (see Figs. E8.1 through E8.6). In patients with mandibular prognathism, it is best to wait until completion of growth for a mandibular setback orthognathic procedure. This eliminates the possibility of a second surgery due to late or excessive growth of the mandible in the late teens or early twenties, especially in boys. In the event that any dental problem exists, orthodontic therapy alone may be undertaken (depending on the case), followed by retainers (Figs. F4.97 through F4.115).

Text continued on page 304.

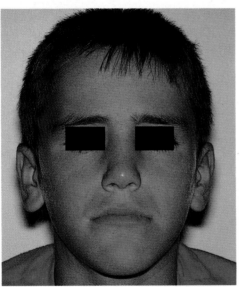

F4.97

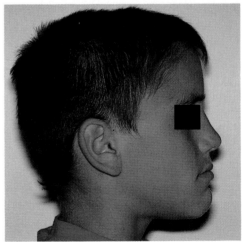

F4.98

Figures F4.97 through F4.102 This class III malocclusion patient has severe crowding of the upper arch (14 mm) and minor crowding in the lower. Note the fullness of the lower third of the face, indicating mandibular prognathism. Also note the end-to-end relationship of the retroclined incisors, also indicative of a class III malocclusion. In order to avoid possible impaction of the upper cuspids (note that the upper first bicuspids have erupted next to the lateral incisors), extraction of all first bicuspid teeth was done (the lower first bicuspids were extracted in order to achieve a class I cuspid relationship).

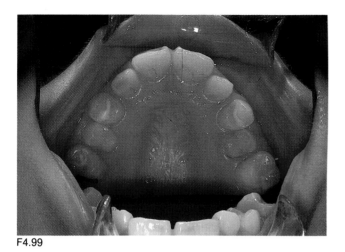

F4.99

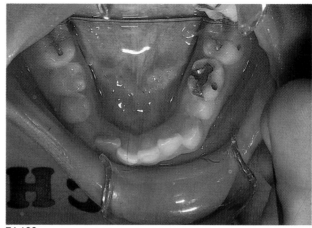

F4.100

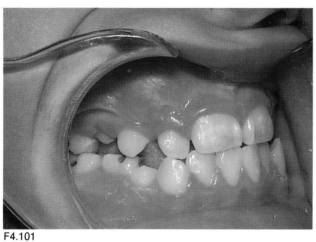

F4.101

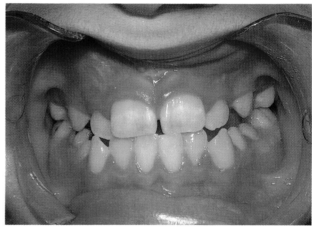

F4.102

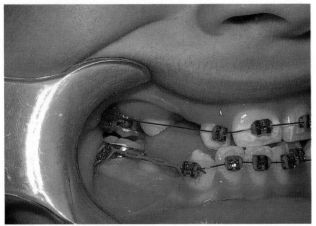

F4.103

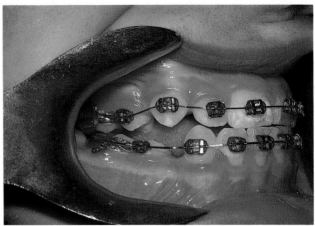

F4.104

Figures F4.103 and F4.104 The upper cuspids erupted within 2 months into the space that was provided for them. Fixed appliances were placed to align and level the arches. As soon as this is done, retainers will keep the teeth in their position in the arches until completion of any further mandibular growth. The class III problem of this patient may remain mild; then again, it may turn out that his mandible will grow excessively. His present mild condition justifies an attempt to finish this case with a positive overbite relationship. A conservative approach will include class III elastics (3/4-inch, 2-oz) during the day, followed by chin-cup therapy at night. The objective of the conservative orthodontic mechanotherapy would be to obtain a positive overbite of at least 1 mm (from the present end-to-end anterior occlusion). The fixed appliance treatment should last about 1 year. The chin cup should be worn at night until well after the patient's pubertal growth spurt. No attempt should be made to retain the teeth in a positive OB/OJ relationship with fixed appliances and class III elastics past 1 year of treatment because if the mandible grows abnormally, the dental compensations would be too great of a compromise with extrusion of the lower anterior teeth and severe periodontal problems.

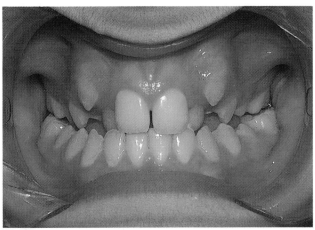

F4.105

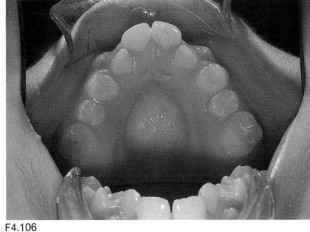

F4.106

Figures F4.105 through F4.107 This is a typical class III 50% malocclusion with a minimum overbite relationship. A constricted upper arch and a normal wide mandibular arch resulted in a bilateral end-to-end posterior crossbite. The patient is circumpubertal.

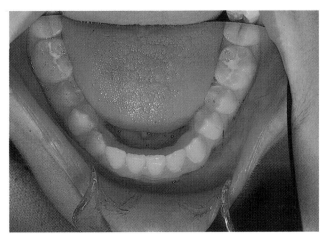

F4.107

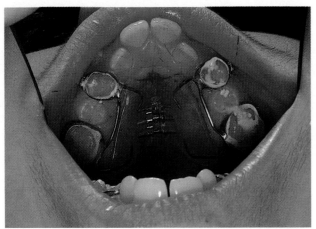

F4.108

Figure F4.108 An RME appliance was used to expand the upper arch to correct the crossbite and at the same time provide space for the upper cuspids.

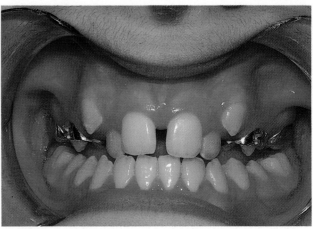

F4.109

Figures F4.109 and F4.110 The expansion was discontinued prematurely (after 12 days) because the acrylic was embedded in the soft tissue of the palate as it moved laterally from the activation of the screw of the appliance.

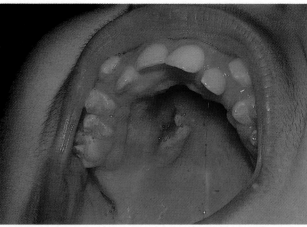

F4.110

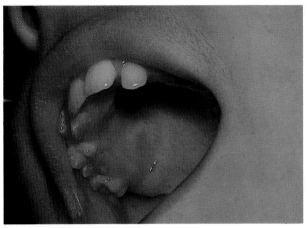

F4.111

Figure F4.111 The palatal soft tissue healed within a week after appliance removal. The expansion was held in the molar region only with a TPA.

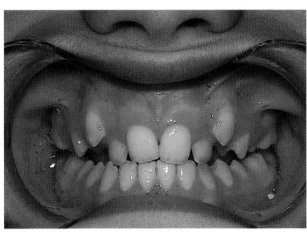

F4.112

Figure F4.112 Two weeks later, the midline diastema had closed from the pull of the transeptal fibers.

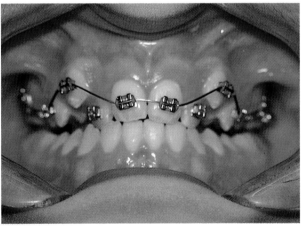

F4.113

Figure F4.113 After bracket placement, a 0.016 × 0.092 inch² Neosentalloy (GAC) rectangular NiTi wire was inserted in all teeth, with the exception of the lateral incisor teeth, to avoid any unnecessary tipping.

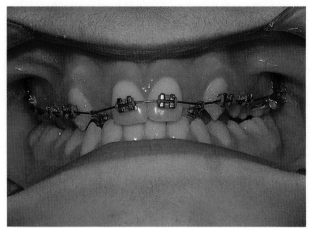

F4.114

Figure F4.114 Within 5 weeks, the cuspids had reached the occlusal plane. At this point, the laterals were wire tied to the archwire.

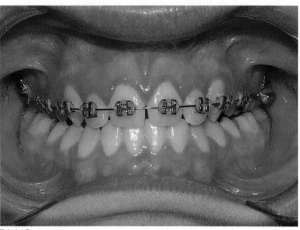

F4.115

Figure F4.115 After 2 months, the laterals were out of crossbite. Note the increase in the overbite relationship by 1 mm as a result of the RME. Also note the residual construction in the posterior region, especially in the bicuspid area. An RME appliance for a second time would be indicated at this point. It may not be necessary to place appliances in the lower arch in some of these cases.

If the crowding is in both arches, extraction of all bicuspids would lead to a class I cuspid and molar relationship[1-4] (Fig. F4.116). If it is in the upper arch only, extractions of the upper first bicuspids would alleviate the crowding but worsen the class III situation (because the anterior teeth would have to be retracted further posteriorly). Thus, the options available to us are (1) maxillary advancement or mandibular setback surgery[8] to obtain a class I cuspid relationship, or (2) lower first bicuspid extractions to end up with a class I occlusion.

The above situation is exactly the opposite, in terms of extraction patterns, to the class II lower severe crowded case. If the crowding is in the lower arch only, extraction of the lower first bicuspids will result in a class I cuspid and a class III molar relationship (Fig. F4.117).

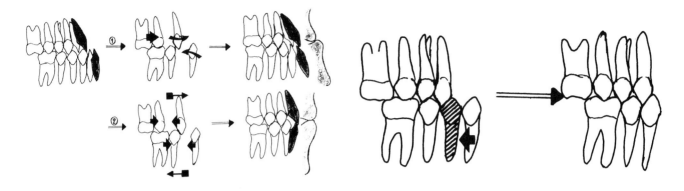

F4.116

F4.117

Figure F4.116 Class III malocclusion with crowding in both arches. (1) If the case is treated with orthodontic means alone, providing that the skeletal problem is minor, then the anterior teeth would have to be tipped *(curved arrows)* and the upper posteriors protracted anteriorly to secure a class I cuspid relationship. Note the compromised concave profile and the compensating inclinations of the anterior teeth. (2) If the case is treated with orthognathic surgery, no compensating dental tipping needs to take place. In fact decompensation of possible existing tipped positions of teeth may need to take place. The teeth can be moved bodily to their positions with either a maxillary or mandibular surgical procedure (or both) to provide the patient with an orthognathic profile.

Figure F4.117 Class III malocclusion with crowding in the lower arch only. Extraction of the lower first bicuspids will allow for a class I cuspid relationship after treatment.

References

1. Graber TM, and Swain BF: *Orthodontics: Current Principles and Techniques.* St. Louis, MO: C.V. Mosby Co., 1985.
2. Johnston LE: *New Vistas in Orthodontics.* Philadelphia: Lea & Febiger, 1985.
3. Proffit WR: *Contemporary Orthodontics.* St. Louis, MO: C.V. Mosby Co., 1986.
4. Graber LW: *Orthodontics: State of the Art, Essence of the Science.* St. Louis, MO: C.V. Mosby Co., 1986.
5. Alexander RG: *The Alexander Discipline. Contemporary Concepts and Philosophy.* Glendora, CA: Ormco Co., 1986.
6. Proffit WR, and White RP: *Surgical–Orthodontic Treatment.* St. Louis, MO: Mosby-Year Book, 1991.
7. Miura F, Masakuri M, and Yasuo O: New application of the superelastic NiTi rectangular wire. J Clin Orthod 24:544–548, 1990.
8. Bell WH: *Surgical Correction of Dentofacial Deformities,* vol. II. St. Louis, MO: C.V. Mosby Co., 1986.
9. Burstone CR: Deep overbite correction by intrusion. Am J Orthod 72:1–22, 1977.
10. McLaughlin RP, and Bennett JC: Anchorage control during leveling and aligning with a preadjusted appliance system. J Clin Orthod 25:687–696, 1991.
11. Drobocky OB, and Smith RJ: Changes in facial profile during orthodontic treatment with extraction of four first bicuspids. Am J Orthod Dentofacial Orthop 95:220–230, 1989.
12. Arvystas MG: Nonextraction treatment of severe class II, division 2 malocclusions. Am J Orthod Dentofacial Orthop 97:510–521, 1990.
13. Arvystas MG: Nonextraction treatment of severe class II, division 2 malocclusions. Am J Orthod Dentofacial Orthop 99:74–84, 1991.
14. Litt RA, and Nielsen IL: Class II, division 2 malocclusion: To extract or not extract? Angle Orthod 54:123–138, 1984.
15. Selwyn-Barnett BJ: Rationale of treatment for class II, division 2 malocclusion. Br J Orthod 18:173–181, 1991.
16. Ellis EE III, and McNamara JA, Jr.: Components of adult class III malocclusion. J Oral Maxillofac Surg 42:295–305, 1984.
17. Guyer EC, Ellis EE III, McNamara JA, Jr., and Behrents RG: Components of Class III malocclusion in juveniles and adolescents. Angle Orthod 56:7–30, 1986.

Chapter 5

Incisor Extraction/Missing Incisor/ Second Molar Extraction Therapy

The intentional extraction of a lower incisor can enable the orthodontist to produce enhanced functional occlusal and cosmetic results with minimal orthodontic manipulation[1] (Figs. F5.1 through F5.20). If the Bolton analysis shows a lower anterior excess, the extraction of a lower incisor might have a positive effect (see Figs. F4.21 through F4.28).

Enamel removal can be distributed among 10 maxillary interproximal surfaces (the mesial surfaces of both cuspids and proximal surfaces of the four incisors) to compensate for lower incisor extraction and reduce any excess overjet at the end of treatment. The proximal enamel is usually thickest on the mesial surfaces of the cuspids and the distal surfaces of the central incisors, whereas the mesial surfaces of lateral incisors may have only 0.5 mm of enamel.[1] If the interproximal surface is indiscriminately flattened, the interproximal contact will be lengthened gingivally, further reducing the space for the gingival papilla.[1]

Extruding the lower incisors to maintain occlusal contact in centric occlusion is advised.[1] If the maxillary anterior tooth size excess is managed successfully, one can usually still achieve a cuspid-protected occlusion. In some cases it is impossible to adequately compensate for the tooth size imbalance, so it may not be possible to achieve a cuspid rise. In these cases, group function may be produced orthodontically and by equilibration to eliminate cross-arch balancing interferences.

Often, patients present with congenitally missing upper lateral incisors (Figs. F5.17 through F5.53). The treatment approaches in such cases are (1) movement of the cuspid teeth in place of the laterals, followed by recontouring of their surfaces to appear like laterals, while at the same time the upper first bicuspids are placed in a class I relation with the lower cuspid teeth (group function is suggested for such cases); and (2) attainment of a full class I cuspid relation by opening up the spaces for bridgework or implants to substitute the lateral incisor teeth.

A number of orthodontists consider extraction of second molars to be unjustified because tooth material is being removed away from the area in which crowding occurs (usually the incisor) and space is created at the end in the dental arch.[2-4] Extraction of second molars assumes not only that the mesioangularly erupting third molar will erupt, but also that it will do so without an abnormal mesial inclination.[4] Even if excellent root parallelism exists, an acceptable contact relation is unlikely between first and third molars.[4-6] The differences would allow for food impaction and increased plaque. Marginal ridge discrepancies and faulty contacts create high-risk areas that are more susceptible to destructive periodontal disease.[4,6] The alveolar ridge is not as wide buccolingually at the bicuspid area and does not lead to food impaction as readily as the wider interproximal bone, located more distally in the arch.[4,6] The effect of the extractions on the third molars cannot be evaluated until the patients are older.[4,6]

First molars can be moved distally in second molar extraction cases with traditional fixed appliance mechanics with as much as 4 to 6 mm of distal movement, with an average of 2 mm on each side. A study of patients treated with functional appliances showed virtually no distal movement of the first molar.[3] The resulting facial profile after extraction of second molars appears to be no different from that obtained after extraction of first bicuspids.[7]

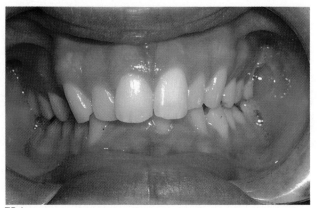

F5.1

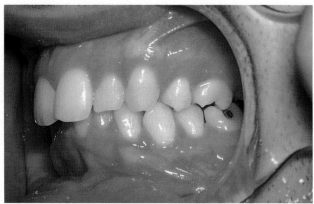

F5.2

Figures F5.1 through F5.4 This is a class II molar occlusion with previous extraction of the upper first bicuspids and a deep overbite. Due to the significant crowding in the lower arch (7 mm) and the already existing class I cuspid relation (which should be preserved), the only treatment option was extraction of one lower incisor and leveling of the arches to decrease the overbite.

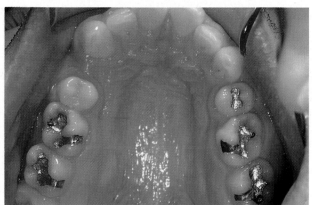

F5.3

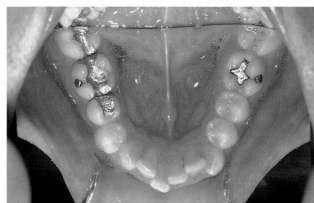

F5.4

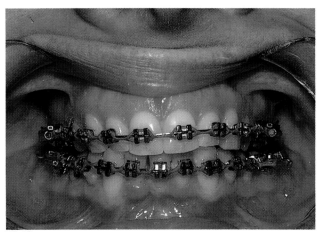

F5.13

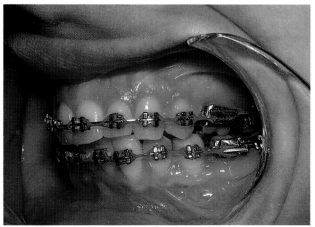

F5.14

Figures F5.13 and F5.14 After the sequence of round wires described in previous cases, and a few months into treatment with the alignment and leveling completed, finishing 0.016 × 0.022 inch² rectangular stainless steel archwires were placed with elastic chains to close any remaining spaces. It must be emphasized that closure of the lower incisor extraction space was initiated on the initial round wires (*i.e.,* 0.014-inch). We want to prevent the collapse of the thin buccal and lingual cortical plates in this area and also prevent the formation of a thin alveolar ridge that may not resorb as easily later on. This may lead to the creation of a gingival cleft that is very unesthetic when the patient smiles.

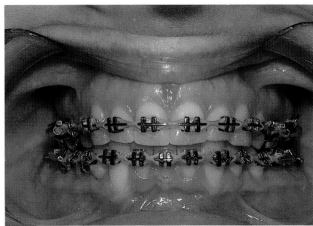

F5.15

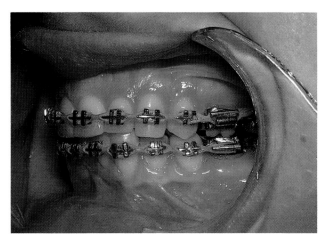

F5.16

Figures F5.15 and F5.16 After space closure. Note the tight contacts of the lower anterior teeth.

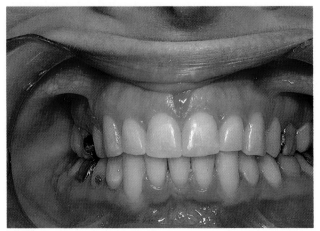

F5.17

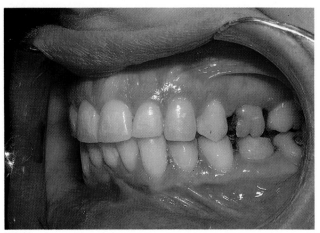

F5.18

Figures F5.17 through F5.20 After appliance removal. Note that a class I occlusion of the cuspids has been achieved (the cuspid is 20% class III), thus reducing the overjet that would have otherwise existed due to the tooth size discrepancy (see previous case).

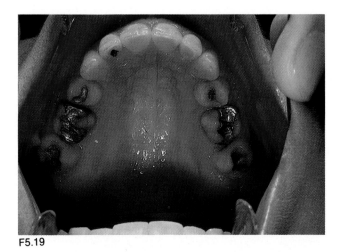

F5.19

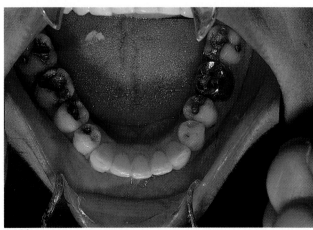

F5.20

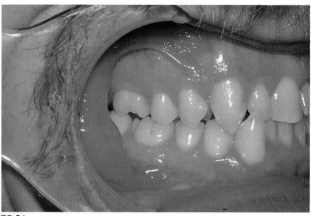

F5.21

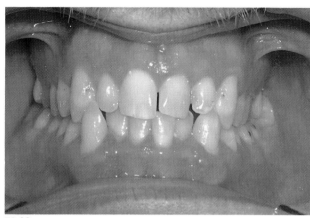

F5.22

Figures F5.21 through F5.25 This adult patient has a class III 50% molar relation with class I cuspids and small upper laterals. The pointed cuspid teeth gave the patient a displeasing appearance. The crowding was moderate for both arches, 3 mm for the upper and 5 mm for the lower.

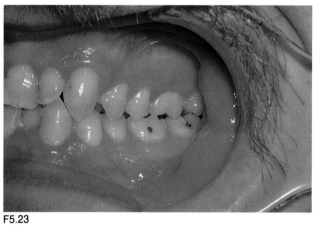

F5.23

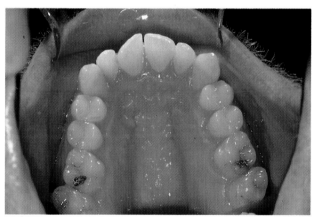

F5.24

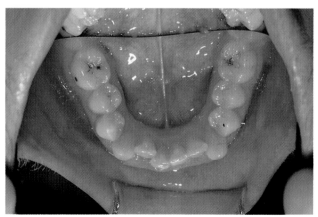

F5.25

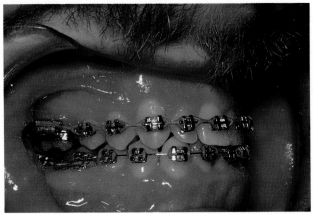

F5.26

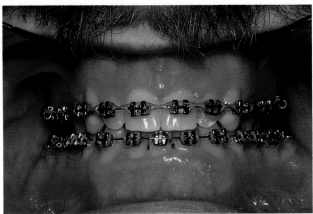

F5.27

Figures F5.26 through F5.28 A lower central incisor extraction (5 mm in width) pattern resulted in an acceptable occlusion. The small upper laterals contributed to the attainment of a normal overjet relationship (had they been of normal size, we would have ended up with excess overjet). The same sequence of wires was followed as shown previously.

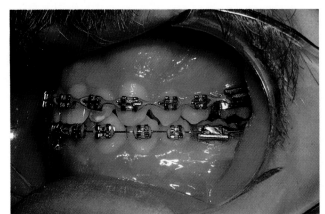

F5.28

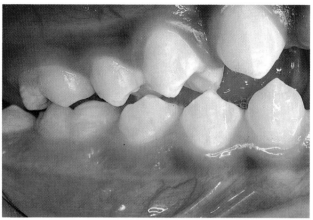

F5.29

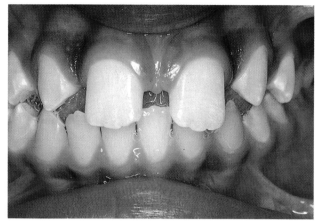

F5.30

Figures F5.29 through F5.32 This child is bimaxillary protrusive and is missing the two upper laterals in the permanent dentition. If she were to have a full complement of teeth, extractions of the first bicuspids would be indicated. Because she is already missing two teeth in the maxillary arch, extraction of the lower first bicuspids would help us reach the same goal. The cuspids will be recontoured toward the end of treatment to make them look like laterals and the upper first bicuspids will occlude in a class I relation with the lower cuspids. (Extensive cuspal, labial, lingual, and interproximal recontouring by the grinding of young teeth associated with orthodontic treatment can be performed without discomfort to the patients and with only minor or no long-term clinical and radiographic reactions: Thordarson A, Zachrisson BV, and Mjör IA: Remodeling of cuspids to the shape of lateral incisors by grinding: A long-term clinical and radiographic evaluation. Am J Orthod Dentofacial Orthop 100:123–132, 1991.)

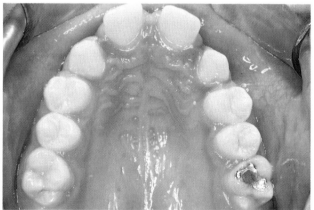

F5.31

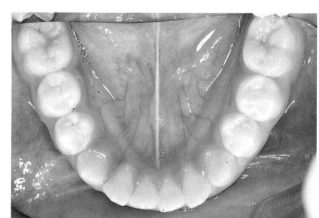

F5.32

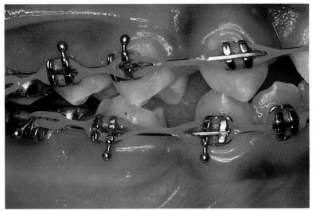

F5.33

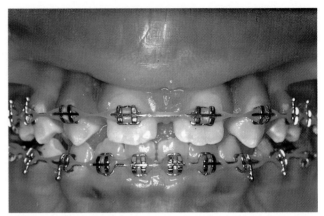

F5.34

Figures F5.33 through F5.36 The patient was given fixed appliances, and a set of 0.016×0.022 inch^2 superelastic Neosentalloy (GAC) NiTi rectangular archwires were inserted for initial alignment and leveling, as well as elastic chains to initiate space closure.

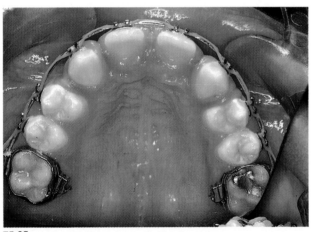

F5.35

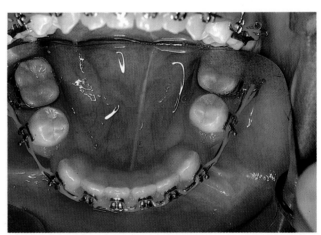

F5.36

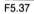

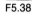

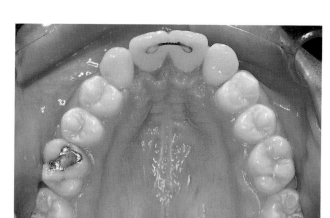

F5.37

F5.38

Figures F5.37 through F5.40 At the end of treatment, the cuspids have been recontoured to resemble lateral incisors. Note the class I upper bicuspid–lower cuspid relation. Group function (in order to avoid excessive forces along the first bicuspid root) guides the occlusion in excursive movements.

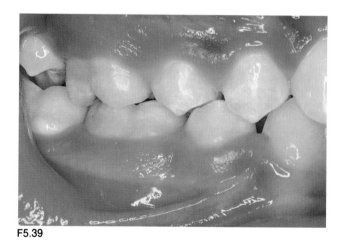

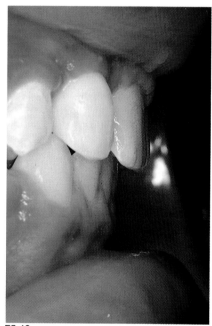

F5.39

F5.40

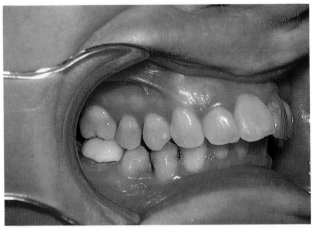

F5.41

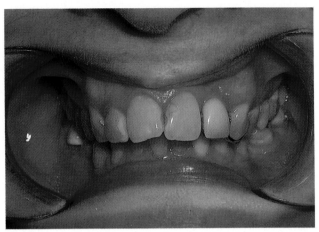

F5.42

Figures F5.41 through F5.43 This adult patient has a class I molar occlusion but a class II 50% cuspid relation and mild upper and lower crowding with excess overjet, deep overbite, and a deep curve of Spee on the mandibular arch. The upper left lateral incisor along with the lower left second bicuspid had been extracted previously. Treatment objectives included moving the upper left cuspid into the position of the previously extracted left lateral incisor and, after termination of treatment, placing a porcelain crown on the cuspid with the morphology of a lateral incisor. The upper left first bicuspid would then occlude in a class I relation with the lower left cuspid.

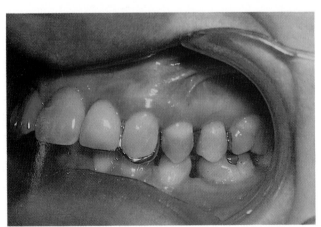

F5.43

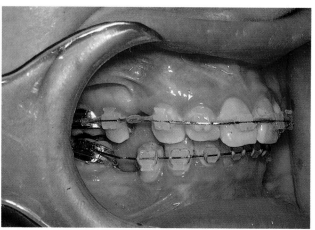

F5.44

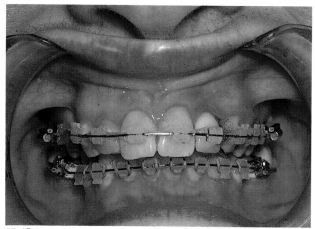

F5.45

Figures F5.44 through F5.47 All teeth were bonded with ceramic appliances with the exception of the first molars, which were cemented with stainless steel bands. The regular stainless steel wire sequence mentioned previously was followed here as well. Due to her deep bite, this patient had clinically visible abrasion of the left first bicuspid cusp tip from contact with the opposing ceramic bracket. The upper left lateral incisor pontic was gradually reduced mesiodistally as the spaces were closed with the elastomeric chain.

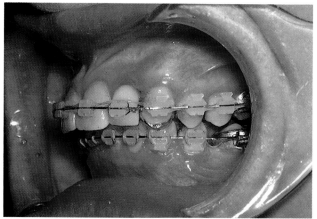

F5.46

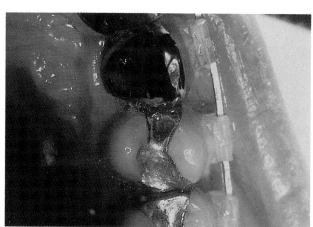

F5.47

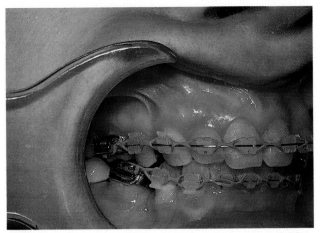

F5.48

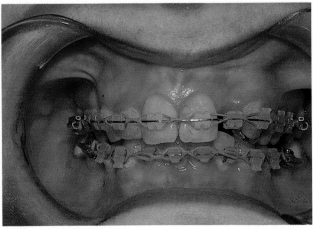

F5.49

Figures F5.48 through F5.50 A year into treatment, the elastomeric chain space closure is continued. Note that due to the small size of the lower incisor ceramic appliances, the elastic modules slip off the brackets. As the lateral incisor space closure continues, bodily movement of the cuspid occurs very slowly (3 mm of movement up to this point). The pontic was removed but the esthetic bracket was left tied to the wire. Also note the improved overbite relation as the occlusion is leveled.

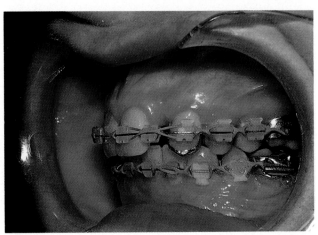

F5.50

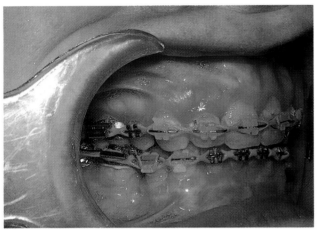

F5.51

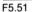

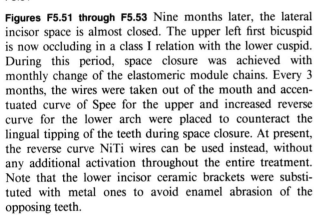

F5.52

Figures F5.51 through F5.53 Nine months later, the lateral incisor space is almost closed. The upper left first bicuspid is now occluding in a class I relation with the lower cuspid. During this period, space closure was achieved with monthly change of the elastomeric module chains. Every 3 months, the wires were taken out of the mouth and accentuated curve of Spee for the upper and increased reverse curve for the lower arch were placed to counteract the lingual tipping of the teeth during space closure. At present, the reverse curve NiTi wires can be used instead, without any additional activation throughout the entire treatment. Note that the lower incisor ceramic brackets were substituted with metal ones to avoid enamel abrasion of the opposing teeth.

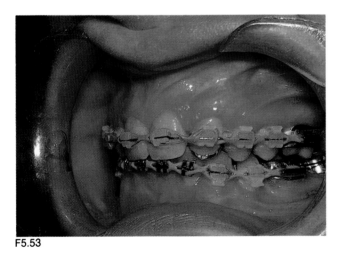

F5.53

References

1. Kokich VG, and Shapiro PA: Lower incisor extraction in orthodontic treatment. Angle Orthod 54:139–154, 1984.
2. Liddle DW: Second molar extraction in orthodontic treatment. Am J Orthod 72:599–616, 1977.
3. Whitney E, and Sinclair P: Combination second molar extraction and functional appliance therapy. Am J Orthod Dentofacial Orthop 91:183–192, 1987.
4. Vanarsdall RL, and White RP, Jr.: Second molar extraction? Int J Adult Orthod Orthog Surg 6:3, 1991.
5. Romanides N, Servoss JM, Kleinrock S, and Lohner J: Anterior and posterior dental changes in second molar extraction cases. J Clin Orthod 24:559–563, 1990.
6. Proffit WR: *Contemporary Orthodontics.* St. Louis, MO: C.V. Mosby Co., 1986.
7. Staggers JA: A comparison of results of second molar and first bicuspid extraction treatment. Am J Orthod Dentofacial Orthop 98:430–436, 1990.

Chapter 6

Intrusion Mechanics/Compromised Periodontium Therapy

Incisor intrusion mechanics can be implemented in a number of ways.[1-4] The simplest approach is with the 2×6 appliance (bands on the molars and 6 brackets on the anterior teeth)[4] (Figs. F6.1 through F6.7) or the base-arch appliance[3,4] (Figs. F6.8 through F6.11). It is possible to intrude teeth with periodontal bone loss as long as regular curettage during treatment takes place. A meticulous oral hygiene and a healthy gingival status are preconditions for a favorable result.[5] The mechanotherapy of choice for such cases is the 2×6 appliance with a slight intrusive component in the anterior region.[1-4] In a recent study on the intrusion of incisors in adult patients with marginal bone loss, it was concluded that the utility and base arches monitor the appliance to a low and constant force, ranging from 10 to 25 g per tooth. The clinical crown length is generally reduced by 0.5 to 1.0 mm. Intrusion in such cases is best performed when the line of force passes through the center of resistance of the incisors (slightly behind the centrals, at the line of the cuspids)[1-4] (Figs. F6.12 through F6.22).

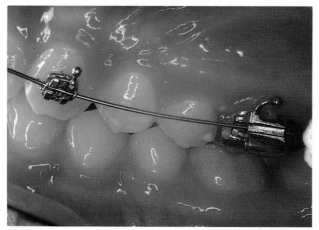

F6.1

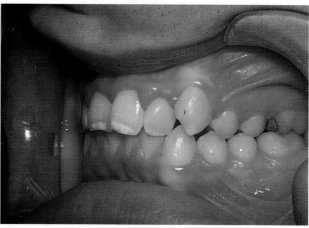

F6.2

Figure F6.1 The 2 × 6 appliance (two bands on the two first molars with six brackets on the six anterior teeth) is used primarily when the anterior teeth are malaligned and while at the same time the bicuspids are in an already excellent intercuspation position.

Figures F6.2 through F6.4 This patient, with a class I occlusion and good posterior occlusion, demonstrated minor (3 mm) upper and lower crowding.

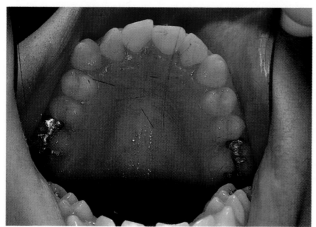

F6.3

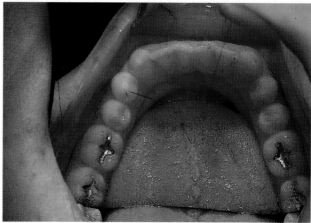

F6.4

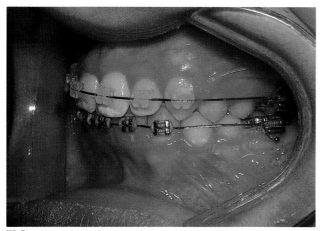

F6.5

Figure F6.5 Upper and lower 2 × 6 appliances corrected the malalignment of teeth in 6 months. Initial .016-inch, round Sentalloy NiTi wires were used for initial alignment and leveling, followed by .016 × .022 inch² stainless steel rectangular finishing wires (shown here).

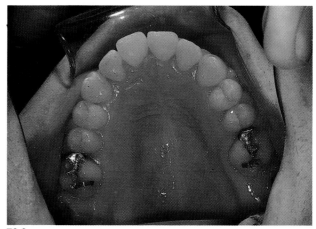

F6.6

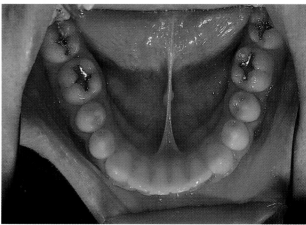

F6.7

Figures F6.6 and F6.7 Maxillary and mandibular arches after treatment.

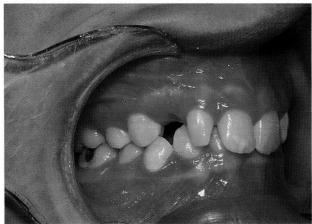

F6.8

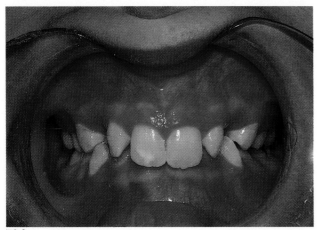

F6.9

Figures F6.8 and F6.9 This patient has a very deep bite and a significant gummy smile that requires intrusion of the upper anterior teeth (as the teeth intrude, the gum line moves upward, thus decreasing the gummy smile).

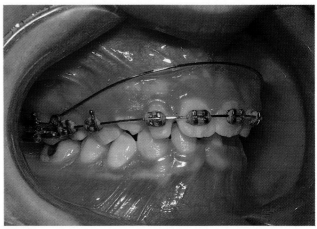

F6.10

Figures F6.10 and F6.11 Intrusion is accomplished with a base arch made of 0.016×0.022 inch² stainless steel wire that is inserted in the auxiliary tube of the molar bands. The main archwire is a rectangular 0.016×0.022 inch² NiTi or stainless steel wire as well. Note the position of the base arch in its passive state: it is over the soft tissue at the level of the middle third of the roots of the anterior teeth. This will produce a total force of 100 to 125 g necessary to intrude the four incisor teeth. It is preferable to intrude the two central incisors to the level of the laterals before intruding all four teeth at once. This should be done with a 2×2 appliance (the wire extending from the two molars to the two centrals). If continuous wires incorporate the lateral incisors, then these teeth will extrude (against air) before the centrals intrude (against bone). When it is activated, it is brought down and wire tied onto the main archwire distal to the laterals on either side. In this manner, the intrusive force should pass through the center of resistance of all four incisors. It is important to tie back the intrusive arch, as well as the main archwire, to prevent the incisors from protruding. The loop of the base arch is used for its activation and increased intrusive effect (if desired) on the anterior segment. Note the significant decrease of the overbite relationship after 6 months of treatment.

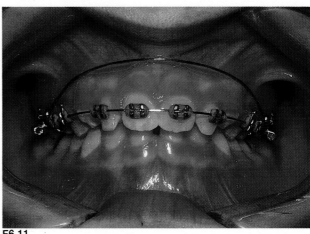

F6.11

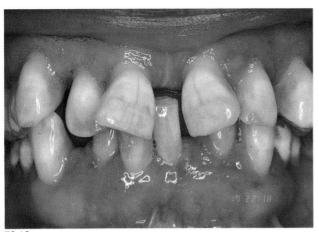

F6.12

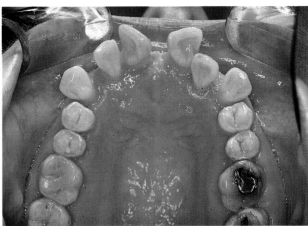

F6.13

Figures F6.12 and F6.13 This patient's occlusion has been severely affected by periodontal disease and significant bone loss. Orthodontic treatment may be attempted only after extensive periodontal treatment has resulted in a healthy periodontium (absence of inflammation, healthy tissues). Note the displaced incisor teeth.

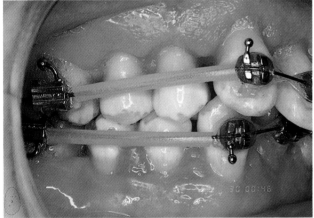

F6.14

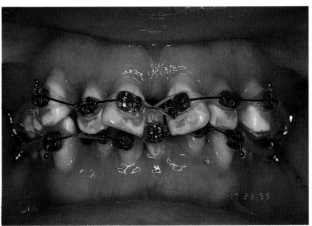

F6.15

Figures F6.14 and F6.15 A 2 × 6 appliance (with brackets instead of bonds on the molar teeth to avoid unnecessary irritation of the tissues) with initial 0.016-inch, round Sentalloy (GAC) very light wires was used. An elastic thread was placed around the brackets in a figure-8 pattern to initiate space closure.

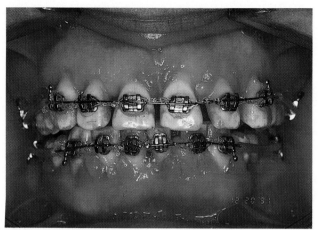

F6.16

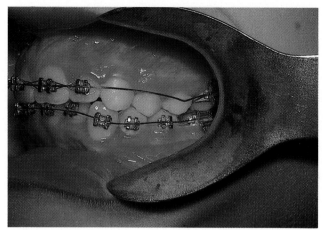

F6.17

Figures F6.16 through F6.18 As soon as the rotations had been corrected (within 3 months), a 0.016-inch round stainless steel archwire was inserted. A slight bend was placed next to the molars (shown here from another patient), which resulted in an intrusive activation in the anterior region. In its passive state, the archwire should lie passively at the level of the CEJ of the incisor teeth. Note the amount of intrusion that was achieved. Forces are kept very low with this slight activation of the wire (40 to 50 g in the whole anterior region or 10 to 15 g per tooth). The spaces were closed with light elastomeric chains.

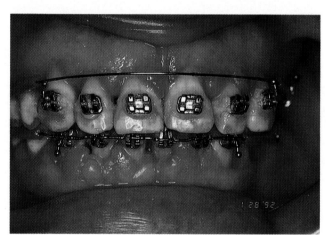

F6.18

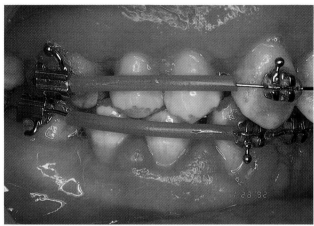

F6.19

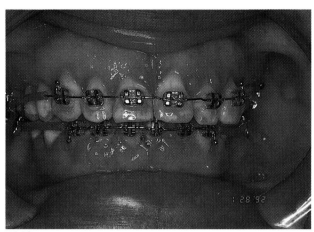

F6.20

Figures F6.19 and F6.20 Toward the end of treatment. Note the slight irritation of the gingiva despite the absence of fixed appliances on the bicuspids. The objectives of this case were simply to align the teeth, improve the overbite relation, and close all spaces. No anteroposterior changes were attempted (the patient will finish with a class II cuspid relation on the right side and a class I on the left, which explains the midline deviation to the left).

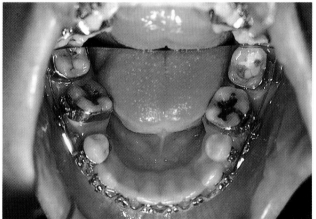

F6.21

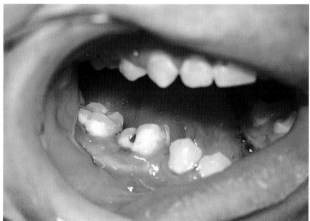

F6.22

Figures F6.21 and F6.22 If a posterior tip-back bend is left in for a long period of time (as in this case, after 6 months), the extrusive effect on the molar tooth will tip the tooth distally and extrude it mesially.

References

1. Melsen B, Agerbaek N, Eriksen J, and Terp S: New attachment through periodontal treatment and orthodontic intrusion. Am J Orthod Dentofacial Orthop 94:104–106, 1988.
2. Melsen B, Agerbaek N, and Markenstam G: Intrusion of incisors in adult patients with marginal bone loss. Am J Orthod Dentofacial Orthop 96:232–241, 1989.
3. Woods MG: The mechanics of lower incisor intrusion: Experiments in nongrowing baboons. Am J Orthod Dentofacial Orthop 93:186–195, 1988.
4. Mulligan T: Common sense mechanics (Parts 1 to 16). J Clin Orthod (Part 1) 13:588–594; (Part 2) 13:676–683; (Part 3) 13:762–766; (Part 4) 13:808–815; (Part 5) 13:53–57; (Part 6) 13:98–103; (Part 7) 13:180–189; (Part 8) 13:265–272; (Part 9) 13:336–342; (Part 10) 13:412–416; (Part 11) 13:481–488; (Part 12) 13:546–553; (Part 13) 13:637–647; (Part 14) 13:716–723; (Part 15) 13:788–795; (Part 16) 13:855–868, 1980.

Retention

Over the past 30 years, a number of studies have dealt with the stability of orthodontic treatment after the retention phase.[1-23] Two thirds of 65 patients examined 10 years postretention, previously treated in the permanent dentition stage with first bicuspid extractions and traditional edgewise mechanics, had unsatisfactory lower anterior alignment after retention.[2] In a follow-up study 20 years postretention, only 10% of the cases were judged to have clinically acceptable mandibular alignment (compared to 30% at the 10-year phase).[1-4] The teeth of patients who had undergone serial extraction plus comprehensive treatment and retention were no better aligned postretention than were those in late extraction cases.[5] There is considerable long-term stability for the majority of cases of mild to moderate malocclusions treated without extractions.[8,20] Arch length shows significant reduction postretention, similar to that of untreated normals and extraction cases (2 to 2.5 mm).[20]

In untreated normals, we see decreases in arch length and intercuspid width; minimal overall changes in intermolar width, overjet, and overbite, and increases in incisor irregularity. Furthermore, no associations or predictors of clinical value are known in regard to assessing stability or relapse. Maturational changes in the permanent dentition of a sample of untreated normals appear, in general, to be similar in nature to those of a postretention sample of treated cases.[15] Orthodontic therapy may temporarily alter the course of the continuous physiologic changes and possibly, for a time, even reverse them; however, following mechanotherapy and the period of retention restraint, the developmental maturation process resumes.[15]

In order to minimize the relapse potential of a case, we should not alter the mandibular arch form; lower incisor apices should be spread distal to the crowns, and the apices of the lower lateral incisors must be spread more than those of the central incisors.[16] The apex of the lower cuspid should be positioned distal to the crown as well.[16] This angulation of the lower cuspid reduces the tendency of the cuspid crown to tip forward into the incisor space. All four lower incisor apices must be in the same labiolingual plane. The lower cuspid root apex must be positioned slightly buccal to the crown. If the apex of the lower cuspid is lingual to the crown at the end of treatment, the forces of occlusion can more easily move the crown lingually toward the space reserved for the lower incisor because of these functional pressures, plus a natural tendency for the crown to upright over its root apex.[16] Even if a lower cuspid with abnormal lingual position of the apex is supported for many years with a fixed retainer, the crown would eventually move lingually when the restraint is removed.[16] If the apex is not moved buccally along with the crown while moving the cuspid distally, lingual relapse of the crown into the incisor area is likely.

There is little doubt that relapse of orthodontically rotated teeth is primarily due to the displaced supra-alveolar connective tissue fibers. A simple surgical method of severing all supracrestal fibrous attachment (circumferential supracrestal fiberotomy; CSF) to a rotated tooth has been demonstrated to significantly alleviate relapse following rotation, with no apparent damage to the supporting structures of the teeth.[10-12]

Following CSF, the most striking feature is an increase in mobility of the teeth. This increased mobility is due to the cutting of transeptal fibers that splint tooth to tooth. However, mobility gradually diminishes within a 2- to 4-week period. A slight overcorrection of tooth rotations should be accomplished at least 6 months before CSF to ensure normal contact point relationships and principal fiber realignment. Reproximation,[13,14] precisely and conservatively performed, increases the long-term stability of the mandibular anterior segment. The majority of all reproximations is performed early in treatment and within 6 months of band removal if no lower retention is employed.[13,14] Serial reproximation during the posttreatment period is often necessary, especially on patients experiencing marked horizontal growth or where the lower arch form has been significantly altered, especially in the mandibular incisor–cuspid areas.

The efficacy of the CSF procedure would appear to be somewhat less in the mandibular anterior segment than in the maxillary anterior segment when observing cases 12 to 14 years after active orthodontic treatment.[11] This observation might be explained by the greater complexity and multifactor potential for relapse inherent in the mandibular anterior arch. The CSF procedure may be more efficient in alleviating pure rotational relapse than in other types of tooth movement.[11] A comparison of electrosurgery with conventional fiberotomies on rotational relapse and gingival tissue in an animal sample showed that there is no significant difference between the two techniques.[21]

Teeth that are orthodontically moved together after extraction of an adjacent tooth do not move through the gingival tissue but appear to push the gingiva ahead to create a fold of epithelial and connective tissues.[12] After the final closure of an extraction site, this excess gingival tissue appears in papillary form buccally and lingually between the approximated teeth. By surgically removing the excess gingiva between properly approximated teeth, relapse can be alleviated.[12]

Third molar absence or presence, impaction, or eruption does not seem to contribute to relapse.[8,17] Neither first nor second bicuspid extraction makes much difference. Arch development, a popular concept today, has only a 10% satisfactory result, with almost all arch-length increase cases worse off in the end than the other samples.[8]

Instability should be assumed, because it is the more likely pattern. Permanent retention, either with fixed or removable retainers, seems to be the logical answer.[8] Patients and parents should be informed of the risk of relapse and the limitations of treatment before treatment begins, and patients should expect to remain in retention long term, with monitoring continuing throughout the patient's adult life.[8]

Bonding a thin, flexible spiral wire lingually to each tooth in a segment is proposed as a simple and effective way to retain anterior teeth.[22] Lingually bonded retainers are made of 0.0195-inch or 0.0215-inch braided spiral wire.[22] Impressions are made with brackets and archwires, and working models are poured in hard stone.[22] Retainer wires are carefully contoured to the working models to provide an intimate adaptation to the critical areas of the lingual surfaces.[22] The retainer wire is then bonded onto the anterior teeth with composite resin. Every patient is instructed to rinse daily with a fluoride solution for as long as the retainer is in place. Excellent long-term success rates for six-unit mandibular and four-unit maxillary retainers have been reported[22] (Figs. F7.1 through F7.3). Wire fatigue fractures could become a problem in the long run, but this could be solved by remaking retainers at, perhaps, 10-year intervals.[22]

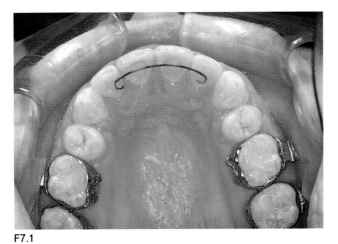

F7.1

Figure F7.1 A bonded 2-2 maxillary retainer wire.

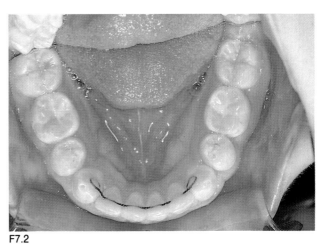

F7.2

Figure F7.2 A bonded 3-3 mandibular retainer wire.

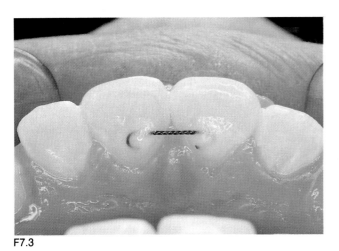

F7.3

Figure F7.3 A bonded 1-1 retainer wire.

The patient is also given a set of Hawley retainers, one maxillary and one mandibular (Figs. F7.4 through F7.6). The maxillary is a wraparound retainer made of 0.036-inch round wire that encompasses all the teeth of the upper arch. The patient is instructed to wear this retainer 24 hr/day for the first 6 months after treatment, followed by 6 months of night-time wear (during sleep hours); after that, twice a week for 6 months, once a week for another 6 months, and, finally, once a month for the rest of the patient's life. Of course, the maxillary bonded wire should also provide lifetime retention of the anterior teeth. The mandibular Hawley retainer should be worn only if the bonded one breaks, until the patient may come to the office for another one. Otherwise, it is not as necessary as the maxillary one because of the minimal changes we may have induced in the mandibular molar and cuspid widths.

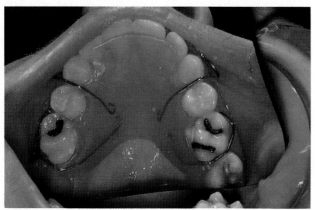

F7.4

Figure F7.4 A maxillary Hawley retainer with circumferential clasps and the cuspid wire over the occlusal surface. This type of retainer is not recommended. A wraparound retainer is preferred because it does not allow for any wires over the occlusal table that may result in premature tooth contacts.

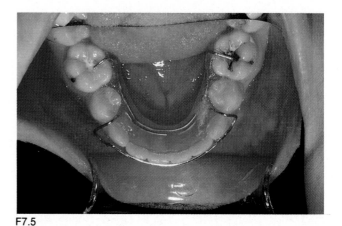

F7.5

Figure F7.5 A mandibular Hawley retainer.

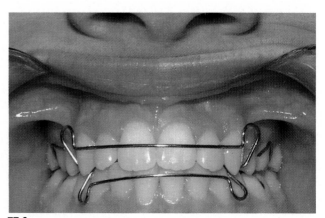

F7.6

Figure F7.6 Anterior view.

In open-bite cases, a tooth positioner may be used for 6 to 8 weeks of night-time wear (or as much as the patient may be able to wear it, depending on his or her daily activities) (Figs. F7.7 through F7.9). This appliance places elastic forces to the teeth and brings them into a predetermined ideal position (the tooth positioner is fabricated to this position). It helps keep the open bite closed as the teeth are pulled in a vertical direction. Bonded fixed and Hawley retainers are also given to these patients for long-term retention. One should make sure, however, that the mandibular anterior teeth do not contact the acrylic of the maxillary Hawley appliance, because this would open the bite in the posterior and promote tooth extrusion, which would open the bite further. On the contrary, if the patient possesses a deep bite at the beginning of treatment, a bite plane is built into the retainer.[23]

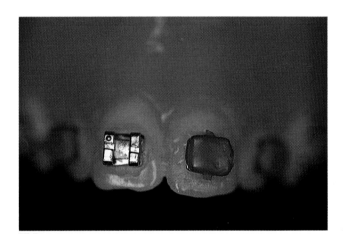

F7.7

Figure F7.7 Plastic caps over the brackets aid in the application of the tooth positioner.

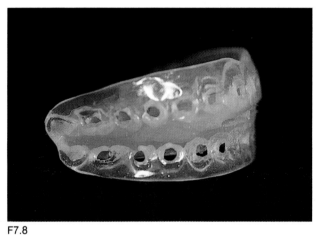

F7.8

Figure F7.8 Tooth positioner (side view).

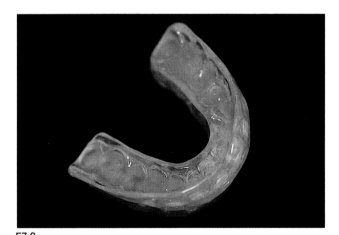

F7.9

Figure F7.9 Tooth positioner (occlusal view).

In most cases, the maxillary second molars are not bonded during treatment. In most instances, provided that the mandibular second molars are in good position and acrylic has been relieved from the lingual side of the retainer, the pressure of the buccinator muscles and normal eruption will move the maxillary second molars into proper position.[23]

Finally, if the patient is suspected of being a tongue thruster, a 5-mm hole should be made with an acrylic bur in the anterosuperior palatal portion of the maxillary Hawley acrylic. The tip of the tongue should rest on this hole as the patient develops a correct swallowing pattern.[23]

The fabrication of the maxillary Hawley wraparound retainer requires step-by-step attention to detail that justifies its long-term purpose (Figs. F7.10 through F7.31). It is very important that the patient leaves the office with a passive appliance that will ensure the retention of the excellent orthodontic result and the beautiful smile that has been attained.

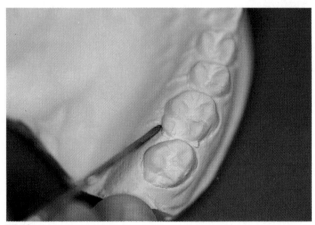

F7.10

Figure F7.10 The finished cast is cleaned of any bubbles or artifacts.

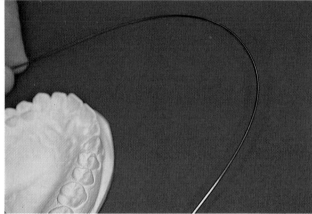

F7.11

Figures F7.11 through F7.14 A 0.036-inch round wire is gently bent crossed over and manipulated with the thumb to obtain the shape of the dental arch.

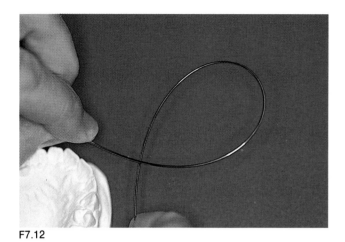

F7.12

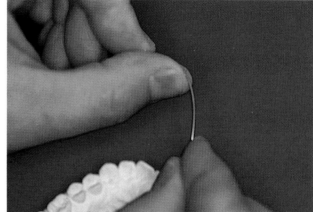

F7.13

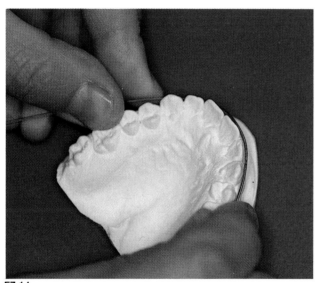

F7.14

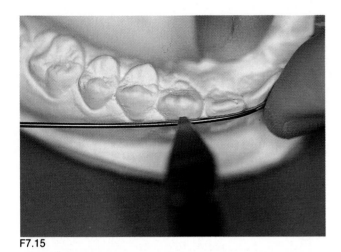

F7.15

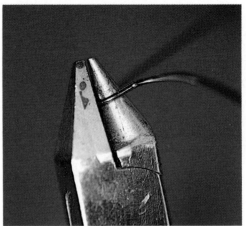

F7.16

Figures F7.15 through F7.17 The wire is marked at the midpoint of the cuspid tooth and a loop is bent around the round part of the birdbeak pliers.

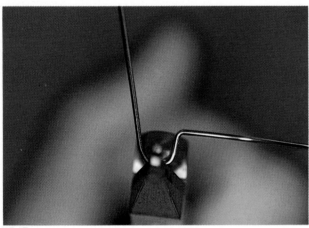

F7.17

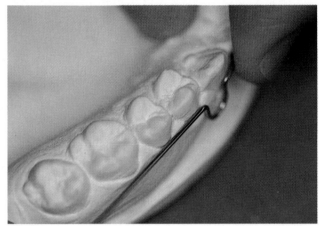

F7.18

Figure F7.18 The wire should contact the bicuspids at the level of the gingival margins.

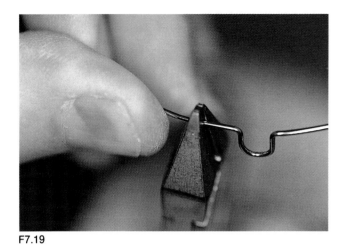

F7.19

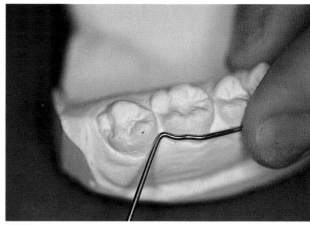

F7.20

Figures F7.19 through F7.23 The wire is bent inward to contact the first molar and curve around the second molar.

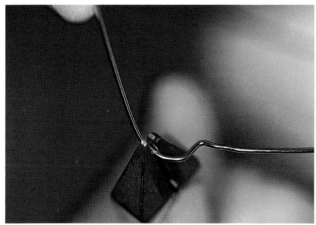

F7.21

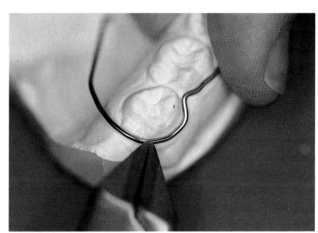

F7.22

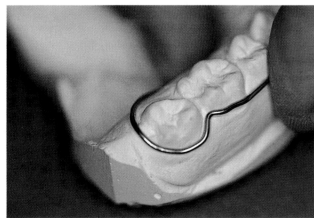

F7.23

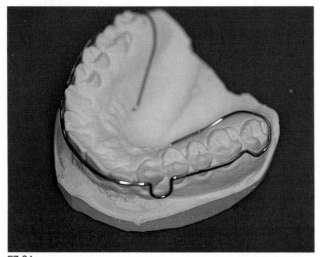

F7.24

Figure F7.24 The wire ends on the palatal side of the bicuspid roots on both sides.

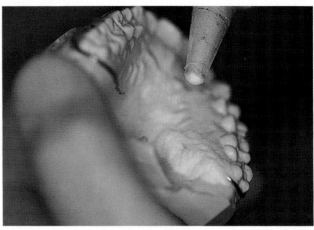

F7.25

Figures F7.25 through F7.27 After the cast is soaked in water for 15 minutes, the "salt-and-pepper" technique is used to place the acrylic over the palatal surface of the wires.

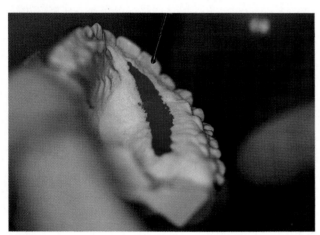

F7.26

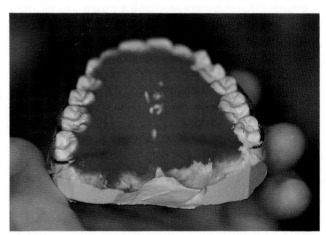

F7.27

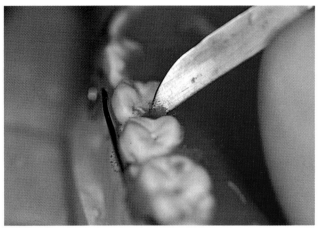

F7.28

Figure F7.28 A sharp instrument is used to define the margins of the acrylic.

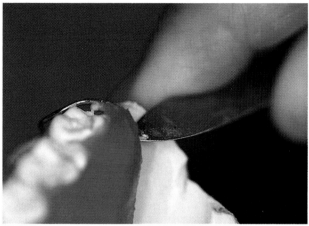

F7.29

Figure F7.29 After the material has set, the retainer is removed from the cast.

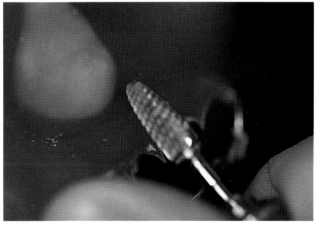

F7.30

Figure F7.30 It is then trimmed with an acrylic bur and thoroughly polished.

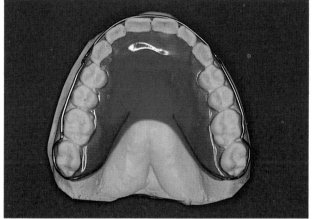

F7.31

Figure F7.31 The finished wraparound maxillary Hawley retainer. A tight fit on the cast ensures a good fit in the patient's mouth as well.

References

1. Little R: Stability and relapse of dental arch alignment. Br J Orthod 17:235–241, 1990.
2. Little R, Waller T, and Riedel R: Stability and relapse of mandibular anterior alignment—First bicuspid extraction cases treated by traditional edgewise orthodontic. Am J Orthod 80:349–365, 1981.
3. Little R, Riedel R, and Artun J: An evaluation of changes in mandibular anterior alignment from 10 to 20 years postretention. Am J Orthod Dentofacial Orthop 93:423–428, 1988.
4. Little R, and Riedel R: Postretention evaluation of stability and relapse—mandibular arches with generalized spacing. Am J Orthod Dentofacial Orthop 95:37–41, 1989.
5. Little R, Riedel R, and Engst D: Serial extraction of first bicuspids—postretention evaluation of stability and relapse. Angle Orthod 60:255–326, 1991.
6. Little R, Riedel R, and Stein A: Mandibular arch length increase during the mixed dentition: Postretention evaluation of stability and relapse. Am J Orthod Dentofacial Orthop 97:393–404, 1990.
7. McReynolds DC, and Little RM: Mandibular second bicuspid extraction—postretention evaluation of stability and relapse. Angle Orthod 61:133–144, 1991.
8. Little RM: Orthodontic stability and relapse. Summary by Bergh HC, Pacific Coast Society of Orthodontists Bulletin 35–38, 1991.
9. Kaplan R: Mandibular third molars and postretention crowding. Am J Orthod 66:411–430, 1974.
10. Edwards J: A surgical procedure to eliminate rotational relapse. Am J Orthod 57:35–46, 1970.
11. Edwards J: A long term perspective evaluation of the circumferential supracrestal fiberotomy in alleviating orthodontic relapse. Am J Orthod 93:380–387, 1988.
12. Edwards J: The prevention of relapse in extraction cases. Am J Orthod 60:128–140, 1971.
13. Boese L: Fiberotomy and reproximation without lower retention, nine years in retrospect: Part I. Angle Orthod 50:88–97, 1980.
14. Boese L: Fiberotomy and reproximation without lower retention, nine years in retrospect: Part II. Angle Orthod 50:169–178, 1980.
15. Sinclair P, and Little R: Maturation of untreated normal occlusions. Am J Orthod 83:114–123, 1983.
16. Williams R: Eliminating lower retention. J Clin Orthod 11:342–349, 1985.
17. Ades R, Joondeph D, Little R, and Chapko M: A long term study of the relationship of third molars to changes in the mandibular dental arch. Am J Orthod Dentofacial Orthop 97:323–335, 1990.
18. Orchin JD: Permanent lingual bonded retainer. J Clin Orthod 24:229–231, 1991.
19. Goldstein RE, and Goldstein CE: Is your case really finished? J Clin Orthod 22:702–713, 1988.
20. Glenn G, Sinclair P, and Alexander RG: Nonextraction orthodontic therapy: Posttreatment dental and skeletal stability. Am J Orthod Dentofacial Orthop 92:321–328, 1987.
21. Fricke LL, and Rankine CAN: Comparison of electrosurgery with conventional fiberotomies on rotational relapse and gingival tissue in the dog. Am J Orthod Dentofacial Orthop 97:405–412, 1990.
22. Dahl EH, and Zachrisson BU: Long term evaluation of bonded retainers. J Clin Orthod 25:619–630, 1991.
23. Alexander RG: *The Alexander Discipline. Contemporary Concepts and Philosophies.* Glendora, CA: Ormco Co., 1986.

Index